Respiratory
Care
Drug
Reference

Mosby's

Respiratory Care Drug Reference

Joseph L. Rau, Jr., Ph.D., RRT

Professor and Chair
Cardiopulmonary Care Science
Georgia State University
Atlanta, Georgia

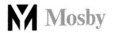 Mosby

St. Louis Baltimore Boston Carlsbad Chicago Naples New York
Philadelphia Portland London Madrid Mexico City Singapore
Sydney Tokyo Toronto Wiesbaden

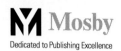

Mosby

Dedicated to Publishing Excellence

A Times Mirror Company

Vice President and Publisher: Don Ladig
Developmental Editor: Anne Gleason
Editor: Jennifer Roche
Project Manager: Deborah Vogel
Editing and Production: Carlisle Publishers Services
Designer: Elizabeth Rohne Rudder
Manufacturing Manager: Theresa Fuchs

A NOTE TO THE READER

The authors and publisher have made every attempt to check dosages and content for accuracy. Because the science of pharmacology is continually advancing, our knowledge base continues to expand. Therefore we recommend that the reader always check product information for changes in dosage or administration before administering any medication. This is particulary important with new or rarely used drugs. At press time we learned that paramethasone acetate and pentaerythritol tetranitrate are no longer available.

Printed in the United States of America

Composition by Carlisle Communications, Ltd.
Printing/binding by Courier Companies, Inc.
Mosby–Year Book, Inc.
11830 Westline Industrial Drive
St. Louis, Missouri 63146.

International Standard Book Number 0-8151-8456-5
96 97 98 99 00 / 9 8 7 6 5 4 3 2 1

Acknowledgment

The author would like to acknowledge and express appreciation to Linda Skidmore-Roth, for her permission to use the *Nursing Drug Reference* computer database for the drug monographs in this book.

This reference text is intended for respiratory care practitioners and those associated with the use of drug therapy in respiratory and critical care medicine. Such individuals often have need for a convenient, practical compendium for prescriptive information on drugs given by aerosol delivery and drugs used in treating cardiopulmonary disorders. This need forms the basis for the selection of drugs in the text. The first three sections offer detailed information on methods of aerosolization and aerosolized drugs for the convenience of those prescribing or administering these drugs. Section IV provides grouping of drugs related to respiratory and critical care medicine, including antiinfective groups, local anesthetics, and central nervous system depressants (barbiturates, narcotics, other sedative-hypnotics, general anesthetics). Aspects of these drug groups, which are relevant to respiratory care, are summarized. The alphabetized listing of individual agents in Section V gives detail on drugs of primary use in patients with cardiopulmonary diseases. This section includes drugs affecting the cardiovascular system or commonly seen in critical care (e.g., antihypertensive agents, antidysrhythmics, antianginal drugs, diuretics, anticoagulants, neuromusclar blocking agents, and corticosteroids). Agents directly targeted at diseases of the respiratory system, such as antituberculosis agents and antihistamines (H_1 antagonists) are also included for reference. Effects on the respiratoryor cardiovascular system or interactions with aerosolized drugs are noted where applicable.

Although every effort has been made to ensure that the information on drug action and dosage is accurate and in accord with the standards accepted at the time of publication, the user is advised to always check the product information on any drugs before administering them.

Joseph L. Rau, Jr., Ph.D., RRT

Georgia State University, Atlanta, Ga.

RESPIRATORY CARE DRUG REFERENCE

TABLE OF CONTENTS

DEVICES FOR AEROSOLIZING DRUGS

The following is a summary of commonly used devices associated with the aerosol delivery of drugs.

Aerosol generating devices: Drugs intended for oral inhalation are marketed for one or more of the following aerosol generating and delivery devices:

Metered dose inhaler (MDI)
Small volume nebulizer (SVN)
Dry powder inhaler (DPI)

Reservoir (spacer) devices: A reservoir apparatus can be combined with an MDI to improve use of the MDI and optimize aerosol drug delivery. Other terms used:

Spacer
Add-on device
Extension chamber (usually lacks valves; open-ended)
Holding chamber (has one-way valves to hold aerosol in chamber)

Ultrasonic nebulizers (USN): An alternative nebulizing device that operates on the principle of the piezoelectric effect (conversion of electrical energy into acoustical, or sound, waves) to aerosolize liquid solutions of drugs. Small, portable units operating on DC 12-volt sources are available. An example of a USN unit is the DeVilbiss AeroSonic.

SPAG unit: The Small Particle Aerosol Generator, or SPAG, is an aerosol device marketed with the drug ribavirin.

Nasal inhalers: A metered dose inhaler formulation with the mouthpiece replaced with a nasal insufflator adaptor for nasal inhalation and local, topical treatment of the nasal passages. *Inhalers are not intended for treatment of the lower respiratory tract.*

Examples of aerosol drugs available in nasal inhaler formulation:

Dexamethasone sodium phosphate (Decadron Phosphate Turbinaire)
Beclomethasone (Beconase, Vancenase)
Flunisolide (Nasalide)
Triamcinolone acetonide (Nasacort)
Budesonide (Rhinocort)
Fluticasone propionate (Flonase)
Cromolyn sodium (Nasalcrom)
Ipratropium (Atrovent Nasal Spray)

AGE GUIDELINES FOR DEVICE USE

General age requirements vary for use of different aerosol drug delivery techniques. These general guidelines must be adapted to individual children, depending on their degree of maturity, cooperation, and ability to use a specific device.

DELIVERY METHOD	MINIMUM AGE
Small-volume nebulizer	Neonate and older
Metered dose inhaler	7 years and older
• With spacer	3 years and older
• With spacer and mask	Infant
• With ETT (endotracheal tube)	Neonate and older
Dry powder inhaler	3 to 4 years and older
Ultrasonic nebulizer	Infant to adult
SPAG	Neonate to child, receiving ribavirin

SMALL-VOLUME NEBULIZER (SVN)

Technical description Small reservoir (holds 3 to 5 ml medication solution), hand-held, gas-powered aerosol generator using a jet-shearing principle of aerosol production. The gas power source can be either a 50 psig pressure source powering a flow meter at 6 to 8 liters per minute (L/min) or an electrically powered compressor directly driving the nebulizer. Small-bore tubing (e.g., oxygen tubing) connects the gas source and the nebulizing device.

Summary of use
- Filling volume—3 to 5 ml
- Power gas flow rate—6 to 8 L/min (most solutions; antibiotics or other liquids may differ)
- Treatment time—less than 10 minutes usually
- Pattern of inhalation—slow deep breaths, occasional inspiratory hold if possible; tidal breathing is effective, as is rapid shallow breathing
- Inspiratory nebulization only—increases efficiency of percent of dose nebulized; may lengthen treatment time unacceptably

Advantages
- Any drug solution or mixture can be aerosolized.
- Minimal coordination for inhalation is required.
- SVNs are useful in very young patients, the very old or debilitated, or those in acute distress.
- This delivery is effective with low inspiratory flows or volumes.
- Inspiratory pause is not required for efficacy.
- Drug concentrations can be modified.

Disadvantages
- Equipment is cumbersome and expensive.
- Treatment time is lengthy relative to MDIs and DPIs.
- Equipment contamination with bacteria is possible.
- Face mask delivery gives a wet, cold spray.

METERED DOSE INHALER (MDI)

Technical description Small pressurized canisters containing a mixture of freon propellant and drug along with other ingredients for dispersion. MDIs give several hundred accurately metered doses of aerosol drug when activated.

Summary of use
- Shake canister, discharge once if not used in 4 hours.
- Inspect mouthpiece for any foreign debris before using.

- Hold actuator vertically, with canister properly placed in mouthpiece/actuator.
- Position MDI 1 to 2 inches in front of open mouth (alternatively, place on lower teeth, mouth open).
- Exhale to end-tidal volume.
- Start inhaling slowly, and actuate canister.
- Inhale slowly to total lung capacity.
- Hold breath 5 to 10 seconds.
- Exhale normally.
- Wait 15 to 30 seconds to ensure adequate refill of metering valve for repeat dose.
- Replace mouthpiece cover on actuator.

Advantages
- MDIs are portable and compact.
- Aerosol dose delivery is efficient and reproducible.
- Treatment time is short.

Disadvantages
- Complex actuation-breathing coordination is required.
- Drug concentrations are fixed.
- Airway irritation from propellant can occur.
- Oropharyngeal impaction and loss can be high without spacer.
- Environmental release of chlorofluorocarbons is a problem until replacement by non-CFC propellants.

EXTENSION OR AUXILIARY (SPACER) DEVICES

Technical description Extension or spacer devices are reservoirs ranging in size from around 80 ml to over 750 ml. An MDI is attached at one end, and the patient inhales aerosol from the other end, or mouthpiece, after the MDI is actuated.

Design variables:
> Volume
> Direction of MDI spray—forward versus reverse plume relative to user's mouth
> Built-in canister nozzle adaptor/actuator versus insertion of MDI mouthpiece
> Presence or absence of one-way valves
> Possibility of rebreathing into chamber

Characterization of selected current chambers:

	VOLUME*	VALVE	SPRAY DIRECTION+	ACTUATOR
ACE	175 ml	One-way inspiratory	Reverse	Built-in
Aerochamber	145 ml	One-way inspiratory	Forward	Accepts MDI mouthpiece
Optihaler	70 ml	No valve	Reverse	Built-in

*Approximate volumes.
+Relative to patient's mouth or artificial airway.

Summary of use
- Follow all manufacturers' instructions for use and cleaning.
- Inspect the mouthpiece of the chamber for any foreign material and remove before to inhalation (keep the mouthpiece cap placed on the chamber when not in use).
- Inhale from the chamber either simultaneously or immediately after actuating the MDI to maximize available dose. Delays in inhaling after actuation can result in less drug available on inhalation.
- A single actuation followed by inhalation maximizes aerosol drug availability. Multiple actuations into a chamber can decrease the amount of drug *per actuation* delivered from the mouthpiece;

Advantages
- The holding volume allows aging of aerosol particles to reduce velocity and size.
- Slower particle velocity and smaller size reduces oropharyngeal drug loss.
- The reservoir holding chamber lessens the need for coordination of actuation and inhalation by the user.

Disadvantages
- These devices can be large and cumbersome.
- Bacterial infection can occur with inadequate cleaning.
- Some assembly may be required.
- Devices add to the time required for an MDI dose because they must be attached to the MDI before use.

DRY POWDER INHALER (DPI)

Technical description This small apparatus, about the size of an MDI, contains a unit dose of powdered drug. The device is breath-actuated, and turbulent air flow during a rapid inspiration creates a microfine aerosol of drug particles. The drug powder may contain carrier agents such as lactose or glucose to improve flow properties and act as a bulking agent.

Indications for use
- Inadequate coordination for MDI use
- Need for a more portable alternative to a SVN
- Patient sensitivity to CFC propellants in MDIs
- Subjects capable of high inspiratory flow rates (> 60 L/min)
    *with DPIs currently available in the United States
- Need for accurate dose monitoring
- Drug available in DPI formulation

Summary of use (cromolyn Spinhaler and albuterol Rotahaler) Note: There is greater variation among DPI devices than among other aerosol devices; manufacturers' literature and instructions should be carefully reviewed before using or instructing patients in their use. These directions may not apply to new devices marketed in the future.
- Load the dispensing device with a gelatin capsule, as instructed.

- Open the capsule:
    Spinhaler—hold device vertically and slide sleeve up and down to pierce the capsule.
    Rotahaler—hold device horizontally and turn the upper portion as far as it will go.
- Exhale fully, away from the DPI, to prevent moisture from accumulating in the device.
- Place lips around mouthpiece, teeth apart, and breathe in quickly (>60 L/min) and deeply.
- If necessary, inhale again to empty capsule of powder.

Advantages
- Small and portable device
- Short preparation and administration times
- No need for hand-breathing coordination or complicated inspiratory maneuvers
- No freon propellants
- No "cold freon" effect to inhibit full inspiration
- Drug dose counting possible

Disadvantages
- Limited drug availability to date
- Possible reaction to lactose or glucose carrier (with current formulations in the United States)
- High inspiratory flow rates are needed with current devices.
- Requirement to load capsule containing powder before use.

SMALL PARTICLE AEROSOL GENERATOR (SPAG)
The following is a summary only of operation of the SPAG unit. The manufacturer's detailed manual *must* be reviewed before operating this unit.

Technical description The SPAG has a large reservoir and gas-powered, jet shearing aerosol generator. It is intended for use in delivering the antiviral drug ribavirin (Virazole).

Summary of use
Assemble the SPAG as directed in the operating manual. In particular:
- Check the three nebulizer capillary tubes for patency.
- Check the drying air hose and the nebulizer hose for correct connections on the reservoir cap.
- Insert the drying chamber in the correct direction as indicated by the arrow.
- Connect the SPAG to a 50 psig powered external flow meter opened to flush.
- Adjust the SPAG pressure regulator, the nebulizer flow meter, and the drying air flow meter to maintain the following values, as suggested by the manufacturer, for initial use:
    pressure regulator—26 psi
    nebulizer flow meter—6 to 10 L/min
    drying air flow meter—2 to 9 L/min
Monitor and adjust settings.
Check that three aerosol spots appear on reservoir wall.

INDICATIONS FOR DIFFERENTIAL CHOICE OF AEROSOL DELIVERY DEVICE

Achieving successful and therefore more efficacious use of an aerosol device can be optimized by matching the advantages/disadvantages of each type of device to the needs or limitations of the individual using the device. Other considerations may include third-party reimbursement or overall cost. The following suggested indications for differential choice of an aerosol delivery device are based on the advantages and disadvantages of each category of device.

Indications for use of small volume nebulizers
- Person unable to follow instructions (due to age or disorientation) or too debilitated to use MDI or DPI
- Poor inspiratory capacity
- Inspiratory hold not possible
- Rapid or unstable respiratory pattern
- Need to nebulize nonstandard drug solutions or concentrations

Indications for use of metered dose inhalers
- Ability to follow instructions
- Ability to mechanically coordinate actuation and breathing
- Adequate inspiratory capacity (>900 ml)
- Inspiratory hold possible
- Stable, calm respiratory pattern

Indications for use of reservoirs with MDIs
- Delivery of an inhaled aerosolized corticosteroid
- Subjects with poor hand-breathing coordination who want to use an MDI
- For all MDI use, as a means of maximizing lung delivery and mimimizing oropharyngeal drug impaction and loss

Indications for use of dry powder inhalers
- Inadequate coordination for MDI use
- Need for a more portable alternative to a SVN
- Patient sensitivity to CFC propellants in MDIs
- High inspiratory flow rates (> 60 L/min) possible
     *with DPIs currently available in the United States
- Need for accurate dose monitoring
- Drug available in DPI formulation

Indication for use of SPAG unit Delivery of the antiviral drug ribavirin

Drugs delivered by oral inhalation or nasal inhalation are intended to provide a local topical treatment for the respiratory tract. The following advantages can be realized by this method and route of delivery:

1. Aerosol doses are smaller than those used for the same purpose and given systemically.
2. Side effects are usually fewer and less severe with aerosol delivery than with oral or parenteral delivery.
3. The onset of action is rapid.
4. Drug delivery is targeted to the respiratory system.
5. The inhalation of aerosol drugs is painless and relatively safe. Convenience depends on the specific delivery device used.

Therapeutic Purposes of Aerosolized Agents

DRUG GROUP	THERAPEUTIC PRUPOSE	AGENTS
Adrenergic agents	Relaxation of bronchial smooth muscle, bronchodilation; reduced R_{AW} and improved ventilatory flow rates in airway obstruction such as COPD, asthma, CF, acute bronchitis. Epinephrine or other alpha-adrenergic drugs—topical vasoconstriction and decongestion.	Epinephrine Isoproterenol Isoetharine Terbutaline Metaproterenol Albuterol Pirbuterol Bitolterol Salmeterol
Anticholinergic agents	Relaxation of cholinergic-induced bronchoconstriction to improve ventilatory flow rates in COPD and asthma.	Ipratropium bromide
Mucoactive agents	Modification of the properties of respiratory tract mucus; current agents lower viscosity and promote clearance of secretions.	Acetylcysteine Dornase alfa
Corticosteroids	Reduce and control the inflammatory response in the airway usually associated with asthma.	Dexamethasone Beclomethasone dipropionate Triamcinolone acetonide Flunisolide Fluticasone* Budesonide* *(nasal inhaler only)
Antiasthmatic agents	To prevent the onset and development of the asthmatic response through inhibition of chemical mediators of inflammation.	Cromolyn sodium Nedocromil sodium
Antiinfective agents	To inhibit or eradicate specific infective agents, such as *P. carinii* (pentamidine), or respiratory syncytial virus (ribavirin).	Pentamidine Ribavirin
Exogenous surfactants	Approved clinical dose is by direct intratracheal instillation for the purpose of restoring a more normal lung compliance in respiratory distress syndrome of the newborn.	Colfosceril palmitate Beractant

This section provides information on currently approved drugs used for oral inhalation, including the exogenous lung surfactants administered by direct tracheal instillation. Practitioners are encouraged to obtain and read the complete drug insert material prior to administering these drugs, particularly if the drug is not familiar to the practitioner.

Abbreviations used:
>   MDI—metered dose inhaler
>   DPI—dry powder inhaler
>   SVN—small volume nebulizer

BETA-ADRENERGIC BRONCHODILATORS

Note: for complete listing of dosage forms other than the inhaled aerosol (if available), see the individual drug listing for each agent.

Agents (alphabetically):

- Albuterol (Proventil, Ventolin)
- Bitolterol (Tornalate)
- Epinephrine (Adrenalin, AsthmaNefrin, Primatene Mist, various)
- Isoetharine (Bronkosol, Bronkometer)
- Isoproterenol (Isuprel, Medihaler-Iso)
- Metaproterenol (Metaprel, Alupent)
- Pirbuterol (Maxair)
- Salmeterol (Serevent)
- Terbutaline (Brethaire)

General indication and use: Relaxation of bronchial smooth muscle to produce bronchodilation in asthma, chronic obstructive pulmonary disease (COPD), bronchiectasis, and other obstructive pulmonary disease states. The exact clinical use is determined by the receptor selectivity of action (alpha, beta-1, beta-2) and the pharmacokinetics, which are described for each individual agent.

General side effects/adverse reactions: Incidence and severity of side effects vary with the receptor selectivity of the individual agent.

- Tremor
- Palpitations
- Tachycardia
- Headache
- Increase in blood pressure
- Nervousness
- Insomnia
- Dizziness
- Hypokalemia
- Nausea
- Paradoxical bronchospasm

Contraindications:
- Hypersensitivity reaction to any component of the aerosol
- Unstable cardiac arrhythmias, especially with less beta-2 preferential agents, such as isoproterenol

Precautions:
- Reactions to freon (chlorofluorocarbon propellants in MDI)
- Reactions to preservatives such as sulfites in nebulizer solutions
- Confirmation that patients can use MDI or DPI delivery form or can assemble and use nebulizer system

Drug interactions with adrenergic aerososl class*	
DRUG OR GROUP	INTERACTION
Beta-blockers	May decrease effect of adrenergic agent
	With epinephrine, an initial hypertensive episode (alpha effect) followed by bradycardia
Guanethidine	May increase the effect of adrenergic agents
	Hypotensive effect of guanethidine may be reversed.
Methyldopa	Possible increased pressor response
MAO inhibitors	Increased effect, possible hypertensive crisis
Oxytocic drugs	Possible hypertension
Rauwolfia alkaloids	Effect antagonized by adrenergic agents
Tricyclic antidepressants	Increased pressor response; possible dysrhythmias
Albuterol	May decrease digoxin serum levels
Theophylline	Enhanced toxicity and decreased theophylline levels
Insulin	Epinephrine-like agents increase glucose levels

*These interactions are most likely when adrenergic agents are given systemically rather than locally to the lung by aerosol; however, systemic absorption is known to occur with inhaled aerosols, and the possibility of interaction should be considered.

Respiratory care assessment of drug therapy:
- Assess effectiveness of drug therapy based on the indication(s) for the aerosol agent: presence of reversible airflow due to primary bronchospasm or other obstruction secondary to an inflammatory response and/or secretions, either acute or chronic.
- Monitor flow rates using office or bedside peak flow meters or laboratory reports of pulmonary function, especially before and after bronchodilator studies, to assess reversibility of airflow obstruction.
- Instruct and then verify correct use of aerosol delivery device (SVN, MDI, reservoir, DPI).
- Assess breathing rate and pattern.
- Assess breath sounds by auscultation before and after treatment.
- Assess pulse before and after treatment.
- Assess patient's subjective reaction to treatment for any change in breathing effort or pattern.
- Assess arterial blood gases or pulse oximeter saturation, as needed, for acute states with asthma or COPD to monitor changes in ventilation and gas exchange (oxygenation).

- Note effect of beta agonists on blood glucose (increase) and K^+ (decrease) laboratory values, if these are available.
- Monitor blood pressure and pulse rate if subject is on other adrenergic agents or tricyclic antidepressants.
- Monitor long-term pulmonary function studies of lung volumes, capacities, and flows.
- Instruct asthmatic patients in use and interpretation of disposable peak flow meters to assess severity of asthmatic episodes.
- Instruct patients in use, assembly, and especially cleaning of aerosol inhalation devices.

Note: death has been associated with excessive use of inhaled adrenergic agents in severe acute asthma crises. Individuals using such drugs should be instructed to contact a physician or an emergency room if there is no response to the usual dose of the inhaled agent.

Albuterol

Proventil, Ventolin, Ventolin Rotacaps

Class: Beta-2 preferential adrenergic bronchodilator

Indication: Relief and prevention of airflow obstruction in individuals with reversible obstructive airway disease (COPD, asthma, acute bronchitis, cystic fibrosis, bronchiectasis), including exercise-induced bronchospasm (EIB).

Action: The saligenin structure of albuterol (salbutamol) is a catecholamine analogue. Stimulation of beta-2 receptors relax and dilate airway smooth muscle through activation of the cyclic AMP system. Increases in airway diameter, improvement in airflow, and adrenergic stimulation of ciliary beat may improve secretion clearance.

Dose and administration:
- Nebulizer: 0.5 ml of 0.5% solution, tid, qid
- MDI: 2 puffs, 90 µg/puff, tid, qid
- DPI: 1 cap, 200 µg per cap, q. 4 to 6 hours

Pharmacokinetics (by inhalation):
- Onset: within 5 minutes
- Peak effect: 30-60 minutes
- Duration: 3-8 hours

Bitolterol mesylate

Tornalate

Class: Beta-2 preferential adrenergic prodrug bronchodilator

Indication: Relief and prevention of airflow obstruction in individuals with reversible obstructive airway disease (COPD, asthma, acute bronchitis, cystic fibrosis, bronchiectasis).

Action: Bitolterol mesylate is inhaled as a prodrug. Once in the airway, the bitolterol molecule is hydrolyzed by esterase enzymes to the active agent colterol, which is a catecholamine. Gradual formation of colterol gives a sustained release effect of 5 to 8 hours. Colterol is beta-2 preferential. Stimulation of beta-2 receptors relax and dilate airway smooth muscle.

Increases in airway diameter, improvement in airflow, and adrenergic stimulation of ciliary beat may improve secretion clearance.

Dose and administration:
- Nebulizer: 1.25 ml of 0.2% solution, bid, tid, qid
- MDI: 2 puffs, 0.37 mg/puff, q. 8 hours

Pharmacokinetics:
- Onset: 3-4 minutes
- Peak effect: approx. 60 minutes
- Duration: 5-8 hours

Epinephrine and racemic epinephrine

Adrenalin Chloride, AsthmaNefrin, microNefrin, Vaponefrin, AsthmaHaler Mist, Medihaler-Epi, Primatene Mist, and others

Class: Nonselective, adrenergic bronchodilator and vasopressor

Indication: Temporary relief of airflow obstruction due to bronchospasm in asthma (beta-2 effect) and treatment of postintubation wheezing or croup (alpha effect). The nebulization solution can be directly instilled through a bronchoscope to control airway bleeding (alpha effect). (Pharmacokinetics and lack of beta selectivity limit epinephrine's usefulness as a maintenance agent in asthma or other chronic airflow obstruction.)

Action: Epinephrine and its synthetic stereoisomer mixture, racemic epinephrine, stimulate alpha, beta-1, and beta-2 adrenergic receptors. Only the levorotatory form is physiologically active. The alpha effect produces vasoconstriction, which in the airway leads to decongestion (shrinkage of engorged capillary beds in the mucosa). The beta-2 effect produces bronchodilation. The beta-1 effect can cause tachycardia.

Dose and administration:

Epinephrine
- Nebulizer: 0.25 to 0.5 ml of 1:100 (1%) solution, qid or as ordered
- MDI: strength varies with brand (0.16 mg/spray, 0.2 mg/spray, and 0.25 mg/spray), qid or as ordered

Racemic epinephrine
- Nebulizer: 0.25 to 0.5 ml of 2.25% solution (equivalent to 1.125% epinephrine base), qid or as ordered

Pharmacokinetics:
- Onset: 1-5 minutes
- Peak effect: 5-20 minutes
- Duration: 1-3 hours

Isoetharine

Bronkosol, Beta-2, Bronkometer

Class: Beta-2 preferential adrenergic bronchodilator

Indication: Relatively short-acting relief and prevention of airflow, obstruction in individuals with reversible obstructive airway disease (COPD, asthma, acute bronchitis, cystic fibrosis, bronchiectasis).

Action: Catecholamine structure stimulates beta-2 receptors to relax and dilate airway smooth muscle through activation of the cyclic AMP system. Increases in airway, diameter, improvement in airflow, and adrenergic stimulation of ciliary beat may improve secretion clearance.

Dose and administration:
- Nebulizer: 0.25 to 0.5 ml of 1% solution (equivalently, 2.5 to 5.0 mg with various solution concentrations available), qid or as ordered
- MDI: 1 to 2 puffs, 340 µg/puff, qid or as ordered

Pharmacokinetics:
- Onset: within 5 minutes
- Peak effect: 15-60 minutes
- Duration: 1-3 hours

Isoproterenol
Isuprel, Isuprel Mistometer, Medihaler-Iso

Class: Nonselective beta (beta-1 and beta-2) adrenergic agonist
Indication: Relatively short-acting relief and prevention of airflow obstruction in individuals with reversible obstructive airway disease (COPD, asthma, acute bronchitis, cystic fibrosis, bronchiectasis).

Action: Stimulation of beta-2 receptors relax and dilate airway smooth muscle through activation of the cyclic AMP system. Increases in airway diameter, improvement in airflow, and adrenergic stimulation of ciliary beat may improve secretion clearance. Beta-1 stimulation can cause tachycardia.

Dose and administration:
- Nebulizer: 0.25 to 0.5 ml of 1:200 (0.5%) solution, qid
- MDI: 2 puffs, 131 µg/puff, qid or as ordered

Pharmacokinetics:
- Onset: 2-5 minutes
- Peak effect: 5-30 minutes
- Duration: 0.5 to 2 hours

Isoproterenol HCl and phenylephrine bitartrate
Duo-Medihaler

Class: Nonselective beta agonist (isoproterenol) and alpha agonist (phenylephrine)
Indication: Relatively short-acting relief and prevention of airflow obstruction in individuals with reversible obstructive airway disease (COPD, asthma, acute bronchitis, cystic fibrosis, bronchiectasis).
Action: The compound provides both alpha and beta receptor activation. Stimulation of beta-2 receptors relax and dilate airway smooth muscle through activation of the cyclic AMP system. Increases in airway diameter, improvement in airflow, and adrenergic stimulation of ciliary beat may improve secretion clearance. Beta-1 stimulation can cause tachycardia. Alpha receptor stimulation may cause decreased swelling or topical mucosal edema in the airway.

Dose and administration:
- MDI: 1 to 2 inhalations with 0.16 mg isoproterenol HCl and 0.24 mg phenylephrine bitartrate per actuation, 4 to 6 times daily

Metaproterenol

Alupent, Metaprel

Class: Beta-2 preferential adrenergic bronchodilator

Indication: Relief and prevention of airflow obstruction in individuals with reversible obstructive airway disease (COPD, asthma, acute bronchitis, cystic fibrosis, bronchiectasis), including exercise-induced bronchospasm (EIB).

Action: The resorcinol structure of metaproterenol is a catecholamine analogue. Stimulation of beta-2 receptors relax and dilate airway smooth muscle through activation of the cyclic AMP system. Increases in airway diameter, improvement in airflow, and adrenergic stimulation of ciliary beat may improve secretion clearance.

Dose and administration:
- Nebulizer: 0.3 ml of 5% solution, tid, qid
- MDI: 2 to 3 puffs, 0.65 mg/puff, q. 4 hours

Pharmacokinetics:
- Onset: 1-5 minutes
- Peak effect: approx. 60 minutes
- Duration: 2-6 hours

Pirbuterol acetate

Maxair

Class: Beta-2 preferential adrenergic bronchodilator

Indication: Relief and prevention of airflow obstruction in individuals with reversible obstructive airway disease (COPD, asthma, acute bronchitis, cystic fibrosis, bronchiectasis), including exercise-induced bronchospasm (EIB).

Action: Pirbuterol is a catecholamine analogue. Stimulation of beta-2 receptors relax and dilate airway smooth muscle through activation of the cyclic AMP system. Increases in airway diameter, improvement in airflow, and adrenergic stimulation of ciliary beat may improve secretion clearance.

Dose and administration:
- MDI: 2 puffs, 0.2 mg/puff, q. 4 - 6 hours

Pharmacokinetics:
- Onset: within 5 minutes
- Peak effect: approx. 30 minutes
- Duration: approx. 5 hours

Salmeterol xinafoate

Serevent

Class: Beta-2 preferential adrenergic bronchodilator

Indication: Long-term, maintenance treatment of asthma (which cannot be controlled by prn use of beta agonists) and bronchospasm with reversible obstructive airway disease; prevention of exercise-induced bronchospasm (EIB). (*Not* for relief of acute bronchospasm: see pharmacokinetics.)

Action: Salmeterol is a saligenin structure with a very large, lipophilic side chain, producing long-acting stimulation of beta-2 receptors. Stimulation of beta-2 receptors relaxes and dilates airway smooth muscle through activation of the cyclic AMP system. In addition, salmeterol possesses some inhibition of the inflammatory response.

Dose and administration:
- MDI: 2 actuations of 21 µg/actuation (25 µg/actuation at nozzle), bid

Pharmacokinetics:
- Onset: within 20 minutes
- Peak effect: 1-2 hours
- Duration: 12 hours

Terbutaline
Brethaire
Class: Beta-2 preferential adrenergic bronchodilator
Indication: Relief and prevention of airflow obstruction in individuals with reversible obstructive airway disease (COPD, asthma, acute bronchitis, cystic fibrosis, bronchiectasis), including exercise-induced bronchospasm (EIB).
Action: The resorcinol structure of terbutaline is a catecholamine analogue. Stimulation of beta-2 receptors relax and dilate airway smooth muscle through activation of the cyclic AMP system. Increases in airway diameter, improvement in airflow, and adrenergic stimulation of ciliary beat may improve secretion clearance.

Dose and administration:
- MDI: 2 puffs, 0.2 mg/puff, q. 4 to 6 hours

(Note: no nebulizer solution is available; the injectable ampule solution with 1 mg/ml has been nebulized in varying doses.)

Pharmacokinetics:
- Onset: 5-30 minutes
- Peak effect: 30-60 minutes
- Duration: 3-6 hours

ANTICHOLINERGIC BRONCHODILATORS
Only one anticholinergic agent, ipratropium bromide, currently has approval from the FDA as an inhaled aerosol. Other drugs, such as atropine sulfate and glycopyrrolate, have been administered as a nebulized solution.

Ipratropium bromide
Atrovent
Class: Anticholinergic (parasympatholytic) bronchodilator
Indication: Maintenance treatment of airflow obstruction in COPD, especially chronic bronchitis and emphysema. Often used in treatment of acute and chronic asthma.

Action: Ipratropium and other anticholinergic agents block vagally mediated reflex bronchoconstriction by competitively antagonizing acetylcholine at the cholinergic airway receptors. Ipratropium is related to atropine sulfate, but is a quaternary ammonium compound which does not cross the blood-brain barrier or other lipid membranes.

Dose and administration:

■ Nebulizer: 2.5 ml of a 0.02% strength solution (500 µg), 3 to 4 times daily

(Additional normal saline diluent of 1 to 2 ml can be added for optimal nebulizer function if needed, since many SVNs require 3 to 4 ml for efficient nebulization, with minimal wasted ("dead") volume.)

The nebulizer solution can be mixed with albuterol if used within one hour. Data not available on compatibility with other drug mixtures.

■ MDI: 18 µg/actuation, 2 actuations inhaled, 3 to 4 times daily

Side effects/adverse reactions: Since ipratropium does not distribute well from the lung, systemic side effects are minimal. The primary local effect is dry mouth due to the antimuscarinic action.

■ Dryness of the oropharynx
■ Cough
■ Irritation from aerosol
■ Symptom exacerbation
■ Palpitations
■ Nervousness
■ Dizziness, headache
■ Blurred vision

Contraindications: Hypersensitivity to ipratropium or atropine-like drugs.

Precautions: Use with caution in subjects with narrow-angle glaucoma, prostatic hypertrophy, or bladder neck obstruction.

Instruct subjects to avoid direct spraying of the drug into the eye, which will produce the topical effect of mydriasis and cycloplegia similar to atropine sulfate.

Due to a slower onset of action than other bronchodilator classes, ipratropium may not be an ideal single agent for relief of acute bronchospasm. Consider use of a beta agonist for initial therapy.

Individuals using such drugs should be instructed to contact a physician or an emergency room if there is no response to the usual dose of the inhaled agent or if breathing becomes more difficult.

Pharmacokinetics:

■ Onset: approx. 15 minutes
■ Peak effect: 1-2 hours
■ Duration: 4-6 hours

(Elimination half-life is about 2 hours after inhalation.)

Drug interactions:
- Directly antagonized by cholinergic agents such as methacholine
- Additive effect with adrenergic (sympathomimetic) agents
- Can be used concomitantly with:
  Adrenergic bronchodilators
  Methylxanthines
  Corticosteroids
  Cromolyn sodium

Respiratory care assessment of drug therapy:
- Assess effectiveness of drug therapy based on the indication(s) for the aerosol agent, such as presence of reversible airflow due to primary bronchospasm or other obstruction secondary to an inflammatory response and/or secretions, either acute or chronic.
- Monitor flow rates using office or bedside peak flow meters or laboratory reports of pulmonary function. Pulmonary function before and after studies performed with a beta agonist may not reliably predict response to an anticholinergic agent such as ipratropium bromide.
- Instruct and then verify correct use of aerosol delivery device (MDI, SVN), including cleaning for home use.
- Assess breathing rate and pattern.
- Assess breath sounds by auscultation before and after treatment.
- Assess pulse before and after treatment.
- Assess patient's subjective reaction to treatment for any change in breathing effort or pattern.
- Assess arterial blood gases or pulse oximeter saturation, as needed, for acute states with asthma or COPD to monitor changes in ventilation and gas exchange (oxygenation).
- Long-term: monitor pulmonary function studies of lung volumes, capacities, and flows.

Other anticholinergic agents given by inhaled aerosol
(not FDA-approved as inhaled aerosol)
  Atropine sulfate
    Adult: 0.025 mg/kg tid, qid
    Child: 0.05 mg/kg tid, qid
  Glycopyrrolate (Robinul)
    Dose: 1 mg, tid, qid

MUCOACTIVE AGENTS
Agents:
- Acetylcysteine (Mucomyst)
- Dornase alfa (Pulmozyme)

Acetylcysteine
Mucomyst, Mucosil-10, Mucosil-20
Class: Mucolytic
Indication: Mucolytic therapy of abnormal, viscid, or inspissated tracheobronchial mucus secretions in acute or chronic

bronchopulmonary disease (COPD, tuberculosis, bronchiectasis, cystic fibrosis, primary amyloidosis of the lung).

Orally, not by aerosol: Antidote therapy to reduce or prevent hepatic injury following overdose of acetaminophen.

Action: The sulfhydril group of acetylcysteine substitutes for the disulfide bonds in the mucoprotein complex, lowering the viscosity as well as elasticity of the mucus.

With oral use as an antidote to acetaminophen overdose and hepatotoxicity, acetylcysteine can cross into liver cells to provide the sulfhydril group to react with the toxic metabolite of the acetaminophen in the liver, thereby inactivating the metabolite and protecting the liver.

Dose and administration:

■ Nebulizer: 3 to 5 ml of a 10% or 20% strength solution, tid or qid (The 10% strength is usually less irritating to the airway.)
■ Direct instillation: 1 to 2 ml instilled directly into an airway segment

Side effects/adverse reactions:

■ Airway irritation and bronchospasm; more likely with the 20% strength than the 10%, and with hyperreactive airways
■ Increased volume of secretions, possibly obstructing the airway (ensure adequate cough or means of suctioning the airway with endotracheal tubes in place)
■ Stomatitis in presence of tracheotomy
■ Nausea or vomiting due to disagreeable odor from hydrogen sulfide
■ Fever
■ Rhinorrhea
■ Drowsiness, clamminess
■ Acquired sensitization to acetylcysteine; rare, but confirmed by several respiratory care practitioners who reported dermatitis after prolonged exposure to the drug
■ Antidotal use: large doses can result in nausea, vomiting, or other GI symptoms, rash, pruritis, angioedema, bronchospasm, tachycardia, hypotension, and hypertension.

Contraindications: Hypersensitivity to acetylcysteine.

Precautions: Administer with caution to asthmatics and monitor for changes in airway resistance (wheezing increase, decreased breath sounds, increased difficulty in breathing, increased peak airway pressure if ventilated).

Use 10% strength with asthmatics and other individuals to reduce airway irritation.

Provide equipment and personnel for mechanical suction if necessary in the presence of large volumes of secretions.

Prepare patient for disagreeable odor.

With face mask use, the aerosol will leave on the patient's face a sticky residue that should be washed off after treatment.

Solution color may change to a slight purplish tinge due to preservative EDTA; this does not impair the drug's efficacy or safety.

Carefully rinse the nebulizer reservoir after each treatment to prevent concentration of the drug due to evaporation, which could increase airway irritation on subsequent treatments.

Pharmacokinetics: The drug acts topically, and presumably immediately, on contact with respiratory tract mucous secretions.

Drug interactions: Acetylcysteine is chemically or physically incompatible when mixed with the following: tetracycline, chlortetracycline, oxytetracycline, erythromycin lactobionate, amphotericin B, sodium ampicillin. If these agents are to be nebulized, they should be administered in separate solutions, not the same nebulizer.

Iodized oil, chymotrypsin, trypsin, and hydrogen peroxide are incompatible with acetylcysteine.

Acetylcysteine will also react with certain metals, such as iron or copper, and rubber. Do not use nebulizing equipment with these materials exposed to the drug. Silver will tarnish, but this does not affect the drug action.

Respiratory care assessment:
- Assess therapy based on indication for drug: mucolysis and improved clearance of secretions.
  - Monitor color, consistency, and amount of sputum produced before and after treatments, using a 24-hour collection system.
  - Monitor airflow changes for improvement.
  - Long-term: monitor number and severity of respiratory tract infections and need for antibiotic therapy.
- Instruct and then verify correct use of aerosol nebulization system, including cleaning.
- Assess breathing rate and pattern.
- Assess breath sounds by auscultation before and after treatment.
- Assess pulse before and after treatment.
- Assess patient's subjective reaction to treatment for any change in breathing effort or pattern.
- Assess patient's adequacy of cough and level of consciousness to determine need for mechanical suctioning to clear airway with treatment.
- Assess patient's ability to clear and expectorate secretions to determine need for adjunct bronchial hygiene such as postural drainage or percussion, PEP therapy, or autogenic drainage.
- Discontinue therapy if patient experiences adverse reactions.

Dornase alfa (recombinant human DNase)
Pulmozyme
Class: Viscolytic enzyme
Indication: Management of cystic fibrosis to reduce the frequency of respiratory infections requiring parenteral antibiotics and to improve overall pulmonary function.
Action: Dornase alfa is a solution of recombinant human deoxyribonuclease I (rhDNase), which can enzymatically degrade DNA. Infected respiratory tract secretions contain cellular debris, including DNA, from neutrophils, which increases the viscosity

of the mucus secretion and reduces clearance. This in turn leads to retained secretions, setting up a cycle of further infection and thick, purulent secretions. By cleaving DNA in purulent secretions, mucus viscosity is lowered, and mucociliary clearance can be more effective. Subsequent airway infection is reduced and pulmonary function can improve.

Dose and administration:
- 2.5 mg in a single use ampule inhaled once daily
- Recommended nebulizer systems:
  Disposable Hudson T Up-draft II, with Pulmo-Aide compressor
  Disposable Marquest Acorn II, with Pulmo-Aide compressor
  Reusable Pari LC Jet, with PARI PRONEB compressor
- Protect ampules from light.

(Data on efficacy of other nebulizing systems was not provided during clinical trials.) Store in protective foil pouch under refrigeration, 2°-8° C, 36°-46° F.

Side effects/adverse reactions: Side effects with dornase were little different from placebo in clinical trials, and discontinuation rate was similar for dornase (3%) and placebo (2%). Anti-DNase antibody production was not found with inhaled rhDNase. Possible side effects include:
- Voice alteration
- Pharyngitis, laryngitis
- Rash
- Chest pain
- Conjunctivitis

Other adverse reactions reported:
- Respiratory—apnea, bronchiectasis, bronchitis, cough increase, dyspnea, hemoptysis, decrease in lung function, nasal polyps, pneumonia, pneumothorax, rhinitis, sinusitis, sputum increase, wheeze
- Body—abdominal pain, asthenia, fever, flu syndrome, malaise, sepsis
- GI—intestinal obstruction, gall bladder disease, liver disease, pancreatic disease
- Metabolic—diabetes mellitus, hypoxia, weight loss

Contraindications: Hypersensitivity to dornase, Chinese Hamster Ovary cell products, or any of the product's components.

Precautions: Monitor for adverse reactions.

Pharmacokinetics (based on 2.5 mg inhaled dose):
- Sputum concentration of 3 µg/ml within 15 minutes
- Sputum concentration declined to 0.6 µg/ml 2 hours after inhalation

Drug interactions: Can be safely used with standard CF therapies:
- Oral, inhaled, parenteral antibiotics
- Bronchodilators
- Enzyme supplements
- Vitamins
- Oral and inhaled corticosteroids
- Analgesics

Do not mix other drugs directly in the nebulizer with dornase.

Respiratory care assessment:
- During treatment:
  Instruct and then verify correct use of aerosol nebulization system.
  Assess breathing rate and pattern.
  Assess breath sounds by auscultation before and after treatment.
  Assess pulse before and after treatment.
  Assess patient's subjective reaction to treatment for any change in breathing effort or pattern.
- Long-term: monitor number and severity of respiratory tract infections and need for antibiotic therapy.
- Monitor pulmonary function for improvement or delayed deterioration.

CORTICOSTEROIDS

Agents:
- Dexamethasone sodium phosphate (Decadron Respihaler)
- Beclomethasone dipropionate (Beclovent, Vanceril)
- Triamcinolone acetonide (Azmacort)
- Flunisolide (AeroBid)

General indication and use: As maintenance, antiinflammatory therapy of asthma. The inhaled aerosol route reduces side effects seen with systemic routes of administration.

Action: The inhaled agents are synthetic, topically active adrenocortical steroids, with the basic glucocorticoid effect of reducing or inhibiting the inflammatory response in the airway. Corticosteroids seem to increase or restore responsiveness to beta-adrenergic agents. Glucocorticoids possess mineralocorticoid (fluid-retaining) properties as well. Because of their degree of topical activity, inhaled aerosols are given in small doses, which have minimal or no systemic effects, such as adrenal suppression.

General side effects/adverse reactions:
- Oropharyngeal and laryngeal fungal infections with *Candida albicans* or *Aspergillus niger*
- Throat irritation, hoarseness, dysphonia
- Coughing
- Dry mouth
- Rash
- Wheezing, bronchoconstriction
- Facial edema
- Adrenal insufficiency following transfer from systemic corticosteroid therapy
- Possible HPA suppression, more significant with doses above recommended levels

Contraindications:
- Not for primary treatment of status asthmaticus or acute asthma crisis
- Hypersensitivity to any component of the aerosol

- Persistent positive sputum culture for *C. albicans*
- Systemic fungal infections

Precautions: Inhaled corticosteroids do not bronchodilate and do not provide rapid relief of bronchospasm.

Use of a reservoir device (spacer, holding chamber) is recommended to reduce the risk of oropharyngeal fungal infection.

Inhaled corticosteroids may not be adequate to control asthma symptoms, and patients should be instructed to seek medical advice if symptoms worsen.

Sufficient weaning from systemic corticosteroids is needed to avoid adrenal insufficiency when transferring to inhaled agents. Death due to adrenal insufficiency can occur during or after transfer from systemic to inhaled aerosol corticosteroids.

During stress or with deterioration, supplementary systemic corticosteroids may be required.

Other agents, such as cromolyn-like drugs, beta agonists, or anticholinergic bronchodilators, may be needed to control symptoms.

Drug interactions with corticosteroid aerosol class*

DRUG OR GROUP	INTERACTION
Beta agonists	Corticosteroids can potentiate the action of beta agonists and restore the responsiveness of beta receptors in the airway
Barbiturates	May decrease the effect of the corticosteroid
Oral contraceptives	Decreased corticosteroid clearance with increased half-life, concentration
Ephedrine	Increased corticosteroid clearance, with decreased half-life
Estrogens	May decrease corticosteroid clearance
Hydantoins (e.g., phenytoin)	May increase corticosteroid clearance, decreased therapeutic effect
Ketoconazole	May decrease corticosteroid clearance, increased therapeutic effect
Macrolide antibiotics	Significant decrease in methlyprednisolone clearance (this is not administered as an inhaled aerosol agent)
Rifampin	May increase corticosteroid clearance, decreased therapeutic effect
Anticholinesterases	Corticosteroids may antagonize in myasthenia gravis
Oral anticoagulants	Corticosteroids may add to or oppose the anticoagulant action
Cyclosporine	Corticosteroids may increase toxicity
Digitalis	Corticosteroids may increase the possibility of toxicity with hypokalemia
Isoniazid	Corticosteroids may decrease serum concentrations of isoniazid
Nondepolarizing muscle relaxants	Corticosteroids can have variable effects: potentiate, antagonize, no effect
Potassium depleting agents	Corticosteroids may aggravate hypokalemia
Salicylates	Corticosteroids may decrease serum salicylate levels and their effectiveness
Theophyllines	Either agent, corticosteroid or theophylline, may show alterations in activity

*Many of the drug interactions listed are based on systemic administration of the corticosteroid. However, the potential for such interaction with the aerosol agent should be considered, based on the mode of action of the drugs involved.

Respiratory care assessment of drug therapy:
- Instruct and then verify correct use of MDI and spacer system, if used.
- Assess breathing rate and pattern.
- Assess breath sounds by auscultation before and after treatment.
- Assess pulse before and after treatment.
- Assess patient's subjective reaction to treatment for any change in breathing effort or pattern.
- Instruct subject in use of a peak flow meter, to monitor baseline PEF and changes. Subject should be clear on when to contact a physician with deterioration in PEF or exacerbation of symptoms.
- Long-term: assess severity of symptoms, number of exacerbations, missed work/school days, and pulmonary function.

Beclomethasone dipropionate
Beclovent, Vanceril
Class: Topically active glucocorticoid
Dose and administration:
- Adult: 2 inhalations of 42 μg/inhalation, 3 or 4 times daily. Alternatively, 4 inhalations twice daily may be effective. Do not exceed 20 inhalations (840 μg) a day.
- Child (6-12 years): 1 or 2 inhalations of 42 μg/inhalation, 3 or 4 times daily. Do not exceed 10 inhalations (420 μg) a day.
Pharmacokinetics: In vitro lung tissue can metabolize beclomethasone dipropionate rapidly to beclomethasone 17-monopropionate and more slowly to free beclomethasone.

The route of excretion of drug and metabolites is in the feces, with less than 10% in the urine. Systemic absorption occurs rapidly with all routes of administration.

Note: the antiinflammatory effect of corticosteroids occurs in hours to days and is not dependent on a single treatment.

Dexamethasone sodium phosphate
Decadron Respihaler
Class: Long-acting glucocorticoid
Dose and administration:
- Adult: 3 inhalations of 84 μg/actuation, 3 or 4 times daily, maximum 12 inhalations/day
- Child: 2 inhalations of 84 μg/actuation, 3 or 4 times daily, maximum 8 inhalations/day
Pharmacokinetics: With 12 inhalations daily, there is absorption of about 0.4 to 0.6 mg dexamethasone.

Flunisolide
AeroBid, AeroBid-M (menthol flavored)
Class: Topically active glucocorticoid
Dose and administration:
- Adult: 2 inhalations of 250 μg/inhalation, twice a day, q. 12 hours, not to exceed 2000 μg a day
- Child (6-15 years): 2 inhalations of 250 μg/inhalation, twice a day, q. 12 hours

Pharmacokinetics: There is approximately 40% systemic availability after inhalation. Absorbed flunisolide is rapidly and extensively metabolized during first pass through the liver. Plasma half-life is approximately 1.8 hours.

Triamcinolone acetonide
Azmacort
Class: Topically active glucocorticoid
Dose and administration: The actuator contains its own reservoir device as part of the mouthpiece assembly; 200 µg released per actuation delivers approximately 100 µg to the patient.
- Adult: 2 inhalations of approximately 100 µg/inhalation, 3 to 4 times daily
- Child (6-12 years): 1 or 2 inhalations of approximately 100 mcg/inhalation, 3 to 4 times daily

Pharmacokinetics: There is rapid disappearance from the lungs. Peak blood levels are seen in 1 to 2 hours. The majority of the dose is eliminated in the feces, with three metabolites identified.

INTRANASAL AEROSOL CORTICOSTEROIDS
Beclomethasone dipropionate
MDI: Beconase, Vancenase
Spray: Beconase AQ, Vancenase AQ
Indication: For seasonal or perennial rhinitis and prevention of recurrence of nasal polyps after surgery.
Dose and administration: 1 inhalation of 42 µg/actuation, in each nostril, 2 to 4 times a day

Budesonide
Rhinocort
Indication: Management of seasonal and perennial allergic rhinitis in adults and children, and nonallergic perennial rhinitis in adults.
Dose and administrations:
- Adults and children > 6 years: 2 sprays of 32 µg/spray, into each nostril morning and evening; or as 4 sprays each nostril in morning only.

Dexamethasone sodium phosphate
Decadron Phosphate Turbinaire
Indication: For allergic or inflammatory nasal conditions and nasal polyps.
Dose and administration:
- Adult: 2 sprays of 84 µg/spray, into each nostril 2 or 3 times a day. Maximum daily dose of 12 sprays.
- Child: 1 or 2 sprays of 84 µg/spray, into each nostril 2 times a day. Maximum daily dose of 8 sprays.

Flunisolide
Nasalide
Indication: For symptoms of seasonal or perennial rhinitis if conventional treatment is unsatisfactory.

Dose and administration:
- Adult: 2 sprays of 25 µg/spray, in each nostril 2 times daily. Maximum daily dose of 8 sprays in each nostril.
- Child: 1 spray of 25 µg/spray, in each nostril 3 times daily, or 2 sprays in each nostril 2 times a day. Maximum daily dose is 4 sprays in each nostril.

Fluticasone propionate
Flonase
Indication: Management of seasonal and perennial rhinitis in patients over 12 years of age.
Dose and administration:
- Adult: 2 sprays of 50 µg/spray in each nostril once daily. Maximum total daily dose not to exceed 200 µg.
- Adolescent, 12 years and older: 1 spray of 50 µg/spray in each nostril once daily. Maximum daily dose should not exceed 200 µg.

Triamcinolone acetonide
Nasacort
Indication: Treatment of seasonal or perennial rhinitis.
Dose and administration:
- Adult and child, 12 and up: 2 sprays of 55 µg/spray, in each nostril once a day.
- May increase dose to 440 µg per day, divided in several ways:
    4 sprays (220 µg) in each nostril once a day;
    2 sprays (110 µg) in each nostril twice a day;
    1 spray (55 µg) in each nostril 4 times a day.

PROPHYLACTIC ANTIASTHMATIC AGENTS
Agents:
- Cromolyn sodium (Intal, Aarane)
- Nedocromil sodium (Tilade)

Cromolyn sodium
Intal; Nasalcrom (nasal solution for rhinitis), Gastrocrom (oral form for mastocytosis)
Class: Mast cell stabilizing prophylactic antiasthmatic agent
Indication: Prophylactic management of asthma of sufficient severity to warrant continual maintenance therapy. Prevention of exercise-induced bronchospasm.
Action: Cromolyn sodium inhibits the degranulation of mast cells which occurs after antigen exposure, thereby inhibiting the release of chemical mediators of inflammation including histamine and SRS-A in the lung.
Dose and administration:
- Nebulizer: Adults and children, 1 ampule solution of 20 mg/ 2 ml ampule, 4 times a day
- DPI: Adults and children, 1 capsule of 20 mg/cap, 4 times a day, in Spinhaler
- MDI: 2 actuations inhaled of 0.8 mg per actuation, 4 times a day.
Side effects/adverse reactions:
- Cough (especially with dry powder)

- Bronchospasm
- Throat irritation
- Dry mouth
- Nasal congestion, sneezing, nasal itching or burning (SVN)
- Lacrimation, swollen parotid gland
- Dysuria, urinary frequency
- Dizziness, headache
- Rash, urticaria, angioedema

Contraindications: Hypersensitivity to cromolyn or any ingredient in the formulations.

Precautions: Cromolyn sodium is not indicated for use during an acute asthma episode, because it has no bronchodilating effect.

Instruct the patient not to swallow the dry powder capsule used with the DPI.

Spinhaler (DPI) requires high flow rates of more than 50 L/min to deliver an adequate dry powder aerosol dose; children below 5 years of age may not be able to achieve adequate inspiratory flows, requiring the nebulizer or MDI formulation.

With renal or hepatic dysfunction, the dose may need to be decreased or discontinued because of impaired clearance and elimination through these systems.

Consider use of a bronchodilator prior to cromolyn use if wheezing or bronchospasm occurs, despite changing from the powder to the MDI or SVN form.

Evaluate patients for reaction to the freon propellants found in the MDI formulation.

Pharmacokinetics: The dose to the lung is absorbed and rapidly excreted unchanged in the bile and urine. The portion of the dose reaching the stomach is excreted.

Drug interactions: None known when given by the inhaled aerosol route. High doses given parenterally in combination with high dose isoproterenol show adverse fetal effects in animal studies. The combination of cromolyn with theophylline gave no additional benefit in children 1 to 6 years old.

Respiratory care assessment:
- Evaluate patient for optimal aerosol delivery formulation (SVN, MDI, DPI). See Section I on methods of aerosol delivery. Note age, ability to inspire sufficiently for DPI, and need for reservoir with MDI.
- Initially:
  Instruct and then verify correct use of MDI and spacer system, if used, or SVN or DPI.
  Assess breathing rate and pattern.
  Assess breath sounds by auscultation before and after treatment.
  Assess pulse before and after treatment.
  Assess patient's subjective reaction to treatment for any change in breathing effort or pattern.

- Evaluate need for prior use of a bronchodilator if wheezing occurs after inhalation of cromolyn. Consider change of delivery form first, especially if DPI causes coughing or wheezing.
- Instruct subject in use of a peak flow meter to monitor baseline PEF and changes. Subject should understand when to contact a physician with deterioration in PEF or exacerbation of symptoms.
- Long-term: assess severity of symptoms, number of exacerbations, missed work/school days, and pulmonary function.

Nedocromil sodium

Tilade

Class: Prophylactic antiinflammatory (mediator inhibitor) for asthma

Indication: Prophylactic maintenance therapy of mild to moderate asthma

Action: Nedocromil is an antiinflammatory agent (not related to corticosteroids or traditional NSAIDS) that inhibits the activation and mediator release of a variety of inflammatory cell types, including eosinophils, neutrophils, macrophages, mast cells, monocytes, and platelets. Its action inhibits the early- and late-phase asthmatic reactions.

Dose and administration: MDI: 2 actuations of 1.75 mg/actuation, 4 times a day

Side effects/adverse reactions:
- Generally well tolerated
- Unpleasant taste
- Cough, pharyngitis
- Rhinitis
- Headache
- Bronchospasm
- Chest pain
- Nausea
- Dyspnea
- Upper respiratory tract infection

Contraindications: Hypersensitivity to nedocromil or ingredients in the formulation.

Precautions: Nedocromil sodium is not indicated for use during an acute asthma episode because it has no bronchodilating effect.

If coughing or bronchospasm occurs consider alternative therapy or use of a bronchodilator.

Monitor patients carefully for adequate adrenal function if transferring or reducing a corticosteroid dose in asthma.

Pharmacokinetics: Following an inhaled dose of 3.5 mg, peak serum levels averaged 28 minutes, and the mean half-life was 3.3 hours. The drug is eliminated primarily in the urine.

Drug interactions: No interactions with the inhaled aerosol are noted.

Respiratory care assessment:
- Initially:

  Instruct and then verify correct use of MDI and spacer system, if used.

  Assess breathing rate and pattern.

  Assess breath sounds by auscultation before and after treatment.

  Assess pulse before and after treatment.

  Assess patient's subjective reaction to treatment, for any change in breathing effort or pattern.

  Evaluate need for prior use of a bronchodilator if wheezing occurs after inhalation of nedocromil. Consider need to change medication.

  Instruct subject in use of a peak flow meter to monitor baseline PEF and changes. Subject should be clear on when to contact a physician with deterioration in PEF or exacerbation of symptoms.
- Long-term: assess severity of symptoms, number of exacerbations, missed work/school days, and pulmonary function.

ANTIINFECTIVE AGENTS
Agents:
- Pentamidine isethionate (NebuPent)
- Ribavirin (Virazole)

Pentamidine isethionate
Nebupent

Class: Antiprotozoal agent

Indication: Pentamidine isethionate delivered by inhaled aerosol is indicated for the prophylactic therapy of *P. carinii* pneumonia (PCP) in subjects with either a prior history of PCP or a peripheral CD4+ cell count of less than $200/cu^3$.

Action: Pentamidine isethionate is an aromatic diamidine with antiprotozoal activity. It is effective against *Pneumocystis carinii,* although the mode of action is not fully understood. Pentamidine blocks RNA and DNA synthesis, interfering with nuclear metabolism and protein synthesis.

Dose and administration: Nebulizer: 300 mg of powdered drug, reconstituted in 6 ml sterile water for injection, given monthly with the Respirgard nebulizer system.

(Other nebulizer systems may not deliver an equivalent dose to that with the Respirgard, and may require dose modification. See Smaldone et al: *J Aerosol Med* 1:113-126, 1988, and Vinciguerra and Smaldone, *Respir Care* 35:1037-1041, 1988.)

Continue nebulizer delivery until the chamber no longer nebulizes. Use a 5 to 7 L/min flow rate to the nebulizer with a 40 to 50 psi source of pressure (wall gas or compressor), or power the nebulizer with a compressor set to deliver a pressure of 22 to 25 psi. Lower pressure compressors (below 20 psi) should not be used.

Side effects/adverse reactions:
- Cough, bronchial irritation
- Shortness of breath, fatigue
- Bad or metallic taste
- Decreased appetite
- Bronchospasm and wheezing
- Dizziness, rash, nausea
- Pharyngitis
- Chest pain
- Night sweats, chills
- Spontaneous pneumothoraces
- Conjunctivitis and rash
- Neutropenia
- Pancreatitis
- Renal insufficiency
- Hypoglycemia
- Digital necrosis
- Possible extrapulmonary infection with *P. carinii*

Contraindications: Presence or history of anaphylactic reaction to inhaled or parenteral pentamidine isethionate.

Precautions: The recommended dose of pentamidine for prophylaxis of PCP is not adequate to treat acute PCP. The possibility of developing acute PCP exists in subjects receiving prophylactic pentamidine.

An inhaled bronchodilator should be available to treat bronchospasm if it occurs.

Administer with caution in subjects who are hypoglycemic, hypotensive or hypertensive.

Environmental containment precautions must be taken to prevent exposure to both the aerosol drug and tuberculosis organisms which may be present in exhaled droplet nuclei of patients on pentamidine. The following safeguards are suggested in the literature:
- Use a nebulizer system with one-way valves, scavenging filter, and thumb control for inspiratory nebulization only.
- Use a nebulizer system producing small aerosol particles of 1 or 2 microns Mass Median Diameter (MMD) to reduce coughing and increase peripheral drug delivery.
- Screen subjects for cough history and pretreat with a beta agonist.
- Use a negative pressure room with at least six air changes per hour, or use an isolation booth/hood with an exhaust and filtration.
- Use personnel barrier protection (mask, gown, gloves, goggles).
- Screen HIV subjects for tuberculosis.
- Keep treatment subjects from others until any coughing subsides.
- Health-care workers should monitor themselves for TB.

Pharmacokinetics: Bronchoalveolar lavage fluid showed 23.2 ng/ml 18 to 24 hours after a single 300 mg dose using the Respirgard II nebulizer. Peak plasma levels were below the lower limit of detection (2.3 ng/ml). Approximately a third of the dose is excreted unchanged in urine within 6 hours. Tissue binding delays clearance of the drug, and small amounts are found in the urine 6 to 8 weeks after a dose. Plasma accumulation with chronic aerosol dosing is not known.

Drug interactions: Pentamidine isethionate should not be mixed in solution for nebulization with any other drug unless physical and chemical compatibility has been verified.

Respiratory care assessment:

- Initially:

  Review isolation and containment system (booth, negative pressure room) and personnel barrier protection when treating patient or instructing in use of aerosol delivery of drug. Screen HIV subjects for tuberculosis.

  Instruct and then verify correct use of the nebulizer system. Ensure use of a system with one-way valves and scavenging expiratory filters, such as the Respirgard, and a system capable of producing a MMD of 1 or 2 microns for peripheral lung deposition.

  Assess breathing rate and pattern.

  Assess breath sounds by auscultation before and after treatment.

  Assess pulse before and after treatment.

  Assess patient's subjective reaction to treatment for any change in breathing effort or pattern.

- Evaluate need for prior use of a bronchodilator if symptoms of bronchospasm or coughing occur after inhalation of pentamidine.

- Monitor subjects for onset of adverse reactions noted.

- Instruct subjects that the development of symptoms such as cough, dyspnea, and fever are suggestive of a pulmonary infection such as PCP. If they develop those symptoms, they should be evaluated by their health care practitioner.

- Long-term: monitor efficacy of pentamidine prophylaxis in preventing episodes of PCP.

Ribavirin

Virazole

Class: Antiviral agent

Indication: For use in treatment of selected hospitalized infants and children with severe lower respiratory tract infections of respiratory syncytial virus (RSV). Infants and children with congenital heart disease or other cardiopulmonary disease, immunosuppression, or prematurity are at increased risk for severe RSV infection.

Action: Exact mode of action is not known. Ribavirin exerts a virostatic effect, probably due to its structural resemblance to nucleosides such as guanosine, which are used in viral synthesis and replication. The nucleoside may be replaced by the ribavirin molecule, which prevents construction of viable viral particles.

Dose and administration: Note: review the manual of operation for the Small Particle Aerosol Generator (SPAG) before administering the drug.

Supplied as 6 g of powdered drug. Dissolve drug in a total of 300 ml of sterile USP water for injection or inhalation, giving a final concentration of 20 mg/ml, placed in the reservoir flask of the SPAG unit. Solution is nebulized with the SPAG aerosol generator unit and administered 12 to 18 hours per day for not less than 3 days and not more than 7 days.

Side effects/adverse reactions:
- Pulmonary function deterioration
- Pneumothorax
- Apnea
- Bacterial pneumonia
- Cardiovascular instability (hypotension, cardiac arrest)
- Rash, eyelid erythema, and conjunctivitis
- Drug precipitation causing occlusion of the endotracheal tube, high inspiratory pressures
- Drug precipitation causing ventilator malfunction and/or expiratory valve obstruction

Contraindications: Females who are or may become pregnant during exposure to the drug should not take it. RSV is not usually a severe infection in this population. Ribavirin has been found to be teratogenic or embryolethal in test dosages of 1 to 10 mg/kg in almost all species studied.

Precautions: Health care workers should avoid exposure to the drug by use of environmental containment measures and barrier protection (masks, gowns, glasses, gloves).

Use filters to prevent contamination and malfunction of ventilator expiratory valves and sensors.

With oxyhood or tent administration, use a secondary wrap with exhaust filtration of the system. Turn off the SPAG unit and replace the FI_{O_2} with an alternate source when breaking containment.

Pharmacokinetics: Ribavirin is absorbed from the lung when administered as an inhaled aerosol. With 8 to 20 hours of aerosol treatment, peak plasma levels are 1 to 3 µg/ml, and respiratory secretions show levels of 1000 µg/ml or greater. Plasma half-life of ribavirin is approximately 9 hours; in respiratory secretions the half-life is 1 to 2 hours.

Drug interactions: Potential for digitalis toxicity.

Respiratory care assessment:
- Check the SPAG unit for proper assembly and function prior to treatment use.
- Assess breathing rate and pattern.

- Assess breath sounds by auscultation before and after treatment.
- Assess pulse before and after treatment.
- Assess patient's subjective reaction to treatment for any change in breathing effort or pattern.
- If mechanically ventilated, monitor machine pressures and sensor functions; exchange filters in the ventilator breathing circuit as needed to prevent gas flow obstruction.
- Monitor the airway for any indication of obstruction or occlusion (increases in peak airway pressure, change in vital signs, distress, color of infant).
- Monitor infants for drug precipitation on the face, eyes, or skin, and for conjunctivitis, erythema, or rash.
- Assess drug effect on RSV infection by ventilatory needs (FIo_2, degree of ventilatory support required, length of ventilatory support).
- Assess and monitor body temperature.

EXOGENOUS LUNG SURFACTANTS
Agents:
- Colfosceril palmitate (Exosurf)
- Beractant (Survanta)

General indication and use: For prevention of respiratory distress syndrome (RDS) in premature infants with very low birth weight (less than 1350g) or with evidence of surfactant deficiency, or rescue treatment of infants with RDS.

Action: Although exogenous lung surfactants have been given experimentally by nebulized aerosol, the route of administration with the approved products is by direct tracheal instillation. The exogenous lung surfactants are either synthetic or modified natural surfactants, which replace natural lung surfactant missing due to prematurity. The primary ingredient is dipalmitoylphosphatidylcholine (DPPC), which forms approximately 85% of natural, endogenous lung surfactant secreted by alveolar type II cells. DPPC can be harvested from natural sources (animals, humans) or synthesized in the laboratory. The drug products contain spreading and adsorption agents to help disperse the solution in the lung. The exogenous product reduces surface tension in the lung, decreasing the work of breathing due to low compliance. The exogenous surfactant is taken up into alveolar type II cells to form a recycled pool of surfactant for subsequent reuse.

General side effects/adverse reactions: Premature birth is associated with high morbidity and mortality, congenital anomalies, and abnormal laboratory values. Side effects due to the drug are difficult to separate from effects due to the infant's condition.
- Reflux into and occlusion of the endotracheal tube
- Oxygen desaturation, bradycardia
- Apnea
- Overventilation, hypocarbia, and hyperoxia

- Pulmonary hemorrhage
- Pulmonary air leak, with pneumothorax, pneumopericardium pneumomediastinum, pulmonary interstitial emphysema
- Mucus plugs and airway occlusion
- Intraventricular hemorrhage

Precautions: Be prepared to adjust mechanical ventilation settings if lung mechanics are changed by the exogenous surfactant. In particular:

- Level of ventilation and peak ventilating pressure or volume
- Inspired oxygen concentration

Respiratory care assessment of drug therapy:

- Monitor pulse and cardiac rhythm during and after administration.
- Monitor airway for patency during administration.
- Monitor color and activity level of infant.
- Monitor chest rise for level of ventilation or use electronic monitor if available.
- Monitor arterial oxygen saturation and adjust FIo_2 accordingly to prevent hyperoxia or hypoxia.
- Monitor transcutaneous Pco_2 if possible and be prepared to adjust level of ventilation as needed to prevent hypercarbia or hypocarbia.
- Assess lung mechanics to determine effectiveness of the exogenous agent in normalizing lung compliance. The instilled drug may cause changes within minutes in some cases.
- Consider the possible adverse effects if pulse, cardiac rhythm, or arterial/transcutaneous blood gas values deteriorate.

Colfosceril palmitate

Exosurf Neonatal

Class: A synthetic lung surfactant

Dose and administration: (See drug insert material for complete dosage and administration description prior to administering the drug; the following is a brief overview of the key points.)

Colfosceril palmitate is supplied as 108 mg of lyophilized powder. Reconstitute each vial with 8 ml of the supplied diluent (preservative-free sterile water for injection).

Each milliliter of reconstituted solution contains:

colfosceril palmitate	13.5 mg
cetyl alcohol	1.5 mg
tyloxapol	1.0 mg

Recommended dose: 5 ml/kg of body weight in two doses of 2.5 ml/kg by tracheal instillation. Each 8 ml vial of solution will treat a maximum body weight of 1600 g (1.6 kg).

Administration: Drug is given through a side port adaptor on the endotracheal tube. Administer the first 2.5 ml/kg half-dose over several minutes with the infant in midline position, then rotated 45° to the right for 30 seconds. Return the infant to the midline position and administer the second 2.5 ml/kg half-dose. Turn the infant 45° to the left for 30 seconds, then return to the midline position. Maintain ventilation throughout. Each dose is given in bursts timed to coincide with inspiration. *Pharmacokinetics:* The drug is administered directly into the trachea, and biophysical effects occur at the alveolar surface. Dipalmitoylphosphatidylcholine, or DPPC, is absorbed from the alveolus into lung tissue to be broken down and recycled for subsequent synthesis and secretion of phospholipids. Rabbit studies show that 90% of alveolar phospholipids are recycled. The alveolar half-life of intratracheally instilled DPPC is approximately 12 hours.

Beractant
Survanta
Class: A modified natural lung surfactant
Dose and administration: (See drug insert material for complete dosage and administration description prior to administering the drug; the following is a brief overview of the key points.)

The drug is supplied as a suspension with 25 mg phospholipids per ml in 8 ml of 0.9% saline solution. Inspect for discoloration (normal color is white to light brown). Swirl gently (do not shake to avoid frothing) to redisperse suspension if settling has occurred.

Recommended dose: 100 mg of phospholipids/kg birth weight (4 ml/kg). Each 8 ml vial will treat a maximum birth weight of 2 kg.

Administration: The calculated dose is given in fourths (quarters); each quarter-dose is given through a 5 French end-hole catheter inserted through the endotracheal tube, with the infant in the following sequence of supine positions:

Head and body slightly down, head turned to the right;
Head and body slightly down, head turned to the left;
Head and body inclined slightly up, head turned to the right;
Head and body inclined slightly up, head turned to the left.
Remove the catheter and ventilate the infant after each quarter-dose is given for at least 30 seconds or until stable.
Pharmacokinetics: The drug is administered directly to the trachea, and biophysical effects occur at the alveolar surface. In surfactant-deficient animals (rabbits and lambs), alveolar clearance of phospholipids is rapid. Within hours of administration, the phospholipids enter endogenous surfactant pathways and form a recycled pool of reutilized surfactant.

This section reviews drug groups that are important in critical and respiratory care, and identifies considerations appropriate to respiratory care.

ANTIINFECTIVE AGENTS

Hypersensitivity reactions may require ventilatory assistance, including oxygen, airway maintenance, and ventilatory support. Such reactions may be more likely in patients with history of allergy, asthma, hay fever, or urticaria.

Maintain sterility during procedures such as tracheal aspiration (suctioning) and asepsis with equipment to avoid infection with nonsusceptible organisms, leading to overgrowth or superinfection.

Check general indices of infection to assess efficacy, including white blood count and differential and temperature.

To monitor respiratory infections, evaluate respiratory status, including rate, pattern, breath sounds on auscultation, dyspnea, cough, sputum production (color, consistency, amount), and chest radiograph with respiratory involvement. Note risk of septicemia and septic shock with the possibility of acute respiratory distress syndrome if infections are not controlled, requiring ventilatory support.

Penicillins

There may be increased risk of allergic reaction if the patient is allergic to cephalosporins (cross-allergy).

Agents

Natural penicillins

Penicillin G (various brand names)
Penicillin V (various brand names)

Penicillinase-resistant

Cloxacillin (Cloxapen, Tegopen)
Dicloxacillin (Dynapen, Pathocil, others)
Methicillin (Staphcillin)
Nafcillin (Unipen, Nafcil, others)
Oxacillin (Bactocill, Prostaphlin)

Aminopenicillins

Amoxicillin (Amoxil, Biomox, Polymox, Trimox, Wymox)
Amoxicillin/potassium clavulanate (Augmentin)
Ampicillin (Omnipen, others)
Ampicillin/sulbactam (Unasyn)
Bacampicillin (Spectrobid)

Extended spectrum

Carbenicillin (Geocillin)
Mezlocillin (Mezlin)
Piperacillin (Pipracil)
Piperacillin/tazobactam sodium (Zosyn)
Ticarcillin (Ticar)
Ticarcillin/potassium clavulanate (Timentin)

Cephalosporins

There may be increased risk of allergic reaction if the patient is allergic to penicillins (cross-allergy).

Agents
  First generation
    Cephalexin (Keflex)
    Cefadroxil (Duricef)
    Cephradine (Velosef)
    Cephalothin (Keflin)
    Cephapirin (Cefadyl)
    Cefazolin (Ancef)
  Second generation
    Cefaclor (Ceclor)
    Cefamandole (Mandol)
    Cefoxitin (Mefoxin)
    Cefuroxime (Zinacef)
    Cefonicid (Monocid)
    Cefmetazole (Zefazone)
    Cefotetan (Cefotan)
    Cefprozil (Cefzil)
    Cefpodoxime (Vantin)
    Loracarbef (Lorabid)
  Third generation
    Cefixime (Suprax)
    Cefoperazone (Cefobid)
    Cefotaxime (Claforan)
    Ceftizoxime (Cefizox)
    Ceftriaxone (Rocephin)
    Ceftazidime (Fortaz)

Carbapenem
Imipenem-cilastatin (Primaxin)

Monobactam
Aztreonam (Azactam)

Aminoglycosides
Neurotoxicity may occur, aggravating muscle weakness, including the diaphragm, due to potential curare-like effect on the
neuromuscular junction. Evaluate effect on readiness to wean
in patients on mechanical ventilation. Muscle weakness can
complicate weaning from ventilatory support. Assess effect on
subjects with neuromuscular disorders (e.g., myasthenia gravis,
Guillain-Barré, botulism, etc.)
    Use neuromuscular blockade cautiously if at all in patients
receiving aminoglycosides.
Agents
    Amikacin (Amikin)
    Gentamicin (Garamycin)
    Kanamycin (Kiantrex)
    Netilmicin (Netromycin)
    Streptomycin
    Tobramycin (Nebcin)
    Neomycin sulfate
    Paromomycin sulfate (Humatin)

Tetracyclines
Avoid use in children under 8 years of age, because use of these drugs results in permanent tooth discoloration of a yellow-gray-brown appearance. Tetracyclines form a complex with calcium in bone-forming tissue.

Tetracyclines should not be taken simultaneously with dairy products or antacids.

Tetracyclines have been noted to produce muscle weakness and neuromuscular impairment.
Agents
> Tetracycline (various)
> Demeclocycline (Declomycin)
> Doxycycline (Vibramycin)
> Methacycline (Rondomycin)
> Minocycline (Minocin)
> Oxytetracycline (Terramycin)

Macrolides
GI irritation is common. Monitor for diarrhea and avoid dehydration, especially in COPD patients.
Agents
> Clarithromycin (Biaxin)
> Azithromycin (Zithromax)
> Dirithromycin (Dynabac)
> Erythromycin (various)
> Troleandomycin (Tao)

Fluoroquinolones
Agents
> Ciprofloxacin (Cipro)
> Norfloxacin (Noroxin)
> Ofloxacin (Floxin)
> Enoxacin (Penetrex)
> Lomefloxacin (Maxaquin)

Lincosamides
Agents
> Lincomycin (Lincocin)
> Clindamycin (Cleocin)

Antifungals
Agents
> Flucytosine (Ancobon)
> Nystatin (Mycostatin)
> Miconazole (Monistat)
> Ketoconazole (Nizoral)
> Amphotericin B
> Griseofulvin (Fulvicin, various)
> Fluconazole (Diflucan)
> Itraconazole (Sporanox)

Sulfonamides
Agents
> Sulfadiazine

Sulfisoxazole (Gantrisin)
Sulfamethoxazole (Gantanol)
Sulfamethizole (Thiosulfil Forte)
Sulfasalazine (Azulfidine)

Miscellaneous Antiinfective Agents

Agents

Chloramphenicol (Chloromycetin)
Spectinomycin (Trobicin)
Vancomycin (Vancocin)
Colistin sulfate (Polymixin E; Coly-Mycin S)
Polymyxin B sulfate (Aerosporin)
Bacitracin
Novobiocin (Albamycin)
Metronidazole (Flagyl)

Antiviral Agents

Agents used to treat HIV

- Practice infection control to prevent opportunistic infection in subjects.
- Monitor subject for respiratory infections, especially *P. carinii* pneumonia (PCP).
- Assess and screen for concomitant TB infection.
- Use isolation techniques (negative pressure booth or hood, etc.) for aerosol treatments.
- Nebulizers with one-way valves and expiratory filtration are preferred for concomitant aerosol drug delivery to control risk of TB transmission to other patients or health care personnel.

Agents

Zidovudine, AZT (Retrovir)
Didanosine, ddI (Videx)
Zalcitabine (Hivid)
Lamivudine, 3TC (Epivir)
Saquinavir mesylate (Invirase)
Stavudine, d4T (Zerit)

Other antiviral agents

Famciclovir (Famvir)
Valacyclovir (Valtrex)
Ribavirin (Virazole)
Amantadine (Symmetrel)
Foscarnet sodium (Foscavir)
Acyclovir (Zovirax)
Ganciclovir (Cytovene)
Rimantadine (Flumadine)

ANTIDEPRESSANT AGENTS

Tricyclic compounds

Tricyclic antidepressants (TCAs) exert three major pharmacological activities: inhibition of presynaptic reuptake of norepinephrine and serotonin, sedation, and peripheral/central anticholinergic effects.

These agents should be used with extreme caution in subjects with coronary artery disease or other cardiovascular disease, including heart failure, angina pectoris, paroxysmal tachycardia, or conduction disturbances. TCAs can produce arrhythmias and prolong conduction time. Hypertension and orthostatic hypotension can occur. Syncope, palpitations, and myocardial infarction have been reported as adverse effects.

Evaluate response of blood pressure if administering beta agonists. Consider use of nonadrenergic bronchodilators such as ipratropium bromide (Atrovent).

Smoking may increase the metabolic transformation of TCAs.

Agents

Amitriptyline (Elavil)
Clomipramine (Anafranil)
Imipramine (Tofranil)
Doxepin (Sinequan)
Trimipramine (Surmontil)
Nortriptyline (Aventyl)
Desipramine (Norpramin)
Protriptyline (Vivactil)
Amoxapine (Asendin)

Monoamine oxidase inhibitors (MAOIs)

Drugs that inhibit the MAO enzyme system cause an increase in endogenous epinephrine, norepinephrine, and serotonin in storage sites in the nervous system. Increased levels of monoamines in the central nervous system are responsible for the antidepressant effect. Hypertensive crises are the most serious reactions. Headache may be the first symptom.

Consider alternative bronchodilators to the beta agonists, such as the anticholinergic, ipratropium, and monitor blood pressure.

Cold agents that contain adrenergics (e.g., ephedrine, phenylephrine, phenylpropanolamine) should not be used without physician approval.

Agents

Phenelzine (Nardil)
Tranylcypromine (Parnate)

ANTIPSYCHOTIC AGENTS

Monitor for sedative effect and CNS depression, leading to hypoventilation.

If hypotension occurs, minimize ventilating and thoracic pressures if the patient is on positive pressure ventilatory support to decrease impeded venous return and maintain adequate cardiac output.

Evaluate efficacy of beta-adrenergic bronchodilator therapy in asthmatics or chronic obstructive pulmonary disease; effect may be lessened by antiadrenergic effect of drug decreasing catecholamine levels.

Beta agonists, especially systemic formulations, may increase hypotensive effect in presence of alpha-adrenergic blocking activity; monitor blood pressure if initiating beta-adrenergic bronchodilator.

Note: bronchopneumonia may occur; lethargy and decreased sense of thirst can cause dehydration, hemoconcentration, and decreased ventilation. Use with caution in patients with chronic respiratory impairment, especially asthma, or the elderly; "silent pneumonia" may develop.

Caution patients to avoid hazardous activities or those requiring alertness.

Patients taking phenothiazines should use sunscreen during sun exposure to prevent burns.

Orthostatic hypotension occurs often; caution patients to rise from sitting or lying position gradually until stabilized on medication.

Patients should avoid over-the-counter preparations (cough, hay fever, cold) unless approved by physician, since serious drug interactions may occur. They should avoid use with alcohol or CNS depressants because increased drowsiness may occur.

Agents
  Phenothiazines
    Chlorpromazine (Thorazine)
    Promazine (Sparine)
    Triflupromazine (Vesprin)
    Thioridazine (Mellaril)
    Mesoridazine (Serentil)
    Acetophenazine (Tindal)
    Perphenazine (Trilafon)
    Prochlorperazine (Compazine)
    Fluphenazine (Prolixin)
    Trifluoperazine (Stelazine)
  Thioxanthenes
    Chlorprothixene (Taractan)
    Thiothixene (Navane)
  Other
    Haloperidol (Haldol)
    Molindone (Moban)
    Loxapine (Loxitane)
    Clozapine (Clozaril)
    Risperidone (Risperdal)
    Pimozide (Orap)

BARBITURATES

Barbiturates are used both as sedative-hypnotics (sleeping aids) as well as for general anesthesia, depending on the specific agent. All barbiturates share the following characteristics:

- Respiratory depression, which is dose dependent, is possible.
- Caution is advised when using for sedative effect in patients with COPD or sleep apnea.

- Barbiturates do not provide analgesia.
- Other CNS depressants, including alcohol, narcotic analgesics, sedatives, cough preparations, and antihistamines, may increase CNS depressant effect, including respiratory depression.
- Airway control/protection, oxygenation, and ventilatory support should be provided to help patients recover from respiratory depression resulting from barbiturate use.
- Cardiovascular status, including blood pressure and pulse, should be monitored for circulatory depression. Overdose can cause cardiovascular collapse.

Agents

    Phenobarbital sodium (Luminal Sodium)
    Mephobarbital (Mebaral)
    Metharbital (Gemonil)
    Amobarbital (Amytal)
    Aprobarbital (Alurate)
    Butabarbital (Butisol)
    Talbutal (Lotusate)
    Secobarbital (Seconal)
    Pentobarbital (Nembutal)
    Thiopental sodium (Pentothal)
    Thiamylal sodium (Surital Sodium)
    Methohexital sodium (Brevital Sodium)

BENZODIAZEPINES

These agents are commonly used as antianxiety or sedative-hypnotic (sleeping) agents. Monitor for possible respiratory depression, which is dose dependent, and use with caution in patients with COPD, or sleep apnea.

Increased CNS depression occurs with the use of alcohol, tricyclic antidepressants, narcotics, barbiturates, sedatives, and hypnotics. Caution individuals that other CNS depressants, including alcohol, narcotic analgesics, cough preparations, and antihistamines, may increase effect, including respiratory depression.

Caution individuals to avoid hazardous activities if drowsiness or dizziness occurs.

Flumazenil (Romazicon) is a benzodiazepine receptor antagonist, which is indicated for the partial or complete reversal of the sedative effects of benzodiazepines when they are used for sedative effect or in the case of overdose.

Agents

    Estazolam (ProSom)
    Flurazepam HCl (Dalmane)
    Temazepam (Restoril)
    Triazolam (Halcion)
    Quazepam (Doral)
    Oxazepam (Serax)
    Prazepam (Centrax)
    Lorazepam (Ativan)

Alprazolam (Xanax)
Chlordiazepoxide (Librium)
Diazepam (Valium)
Halazepam (Paxipam)
Chlorazepate dipotassium (Tranxene)
Midazolam (Versed)

GENERAL ANESTHETIC AGENTS

Note that concomitant administration of narcotic analgesics, antidepressants, or barbiturates will increase sedative effect and CNS depression, including respiratory depression, apnea, and muscle rigidity. Assess sensorium, respiratory rate, and pattern.

Assess degree of recovery before instituting weaning or removing patient from mechanical ventilation.

Use deep breathing, turning, coughing, or other lung inflation techniques (incentive spirometry, intermittent positive pressure breathing) after surgery to prevent increased secretions and atelectasis in lungs.

Nonbarbiturate agents
Ketamine HCl (Ketalar)
Etomidate (Amidate)
Propofol (Diprivan)
Droperidol (Inapsine)

Anesthetic gases
Nitrous oxide
Cyclopropane
Ethylene
Halothane (Fluothane)
Methoxyflurane (Penthrane)
Enflurane (Ethrane)
Isoflurane (Forane)

LOCAL ANESTHETICS

Monitor cardiovascular status, respiratory rate/pattern, and level of consciousness. Twitching, drowsiness, dizziness, tremors, or blurred vision can all indicate early signs of CNS toxicity. Toxicity or overdose can cause convulsions requiring airway and possibly ventilatory support.

Hypersensitivity can result in anaphylaxis, requiring airway/ventilatory support or resuscitation.

Some solutions contain sulfites which may trigger bronchospasm in asthmatic subjects.

Agents
Bupivacaine (Marcaine)
Chloroprocaine (Nesacaine)
Etidocaine (Duranest)
Lidocaine (Xylocaine)
Mepivacaine (Carbocaine)
Procaine (Novocain)
Tetracaine (Pontocaine)
Prilocaine (Citanest)

NARCOTIC ANALGESICS

Evaluate patient for respiratory depression, which is dose dependent. Respiratory depression effect can complicate or prolong weaning from mechanical ventilation; attempts to decrease IMV rates can result in hypoventilation. Nausea and vomiting can also occur, leading to possible aspiration and pneumonitis.

Symptoms of opioid overdose include pinpoint pupil, marked respiratory depression, and ultimately coma. The skin is clammy and subsequently cyanotic. Respirations are slow, shallow, and irregular. Provide control/protection of airway, adequate oxygenation, and support of ventilation until effect of drug subsides.

Other CNS depressants, such as alcohol or barbiturates, can increase the depressant effect of opioids.

The therapeutic response is a decrease in symptoms or report of pain.

Note: opioids can increase airway resistance. Evaluate asthmatics for wheezing indicating bronchoconstriction.

To treat overdose, the narcotic antagonists naloxone (Narcan), naltrexone (ReVia), or nalmefene (Revex) reverses. O_2, airway, and ventilatory support should be provided as appropriate given respiratory status. If reversal does not occur, consider possibility of presence of nonopioid drugs in patient. Monitor respiratory status, especially rate, and depth of tidal volumes for possible hypoventilation. Maintain airway and support ventilation until adequate spontaneous breathing returns.

Do not attempt aggressive weaning from mechanical ventilatory support until adequate reversal occurs, as determined by spontaneous tidal volumes and rate.

Naloxone is a pure antagonist and does not possess agonist properties (respiratory depression, pupillary constriction). There is no effect in the absence of narcotics or agonistic effects of other narcotic antagonists.

Monitor patient for adequate control of pain if withdrawing narcotics.

Agents

> Opium (Pantopon, Paregoric)
> Morphine
> Codeine
> Oxycodone (Roxicodone)
> Oxymorphone (Numorphan)
> Levorphanol (Levo-Dromoran)
> Pentazocine (Talwin)
> Meperidine (Demerol)
> Methadone (Dolophine)
> Fentanyl (Sublimaze)
> Sufentanil (Sufenta)
> Alfentanil (Alfenta)
> Propoxyphene (Darvon)
> Butorphanol (Stadol)

Nalbuphine (Nubain)
Buprenorphine (Buprenex)
Dezocine (Dalgan)

SEDATIVE HYPNOTIC AGENTS (MISCELLANEOUS)

Monitor for possible respiratory depression, which is dose dependent.

Use with caution in patients with COPD, or sleep apnea.

Increased CNS depression results with use of alcohol, tricyclic antidepressants, narcotics, barbiturates, sedatives/hypnotics, cough preparations, or antihistamines.

Patients should avoid hazardous activities while drug action persists.

Agents

Zolpidem tartrate (Ambien)
Paraldehyde (Paral)
Chloral hydrate (Noctec)
Acetylcarbromal (Paxarel)
Glutethimide (Doriden)
Methyprylon (Noludar)
Ethchlorvynol (Placidyl)
Ethinamate (Valmid)
Propiomazine HCl (Largon)

acebutolol

(ase-bute'-oh-lole)
Monitan,* Sectral
Func. class.:
Antihypertensive
Chem. class.: Selective β_1-blocker

Action: Competitively blocks stimulation of β_1-adrenergic receptors within vascular smooth muscle, produces negative chronotropic, inotropic activity (decreases rate of SA node discharge, increases recovery time), slows conduction of AV node, decreases heart rate, which decreases O_2 consumption in myocardium; also decreases renin-aldosterone-angiotensin system at high doses, inhibits β_2-receptors in bronchial system (high doses)

Uses: Mild to moderate hypertension, sinus tachycardia, persistent atrial extrasystoles, tachydysrhythmias, prophylaxis of angina pectoris

Dosage and routes:
Hypertension
■ *Adult:* PO 400 mg qd or in 2 divided doses, may be increased to desired response
Ventricular dysrhythmia
■ *Adult:* PO 200 mg bid, may increase gradually, usual range 600-1200 mg daily
Available forms: Caps 200, 400 mg, tabs 100, 200, 400 mg (Canada only)

Side effects/adverse reactions:
CV: Profound hypotension, bradycardia, CHF, cold extremities, postural hypotension, 2nd or 3rd degree heart block

CNS: Insomnia, fatigue, dizziness, mental changes, memory loss, hallucinations, depression, lethargy, drowsiness, strange dreams, catatonia
GI: Nausea, diarrhea, vomiting, *mesenteric arterial thrombosis, ischemic colitis*
INTEG: Rash, fever, alopecia
HEMA: Agranulocytosis, thrombocytopenia, purpura
EENT: Sore throat, dry burning eyes
GU: Impotence
ENDO: Increased hypoglycemic response to insulin
RESP: Bronchospasm, dyspnea, wheezing

Contraindications: Hypersensitivity to β-blockers, cardiogenic shock, heart block (2nd, 3rd degree), sinus bradycardia, CHF, cardiac failure

Precautions: Major surgery, pregnancy (B), lactation, diabetes mellitus, renal disease, thyroid disease, COPD, asthma, well-compensated heart failure, aortic, mitral valve disease

Pharmacokinetics:
PO: Onset 1-1½ hr.; peak 2-4 hr; duration 10-12 hr; half-life 6-7 hr, excreted unchanged in urine, protein binding 5%-15%

Interactions/incompatibilities:
■ Increased hypotension, bradycardia: reserpine, hydralazine, methyldopa, prazosin, anticholinergics
■ Decreased antihypertensive effects: indomethacin
■ Increased hypoglycemic effect: insulin
■ Decreased bronchodilation: theophyllines β_2-agonist

Lab test interferences:
Interference: Glucose/insulin tolerance tests
Increase: Uric acid, potassium, triglyceride, lipoproteins

RESPIRATORY CARE CONSIDERATIONS:
Assess/evaluate:

■ Avoid use with reversible airway obstruction or bronchospastic disease such as asthma or chronic bronchitis due to potential for bronchospasm (wheezing, dyspnea, complaints of chest tightness) secondary to beta blockade; consider use of other classes of antihypertensive agents for these patients.
■ Monitor all subjects for symptoms of increased airway resistance (wheezing, tightness in chest, difficulty breathing).
■ Monitor effect on BP as well as pulse, especially if on positive pressure ventilatory support.
■ Assess effectiveness of beta-adrenergic bronchodilator therapy for possible antagonism as well as effect on BP to avoid increasing BP, if used.

Patient education:

■ Do not use OTC products containing α-adrenergic stimulants (nasal decongestants, OTC cold preparations) unless directed by physician.
■ Caution patient that orthostatic hypotension may occur.
■ Report symptoms of CHF: difficulty breathing, especially on exertion or when lying down, night cough, and swelling of extremities.

---

acetazolamide/ acetazolamide sodium

(a-set-a-zole'a-mide)
Acetazolamide, AK-Zol, Cetazol, Dazamide, Diamox, Diamox Sequels, Hydrazol/ Diamox Parenteral
Func. class.: Diuretic; carbonic anhydrase inhibitor
Chem. class.: Sulfonamide derivative

Action: Inhibits carbonic anhydrase activity in proximal renal tubules to decrease reabsorption of water, sodium, potassium, bicarbonate; decreases carbonic anhydrase in CNS, increasing seizure threshold; able to decrease aqueous humor in eye, which lowers intraocular pressure.

Uses: Open-angle glaucoma, narrow-angle glaucoma (preoperatively, if surgery delayed), epilepsy (petit mal, grand mal, mixed), edema in CHF, drug-induced edema, acute mountain sickness.

Dosage and routes:
Narrow-angle glaucoma
■ *Adult:* PO/IM/IV 250 mg q4h or 250 mg bid, to be used for short-term therapy
Open-angle glaucoma
■ *Adult:* PO/IM/IV 250 mg-1g/day in divided doses for amounts over 250 mg
Edema
■ *Adult:* IM/IV 250-375 mg/day in AM
■ *Child:* IM/IV 5 mg/kg/day in AM
Seizures
■ *Adult:* PO/IM/IV 8-30 mg/kg/day, usual range 375-1000 mg/day

---

■ *Child:* PO/IM/IV 8-30 mg/kg/day in divided doses tid or qid, or 300-900 mg/m²/day, not to exceed 1.5 g/day
Mountain sickness
■ *Adult:* PO 250 mg q8-12h
Available forms: Tabs 125, 250 mg; caps sust rel 500 mg; inj IM/IV 500 mg

Side effects/adverse reactions:

GU: Frequency, hypokalemia, polyuria, uremia, glucosuria, hematuria, dysuria, crystalluria, renal calculi
CNS: Drowsiness, paresthesia, anxiety, depression, headache, dizziness, confusion, stimulation, fatigue, *convulsions,* sedation, nervousness
GI: Nausea, vomiting, anorexia, constipation, diarrhea, melena, weight loss, *hepatic insufficiency,* taste alterations
EENT: Myopia, tinnitus
INTEG: Rash, pruritus, urticaria, fever, *Stevens-Johnson syndrome,* photosensitivity
ENDO: Hyperglycemia
HEMA: Aplastic anemia, hemolytic anemia, leukopenia, agranulocytosis, thrombocytopenia, purpura, pancytopenia

Contraindications:
Hypersensitivity to sulfonamides, severe renal disease, severe hepatic disease, electrolyte imbalances (hyponatremia, hypokalemia), hyperchloremic acidosis, Addison's disease, long-term use in narrow-angle glaucoma, COPD

Precautions:
Hypercalciuria, pregnancy (C)

Pharmacokinetics:
PO: Onset 1-1½ hr, peak 2-4 hr, duration 6-12 hr

PO—SUS REL: Onset 2 hr, peak 8-12 hr, duration 18-24 hr
IV: Onset 2 min, peak 15 min, duration 4-5 hr
65% absorbed if fasting (oral), 75% absorbed if given with food; half-life 2 ½-5 ½ hr; excreted unchanged by kidneys (80% within 24 hr), crosses placenta

Interactions/incompatibilities:
■ Increased action of amphetamines, procainamide, quinidine, tricyclics, flecainide, ephedrine, pseudoephedrine
■ Increased excretion of barbiturates, ASA, lithium
■ Toxicity: salicylates
■ Hypokalemia: with other diuretics, corticosteroids, amphotericin B
■ IV compatibility: cimetidine, D_5 W, D_{10} W, NaCl, LR, Ringer's Sol
■ Improvement in CVP q8h
■ Signs of metabolic acidosis: drowsiness, restlessness
■ Signs of hypokalemia: postural hypotension, malaise, fatigue, tachycardia, leg cramps, weakness
■ Rashes, temperature elevation qd
■ Confusion, especially in elderly; take safety precautions if needed

Lab test interferences:
False positive: Urinary protein, 17 hydroxysteroid
Increase: Blood glucose levels, bilirubin, blood ammonia, calcium, chloride
Decrease: Urine citrate, potassium

---

italic = common side effects   **bold** = life-threatening reactions

RESPIRATORY CARE CONSIDERATIONS:
Assess/evaluate:

- Monitor acid-base status: carbonic anhydrase inhibitors can lead to metabolic acidosis due to HCO_3 - loss and inhibited H^+ secretion.
- Monitor rate, depth, and rhythm of respiration for increased levels to detect acidosis.
- Evaluate for dehydration, especially in COPD subjects or those with excess respiratory tract secretions.
- Monitor color and consistency of sputum in chronic bronchitic subjects.

acetylcysteine

(a-se-til-sis'tay-een)
Airbron,* Mucomyst, Mucosil
Func. class: Mucolytic
Chem. class: N-acetyl derivative amino acid L-cysteine

See Section III: Aerosol Agents for Oral Inhalation

activated charcoal

Arm-a-char, Actidose-Aqua, Liqu-Char, Superchar, Charcoaide, Charcocaps, Charcodote, Charcotabs, Digestalin
Func. class.: Antiflatulent/antidote
Chem. class.:

Action: Binds poisons, toxins, irritants; increases adsorption in GI tract; inactivates toxins and binds until excreted

Uses: Flatulence, poisoning, dyspepsia, distention, deodorant in wounds, diarrhea

Dosage and routes:
Poisoning
- *Adult and child:* PO 5 - 10 × weight of substance ingested, minimum dose 30 g/250 ml of water, may give 20 - 40g q6h for 1 - 2 days in severe poisoning
Flatulence/dyspepsia
- *Adult:* PO 520 - 975 mg p.c. up to 4.16 g/day
Available forms: Powder; liq 12.5, 25, 30,50 g; caps 260 mg; tabs 325 mg

Side effects/adverse reactions:
GI: Nausea, black stools, vomiting, constipation, diarrhea

Contraindications: Hypersensitivity to this drug, unconsciousness, semiconsciousness, cyanide poisoning, mineral acids, alkalies

Pharmacokinetics:
PO: Excreted in feces

Interactions/incompatibilities:
- Decreased effectiveness of both drugs: ipecac, laxatives
- Do not mix with dairy products

RESPIRATORY CARE CONSIDERATIONS:
Assess/evaluate:
- If used in OD resulting in respiratory depression or potential for such, monitor respiratory status carefully and be prepared to provide ventilatory and airway support until OD effect terminates adequately.
- Oxygenation will usually be adequate at low or normal FIo_2 once ventilation is reestablished adequately for subjects with normal lungs.

*Available in Canada only

- Monitor for aspiration and resulting pneumonitis or ARDS.
Note: patient stools will be black

---

adenosine
(ah-den'oh-seen)
Adenocard
Func. class.: Antidysrhythmic
Chem. class.: Endogenous nucleoside

Action: Slows conduction through AV node, can interrupt reentry pathways through AV node, and can restore normal sinus rhythm in patients with paroxysmal supraventricular tachycardia (PSVT)

Uses: PSVT

Dosage and routes:
- *Adult:* IV BOL 6 mg; if conversion to normal sinus rhythm does not occur within 1-2 min, give 12 mg by rapid IV BOL; may repeat 12 mg dose again in 1-2 min
Available forms: Inj 3 mg/ml

Side effects/adverse reactions:
GI: Nausea, metallic taste, throat tightness, groin pressure
RESP: Dyspnea, chest pressure, hyperventilation
CNS: Lightheadedness, dizziness, arm tingling, numbness, apprehension, blurred vision, headache
CV: Chest pain, *atrial tachydysrhythmias*, sweating, palpitations, hypotension, *facial flushing*

Contraindications: Hypersensitivity, 2nd or 3rd degree heart block, AV block, sick sinus syndrome, atrial flutter, atrial fibrillation, ventricular tachycardia

Precautions: Pregnancy (C), lactation, children, asthma, elderly

Pharmacokinetics: Cleared from plasma in <30 sec, half-life 10 sec

Interactions/ incompatibilities:
- **Increased effects of adenosine: dipyridamole**
- **Decreased activity of adenosine: theophylline or other methylxanthines (caffeine)**
- **Higher degree of heart block: carbamazepine**
- **Incompatible with any other drug in solution or syringe**

Lab test interferences:
Increase: Liver function tests

RESPIRATORY CARE CONSIDERATIONS:
Assess/evaluate:
Cardiac status: BP, pulse, respiration, ECG intervals (PR, QRS, QT)
Note: inhaled adenosine can induce bronchoconstriction in asthmatic subjects, although not in nonasthmatic individuals. Be aware of the possibility of bronchospasm in patients with a history of asthma, although subjects with asthma have received adenosine by injection with no exacerbation. Respiratory status: for side effects of dyspnea, S.O.B., chest pressure or pain, and hyperventilation.

---

italic = common side effects   **bold** = life-threatening reactions

albumin, normal serum 5%/25%
(al-byoo'min)
Albuminar 5%, Albutein 5%, Buminate 5%, Plasbumin 5%, Albuminar 25%, Albutein25%, Buminate 25%, Plasbumin-25%
Func. class.: Blood derivative
Chem. class.: Placental human plasma

Action: Exerts oncotic pressure, which expands volume of circulating blood and maintains cardiac output

Uses: Restores plasma volume in burns, hyperbilirubinemia, shock, hypoproteinemia, prevention of cerebral edema, cardiopulmonary bypass procedures, ARDS

Dosage and routes:
Burns
■ *Adult:* IV dose to maintain plasma albumin at 30-50 g/L, use 5% sol initially, then 25% sol after 24 hr
Shock
■ *Adult:* IV 500 ml of 5% sol q30 min, as needed
■ *Child:* ¼-½ adult dose in nonemergencies
Hypoproteinemia
■ *Adult:* IV 1000-2000 ml of 5% sol qd, not to exceed 5-10 ml/min or 25-100 g of 25% sol qd, not to exceed 3 ml/min, titrated to patient response
Hyperbilirubinemia / erythroblastosis fetalis
■ *Infant:* IV 1 g of 25% sol/kg before transfusion
Available forms: Inj IV 50, 250 mg/ml; (5%, 25%)

Side effects/adverse reactions:
GI: Nausea, vomiting, increased salivation
INTEG: Rash, urticaria
CNS: Fever, chills, flushing, headache
RESP: Altered respirations, *pulmonary edema*
CV: Fluid overload, hypotension, erratic pulse, tachycardia

Contraindications: Hypersensitivity, CHF, severe anemia, renal insufficiency

Precautions: Decreased salt intake, decreased cardiac reserve, lack of albumin deficiency, hepatic disease, renal disease, pregnancy (C)

Pharmacokinetics: In hyponutrition states, metabolized as protein/energy source.

Lab test interferences:
False increase: Alk phosphatase

RESPIRATORY CARE CONSIDERATIONS:
Assess/evaluate:
■ Therapeutic response should include increased BP, decreased pulmonary edema, increased serum albumin.
■ Assess breath sounds to detect presence of rales. Shortness of breath, anxiety, orthopnea, expiratory rales, frothy blood-tinged cough, cyanosis indicate worsening of pulmonary edema—perhaps due to volume overload.
■ Monitor pulmonary wedge pressure if available, or CVP and neck veins, to evaluate circulatory overload.
■ Monitor ventilatory pressures, especially peak and plateau airway pressures, if on mechanical ventilatory

support, for changes in pulmonary edema and, subsequently, lung compliance.

albuterol

(al-byoo'ter-ole)
Albuterol, Proventil, Proventil Repetabs, Salbutamol,* Ventolin, Ventolin Rotacaps, Volmax
Func. class.: Adrenergic β_2-agonist
Chem. class.: Saligenin, a catecholamine analogue

See also: Section III: Aerosol Agents for Oral Inhalation

Action: Causes bronchodilation by selective action on β_2-(pulmonary) receptors by increasing levels of cAMP, which relaxes smooth muscle; produces bronchodilation, CNS and cardiac stimulation, and increased diuresis and gastric acid secretion; longer acting than isoproterenol

Uses: Prevention of exercise-induced asthma, bronchospasm, production of premature labor

Dosage and routes:
To prevent exercise-induced asthma
■ *Adult:* MDI 2 puffs 15 min before exercising, SVN/IPPB 2.5 mg tid-qid
Bronchospasm
■ *Adult:* MDI 1-2 puffs q4-6h; SVN 2.5 mg (0.5 ml of 0.5% solution) tid, qid; PO 2-4 mg tid-qid, not to exceed 8 mg
Prevention of premature labor
Available forms:
MDI 90 µg/ actuation; SVN solution 0.5% or unit dose; DPI 200 µg Rotacap; tabs 2, 4 mg; syr 2 mg/5 ml, extended release tabs 4 mg

Side effects/adverse reactions:
CNS: Tremors, anxiety, insomnia, headache, dizziness, stimulation, *restlessness,* hallucinations, flushing, irritability
EENT: Dry nose, irritation of nose and throat
CV: Palpitations, tachycardia, hypertension, angina, hypotension, dysrhythmias
GI: Heartburn, nausea, vomiting
MS: Muscle cramps

Contraindications: Hypersensitivity to sympathomimetics, tachydysrhythmias, severe cardiac disease

Precautions: Lactation, pregnancy (C), cardiac disorders, hyperthyroidism, diabetes mellitus, hypertension, prostatic hypertrophy, narrow-angle glaucoma, seizures, exercise-induced bronchospasm (aerosol) in children <12 years

Pharmacokinetics: Well absorbed PO, extensively metabolized in the liver, excreted in urine, crosses placenta, breast milk, blood-brain barrier
PO: Onset ½ hr, peak 2 ½ hr, duration 4-6 hr, half-life 2 ½ hr
PO-ER: Onset ½ hour; peak 2-3 hr; duration 12 hr
INH: Onset 5-15 min, peak 1-1½ hr, duration 4-6 hr, half-life 4 hr

Interactions/incompatibilities:
■ Increased action of aerosol bronchodilators
■ Increased action of albuterol: tricyclic antidepressants, MAOIs, other adrenergics
■ May inhibit action of albuterol: other β-blockers

---

italic = common side effects   **bold** = life-threatening reactions

RESPIRATORY CARE CONSIDERATIONS:
Assess/evaluate:

- Assess effectiveness of drug therapy based on the indication(s) for the aerosol agent: presence of reversible airflow due to primary bronchospasm or other obstruction secondary to an inflammatory response and/or secretions, either acute or chronic.
- Monitor flow rates using office or bedside peak flow meters or laboratory reports of pulmonary function, especially before and after bronchodilator studies, to assess reversibility of airflow obstruction.
- Assess breathing rate and pattern.
- Assess breath sounds by auscultation before and after aerosol treatment.
- Assess pulse before and after treatment.
- Assess patient's subjective reaction to drug for any change in breathing effort or pattern.
- Assess arterial blood gases, or pulse oximeter saturation, as needed, for acute states with asthma or COPD, to monitor changes in ventilation and gas exchange (oxygenation).
- Long-term: monitor pulmonary function studies of lung volumes, capacities, and flows.

Patient/family education:

- Instruct and then verify correct use of aerosol delivery device (MDI, SVN) for inhalation route.
- Instruct subjects with asthma in use and interpretation of disposable peak flow meters to assess severity of asthma attacks.

Note: death has been associated with excessive use of inhaled adrenergic agents in severe acute asthma crises; individuals using such drugs should be instructed to contact a physician or an emergency room if there is no response to the usual dose of the inhaled or oral agent.

Alpha₁-Proteinase Inhibitor (Human)

(al'fa one pro'ta-naase inhibitor)
Prolastin
Func. class: enzyme inhibitor
Chem. class: purified human alpha₁-proteinase inhibitor

Action: Alpha₁-proteinase inhibitor (alpha₁-PI) or alpha₁-antitrypsin is a principal inhibitor of neutrophil elastase, an enzyme which degrades elastin tissues and which is released by inflammatory cells such as neutrophils in the lower respiratory tract. In the hereditary disorder of alpha₁-antitrypsin deficiency, there is a reduced serum level of alpha₁-PI; this biochemical imbalance leads to progressive degradation of elastin tissues in alveolar structures by elastase, resulting in severe, panacinar emphysema. The drug alpha₁-proteinase inhibitor is a sterile, lyophilized preparation of purified human alpha₁-proteinase inhibitor and replaces the deficient alpha$_1$-antitrypsin to slow or stop further tissue deterioration.

Uses: Congenital alpha$_1$-antitrypsin deficiency

Dosage and routes:
For IV use only. May be given at a rate of 0.08 ml/kg/min or greater.
Dosage: 60 mg/kg once weekly.
Available forms: Injection, with at least 20 mg alpha$_1$-PI per ml, when reconstituted; in approx. 500 mg activity/single dose vial w/20 ml sterile water or approx. 1000 mg activity/single dose vial w/40 ml sterile water. (Refrigerate at 2° to 8° C; do not refrigerate unused solution, discard)

Side effects/adverse reactions:
INTEG: Delayed fever occurring up to 12 hours after treatment
CNS: Lightheadedness, dizziness
HEMA: Mild transient leukocytosis several hours after infusion

Precautions: Although alpha$_1$-PI, which is obtained from donor pools of fresh human plasma is heat-treated to reduce transmission of infectious agents, recipients are encouraged to receive hepatitis B vaccine. Pregnancy. Safety and efficacy in children not established. Circulatory overload; loss of efficacy through improper storage or handling.

Pharmacokinetics: The half-life of alpha$_1$-PI in vivo was approximately 4.5 days.

RESPIRATORY CARE CONSIDERATIONS:
Assess/evaluate:
- Monitor for adequate "threshold" level of alpha$_1$-PI in serum = 80 mg/dl.
- Assess progression of emphysema, using chest radiograph, pulmonary function tests including diffusion capacity; perform chest examination, including inspection, palpation, percussion, and auscultation of breath sounds.
- Evaluate arterial blood gases if acute deterioration.

Patient education:
- Avoid smoking or second-hand smoke environments.
- Avoid or minimize risks of respiratory infection in crowds.
- Avoid environmental or occupational lung irritants, such as paint fumes.

alprostadil
(al-pros'ta-dil)
Prostin VR Pediatric
Func. class.: Hormone
Chem. class.: Prostaglandin E$_1$

Action: Prostaglandin E$_1$ relaxes smooth muscles of ductus arteriosus to maintain a patent ductus for infants with congenital heart defects restricting aortic blood flow, such as hypoplastic left-sided heart syndrome or coarctation of the aorta; a PDA allows pulmonary artery blood flow through the aorta, to the body, to improve systemic perfusion.

Uses: To maintain patent ductus arteriosus (temporary treatment)

Dosage and routes:
■ *Infants:* IV INF 0.1 µg/kg/
min, until desired response,
then reduce to lowest effective
amount, 0.4 µg/kg/min not
likely to produce greater
beneficial effects
Available forms: Inj IV 500
µg/ml

**Side effects/adverse
reactions:**
MISC: **Sepsis,** hypokalemia,
peritonitis, hypoglycemia,
hyperkalemia
RESP: **Apnea, bradypnea,
wheezing, respiratory
depression**
HEMA: **DIC** (disseminated
intravascular coagulation),
thrombocytopenia, anemia,
bleeding
CNS: Fever, **convulsions,**
lethargy, hypothermia,
stiffness, hyperirritability,
cerebral bleeding
GI: Diarrhea, regurgitation,
hyperbilirubinemia
GU: Oliguria, hematuria,
anuria
CV: **Bradycardia, tachycardia,
hypotension, CHF, ventricular
fibrillation, shock,** flushing,
cardiac arrest, edema

Contraindications: *Hypersensitivity,* respiratory distress
syndrome (RDS)

Precautions: Bleeding
disorders

Pharmacokinetics: Up to
80% metabolized in lungs,
excreted in urine
(metabolites)

**Interactions/
incompatibilities:**
■ Do not mix in sol or syringe
with other drugs; compatibility not known.

**RESPIRATORY CARE
CONSIDERATIONS:
Assess/evaluate:**
■ Differentiate cyanotic heart
disease (restricted pulmonary
blood flow) indicating use of
drug from respiratory distress
syndrome.
■ Therapeutic effect: ideal
assessment of drug efficacy is
echocardiogram to verify
patency of ductus; doppler
studies may also be used.
■ Auscultation will reveal a
murmur if ductus is open,
allowing blood flow during
systole.
■ Monitor improvement in
PaO_2 of limbs using pulse oximetry, which will be sensitive
to decreases in either oxygen or
tissue perfusion by indicating
drops in saturation readings.
■ Monitor arterial pressure,
continuous ECG; if arterial
pressure decreases, reduce or
stop drug.
■ Monitor breath sounds to
detect rales or crackles indicative of pulmonary edema and
CHF.
■ Apnea is common following
infusion of the drug; monitor
respiratory status, support airway, and provide ventilatory
support.
■ If bradycardia occurs,
discontinue drug.
■ Use alprostadil cautiously in
infants with bleeding tenden-
cies; drug inhibits platelet
aggregation.

alteplase
(al-teep′lase)
Activase
Func. class.: Antithrombotic
Chem. class.: Tissue plas-
minogen activator (TPA)

Action: Produces fibrin conversion of plasminogen to plasmin; able to bind to fibrin, convert plasminogen in thrombus to plasmin, which leads to local fibrinolysis, limited systemic proteolysis

Uses: Lysis of obstructing thrombi associated with acute MI; although not currently approved, alteplase will be used for other conditions requiring thrombolysis (i.e., PE, DVT, unclotting arteriovenous shunts)

Dosage and routes:
■ *Adult:* IV a total of 100 mg; 6-10 mg given IV BOL over 1-2 min, 60 mg given over first hour, 20 mg given over second hour, 20 mg given over third hour; or 1.25 mg/kg given over 3 hr for smaller patients
Available forms: Powder for inj 20 mg (11.6 million IU)/vial, 50 mg (29 million IU)/vial

Side effects/adverse reactions:
SYST: GI, GU, intracranial, retroperitoneal bleeding, surface bleeding
CV: Sinus bradycardia, ventricular tachycardia, accelerated idioventricular rhythm
INTEG: Urticaria, rash

Contraindications: Hypersensitivity, active internal bleeding, recent CVA, severe uncontrolled hypertension, intracranial/intraspinal surgery/trauma, aneurysm

Precautions: Pregnancy (C), lactation, children

Pharmacokinetics: Cleared by liver, 80% cleared within 10 min of drug termination

Interactions/ incompatibilities:
■ Increased bleeding: heparin, acetylsalicylic acid, dipyridamole
■ Do not add other drugs to IV solution

Lab test interferences:
Increase: PT, APTT, TT

RESPIRATORY CARE CONSIDERATIONS:
Assess/evaluate:
■ Bleeding from invasive procedures, such as cutdowns or arterial punctures, is an increased risk with fibrinolytic therapy and is common.
■ Minimize arterial or venous punctures.
■ Use sites accessible to manual compression for arterial punctures.
■ Use pressure dressings for arterial puncture after manual compression.
■ Monitor for bleeding from any puncture sites.
■ Risk of fibrinolytic therapy is increased with hypertension, hemostatic defects, or treatment with anticoagulant agents.

Patient Education:
Instruct patient to notify health care personnel of any swelling, hematoma, or bleeding at a puncture site.

ambenonium chloride
(am-be-noe'nee-um)
Mytelase caplets
Func. class.: Cholinergics, Anticholinesterase
Chem. class.: Synthetic quaternary ammonium compound

italic = common side effects   **bold** = life-threatening reactions

Action: An acetylcholinesterase inhibitor; inhibits destruction of acetylcholine, which increases concentration at sites where acetylcholine is released; this facilitates transmission of impulses across myoneural junction

Uses: Myasthenia gravis when other drugs cannot be used

Dosage and routes:
■ *Adult:* PO 5 mg q3-4h, then gradually increased q1-2 days; usually 5-40 mg per dose is sufficient
Available forms: Tabs 10 mg

Side effects/adverse reactions:
INTEG: Rash, urticaria, sweating
CNS: Dizziness, headache, weakness, *convulsions,* incoordination, *paralysis, loss of consciousness,* drowsiness
GI: Nausea, diarrhea, vomiting, cramps, increased salivary, gastric secretions, dysphagia, increased peristalsis
CV: Tachycardia, dysrhythmias, bradycardia, hypotension, AV block, ECG changes, *cardiac arrest,* sycope
GU: Frequency, incontinence, urgency
RESP: Respiratory depression, bronchospasm, constriction, laryngospasm, respiratory arrest, increased secretions, dyspnea
EENT: Miosis, blurred vision, lacrimation, visual changes

Contraindications: Obstruction of intestine, renal system, hypersensitivity

Precautions: Seizure disorders, bronchial asthma, coronary occlusion, hyperthyroidism, dysrhythmias, peptic ulcer, megacolon, poor GI motility, pregnancy (C), bradycardia, hypotension, lactation, children

Pharmacokinetics:
PO: Onset 20-30 min, duration 3-8 hr

Interactions/ incompatibilities:
■ Decreased action of ambenonium: aminoglycosides, anesthetics, antidysrhythmics, mecamylamine, polymyxin, quinidine, magnesium, corticosteroids
■ Increased action of neuromuscular blockers, succinylcholine

RESPIRATORY CARE CONSIDERATIONS:
Assess/evaluate:
■ Assess respiratory rate and pattern, breath sounds for wheezing, hypoventilation.
■ Monitor vital capacity: > 10 ml/kg to clear secretions, provide adequate cough.
■ Monitor arterial saturation (SaO_2, SpO_2) to ensure adequate oxygenation.
■ Assess ABGs if acute deterioration of diaphragmatic strength and ability to ventilate is detected.
■ Provide airway and ventilatory support as needed.
■ Monitor for exacerbation of asthma or airway resistance in COPD subject, due to parasympathetic induced bronchoconstriction.
■ Assess subjective response of patient, for difficulty in breathing, tightness in chest.
■ Assess pulse for bradycardia and BP for decrease.
Note: use of a cholinergic

agent can intensify and prolong a depolarizing blockade induced by succinylcholine, due to the inactivation of acetylcholine needed for neuromuscular transmission.

amiloride HCl
(a-mill'oh-ride)
Amiloride HCl, Midamor
Func. class.: Potassium-sparing diuretic
Chem. class.: Pyrazine

Action: Acts primarily on distal tubule, secondarily by inhibiting reabsorption of sodium and H_2O and increasing potassium retention

Uses: Edema in CHF in combination with other diuretics, for hypertension, adjunct with other diuretics to maintain potassium

Dosage and routes:
Adult: PO 5 mg qd, may be increased to 10-20 mg qd if needed
Available forms: Tab 5 mg

Side effects/adverse reactions:
GU: Polyuria, dysuria, frequency, impotence
ELECT: Acidosis, hyponatremia, *hyperkalemia*, hypochloremia
CNS: Headache, dizziness, fatigue, weakness, paresthesias, tremor, depression, anxiety
GI: Nausea, diarrhea, dry mouth, *vomiting, anorexia,* cramps, constipation, abdominal pain, jaundice, bleeding
EENT: Loss of hearing, tinnitus, blurred vision, nasal congestion, increased intraocular pressure
INTEG: Rash, pruritus, alopecia, urticaria

MS: Cramps, joint pain
CV: Orthostatic hypotension, dysrhythmias, angina
HEMA: Agranulocytopenia, leukopenia, thrombocytopenia (rare)

Contraindications: Anuria, hypersensitivity, hyperkalemia, impaired renal function

Precautions: Dehydration, pregnancy (B), diabetes, acidosis, lactation

Pharmacokinetics:
PO: Onset 2 hr, peak 6-10 hr, duration 24 hr; excreted in urine, feces, half-life 6-9 hr

Interactions/ incompatibilities:
▪ Enhanced action of antihypertensives; lithium toxicity may be provoked
▪ Hyperkalemia: other potassium-sparing diuretics, potassium products, ACE inhibitors, salt substitutes

Lab test interferences:
Interfere: GTT

RESPIRATORY CARE CONSIDERATIONS:
Assess/evaluate:
▪ Produces an increase in sodium excretion and decrease in potassium excretion, leading to possible hyponatremia and hyperkalemia; monitor serum electrolytes.
▪ Evaluate for dehydration, especially in COPD subjects or those with excess respiratory tract secretions.
▪ Monitor color, consistency of sputum.
▪ Monitor blood pressure.
▪ Evaluate breath sounds and respiratory pattern for pulmonary congestion.

italic = common side effects   **bold** = life-threatening reactions

aminophylline (theophylline ethylenediamine)
(am-in-off'i-lin)
Corophyllin,* Phyllocontin, Truphylline
Func. class.: Bronchodilator
Chem. class.: Xanthine, ethylenediamide

Action: Not currently well understood. Xanthines and theophylline in particular may act by blocking adenosine receptors and inhibiting smooth muscle contraction mediated by adenosine receptors. Xanthines are weak bronchodilators, and exert a therapeutic effect by strengthening diaphragmatic contraction and stimulating central respiratory drive receptors, in addition to their bronchodilating effect.

Uses: Asthma, bronchospasm, COPD, apnea of prematurity, Cheyne-Stokes respirations

Dosage and routes:
- *Adult:* PO 500 mg, then 250-500 mg q6-8h; CONT IV 0.3-0.9 mg/kg/hr (maintenance); RECT 500 mg q6-8h
- *Child:* PO 7.5 mg/kg, then 3-6 mg/kg q6-8h; IV 7.5 mg/kg, then 3-6 mg/kg q6-8h injected over 5 min; do not exceed 25 mg/min; may give loading dose of 5.6 mg/kg over ½ hr; CONT IV 1 mg/kg/hr (maintenance); for children/infants, use drug without preservative of alcohol
- *Neonates:* IV/PO 1 mg/kg initially for plasma increases of each 2 µg/ml, then 1 mg/kg q6h
Available forms: Inj IV, IM, rectal supp 250, 500 mg; rectal sol 300 mg/5 ml; elix 250 mg/5 ml; oral liq 105 mg/5 ml; tabs 100, 200 mg, tabs con-rel 225 mg; tabs sust-rel 300 mg

Side effects/adverse reactions:
CNS: Anxiety, restlessness, insomnia, *dizziness, convulsions,* headache, lightheadedness, muscle twitching
CV: Palpitations, sinus tachycardia, hypotension, flushing, dysrhythmias, increased respiratory rate
GI: Nausea, vomiting, anorexia, diarrhea, bitter taste, dyspepsia, anal irritation (suppositories), epigastric pain
RESP: Increased rate
INTEG: Flushing, urticaria, *rectal supp (irritation)*
GU: Urinary frequency

Contraindications: Hypersensitivity to xanthines, tachydysrhythmias

Precautions: Elderly, CHF, cor pulmonale, hepatic disease, active peptic ulcer disease, diabetes mellitus, hyperthyroidism, hypertension, children, pregnancy (C), glaucoma, prostatic hypertrophy

Pharmacokinetics: Well absorbed PO, extended rel well absorbed slowly, rectal supp is erratic, rectal sol is absorbed quickly; metabolized by liver (caffeine); excreted in urine; crosses placenta; appears in breast milk
Half-life: 3-12 hr; half-life increased in geriatric patients, hepatic disease or CHF

PO: Onset ¼ hr., peak 1-2 hr., duration 6-8 hr
PO-ER: Unknown, peak 4-7 hr., duration 8-12 hr
IV: Onset rapid, duration 6-8 hr
REC: Onset erratic, peak 1-2 hr., duration 6-8 hr

Interactions/ incompatibilities:
■ Incompatible with amikacin, Vit C, bleomycin, cephalothin, cephaprin, chloramphenicol, chlorpromazine, cimetidine, clindamycin, codeine, corticotropin, diphenhydrinate, dobutamine, doxorubicin, epinephrine, erythromycin, fructose sol, heparin, hydralazine, hydroxyzine, insulin, invert sugar, isoproterenol, levarterenol, meperidine, methadone, methicillin, methylprednisolone, morphine, nafcillin, papaverine, penicillin G, pentazocine, phenobarbital, phenytoin, procaine, prochlorperazine, promazine, promethazine, succinylcholine, tetracycline, vancomycin, Vit B with C
■ Increased action of aminophylline: cimetidine, propranolol, erythromycin, troleandomycin
■ Dysrhythmias: halothane
■ May increase effects of anticoagulants
■ Cardiotoxicity: β-blockers
■ Increased elimination: smoking
■ Increased toxicity: erythromycin, influenza vaccine, oral contraceptives, glucocorticoids, disulfiram
■ Decreased effects of lithium
■ Decreased effects of this drug: rifampin, barbiturates, adrenergics, ketoconazole

Lab test interferences:
Increased: Plasma free fatty acids

RESPIRATORY CARE CONSIDERATIONS:
Assess/evaluate:
■ Therapeutic response: decreased dyspnea, respiratory rate, and pattern; respiratory stimulation in infancy.
■ Theophylline blood levels (therapeutic level is 10-20 μg/ml); toxicity may occur with small increase above 20 μg/ml, especially elderly; 10-12 μg/ml may be optimal in COPD patients.
■ Monitor fluid intake, diuresis occurs; dehydration may result in elderly or children.
■ Respiratory rate, rhythm, depth; auscultate lung fields bilaterally; notify physician of abnormalities.
■ Allergic reactions: rash, urticaria; if these occur, drug should be discontinued.
■ Assess side effects reported, and evaluate blood level for toxic range.

Patient Education:
■ Take doses as prescribed, do not skip dose.
■ Check OTC medications, current prescription medications for ephedrine; will increase CNS stimulation; do not drink alcohol or caffeine products (tea, coffee, chocolate, colas) which will increase diuresis or add to the xanthine level (caffeine).
■ Avoid hazardous activities; dizziness may occur.
■ If GI upset occurs, take drug with 8 oz water; avoid food, since absorption may be decreased.

---

italic = common side effects   **bold** = life-threatening reactions

- Notify physician of toxicity: insomnia, anxiety, nausea, vomiting, rapid pulse, convulsions.
- Cigarette smoking will increase metabolism of the drug, lowering blood levels.
- Increase fluid intake if sputum becomes thicker when taking drug.
- Use non-diuresing liquids, such as water, juice, Gatorade, or milk rather than diuretic products such as caffeinated coffee, tea, or colas.

amiodarone HCl

(a-mee'-oh-da-rone)
Cordarone
Func. class.: Antidysrhythmic (Class III)
Chem. class.: Iodinated benzofuran derivative

Action: Prolongs action potential duration, and effective refractory period, noncompetitive α- and β-adrenergic inhibition

Uses: Severe ventricular tachycardia, supraventricular tachycardia, ventricular fibrillation not controlled by first-line agents

Dosage and routes:
- *Adult:* PO loading dose 800-1600 mg/day 1-3 wk; then 600-800 mg/day 1 mo; maintenance 200-600 mg/day
Available forms: Tabs 200 mg

Side effects/adverse reactions:
CNS: Headache, dizziness, involuntary movement, tremors, peripheral neuropathy, malaise, fatigue, ataxia, paresthesias, insomnia

GI: Nausea, vomiting, diarrhea, abdominal pain, anorexia, constipation, *hepatotoxicity*
CV: Hypotension, bradycardia, sinus arrest, CHF, dysrhythmias, SA node dysfunction
INTEG: Rash, photosensitivity, blue-gray skin discoloration, alopecia, spontaneous ecchymosis
EENT: Blurred vision, halos, photophobia, *corneal microdeposits,* dry eyes
ENDO: Hyperthyroidism or hypothyroidism
MS: Weakness, pain in extremities
RESP: Pulmonary fibrosis, pulmonary inflammation
MISC: Flushing, abnormal taste or smell, edema, abnormal salivation, coagulation abnormalities

Precautions: Goiter, Hashimoto's thyroiditis, SN dysfunction, 2nd or 3rd degree AV block, electrolyte imbalances, pregnancy (C), bradycardia, lactation

Pharmacokinetics:
PO: Onset 1-3 wk, peak 2-10 hr; half-life 15-100 days; metabolized by liver, excreted by kidneys

Interactions/incompatibilities:
- Bradycardia: β-blockers, calcium channel blockers
- Increased levels of digitalis, quinidine, procainamide, flecainide, disopyramide, phenytoin
- Increased anticoagulant effects: warfarin
- Bradycardia, arrest: lidocaine

RESPIRATORY CARE CONSIDERATIONS:
Assess/evaluate:
- Therapeutic response: decrease in ventricular tachycardia, supraventricular tachycardia, or fibrillation
- Cardiac rate, respiration: rate, rhythm, character, chest pain
- ECG continuously to determine drug effectiveness, check for PVCs, other dysrhythmias
- For dehydration or hypovolemia
- BP continuously for hypotension, hypertension
- For rebound hypertension after 1-2 hr
- Cardiovascular status in general if on positive pressure ventilatory support and adjust ventilator settings to minimize impeded venous return and decreased cardiac output
- In case of pulmonary toxicity, specifically pneumonitis—dyspnea, fatigue, cough, fever, chest pain—drug should be discontinued

amlodipine besylate
(am-loh-dye′-peen)
Norvasc
Func. class.: Calcium channel blocker
Chem. class.: Dihydropyridine

Action: Inhibits calcium ion influx across cell membrane during cardiac depolarization; produces relaxation of coronary vascular smooth muscle, peripheral vascular smooth muscle; dilates coronary vascular arteries; increases myocardial oxygen delivery in patients with vasospastic angina

Uses: Chronic stable angina pectoris, hypertension, vasospastic angina

Dosage and routes:
Angina
- *Adult:* PO 5-10 mg qd
Hypertension
- *Adult:* PO 5 mg qd initially, may increase up to 10 mg/day
Available forms: Tabs 2.5, 5, 10 mg

Side effects/adverse reactions:
CV: Dysrhythmia, edema, bradycardia, hypotension, palpitations, syncope, AV block
GI: Nausea, vomiting, diarrhea, gastric upset, constipation, abdominal cramps, flatulence, anorexia
GU: Nocturia, polyuria, **acute renal failure**
INTEG: Rash, pruritus, urticaria, hair loss
CNS: Headache, fatigue, dizziness, anxiety, depression, insomnia, paresthesia, somnolence, asthenia
OTHER: Flushing, nasal congestion, sweating, shortness of breath, sexual difficulties, muscle cramps, cough, weight gain, tinnitus, epistaxis

Contraindications: Sick sinus syndrome, 2nd or 3rd degree heart block, hypotension less than 90 mm Hg systolic, hypersensitivity

Precautions: CHF, hypotension, hepatic injury, pregnancy (C), lactation, children, renal disease, elderly

Pharmacokinetics: *PO: Onset not determined, peak 6-12 hr, half-life 30-50 hr; metabolized by liver, excreted in urine (90% as metabolites)*

Interactions/ incompatibilities:
- Increased effects of digitalis, neuromuscular blocking

---

italic = common side effects   **bold** = life-threatening reactions

agents, theophylline, prazosin, β-blockers, fentanyl

RESPIRATORY CARE CONSIDERATIONS:
Assess/evaluate:
- Therapeutic response: corrected arrhythmia, decreased anginal pain, decreased BP.
- Monitor cardiovascular status: BP, pulse, respiration, ECG.
- Check for presence of adverse effects, especially dizziness or other signs of hypotension, bradycardia.
- If on positive pressure ventilatory support, monitor cardiac output and/or BP, and adjust level of positive pressure to extent possible, if necessary, to maintain adequate cardiac output.
- Monitor blood pressure if beta agonists are required to treat airway obstruction.
- Consider use of anticholinergic agent such as ipratropium bromide as an alternative to beta agonists if bronchodilator therapy is needed; aerosol inhalation (MDI, SVN, DPI) of adrenergic bronchodilators will generally give lower systemic levels and fewer cardiovascular effects.

Patient education:
Note: hand tremor can occur, such as seen with beta agonist bronchodilators.
Change position slowly to avoid orthostatic hypotension.

ammonium chloride
Func. class.: Acidifier
Chem. class.: Ammonium ion

Action: Lowers urinary pH, liberates hydrogen and chloride ions in blood and extracellular fluid with decreased pH and correction of alkalosis

Uses: Alkalosis (metabolic), systemic and urinary acidifier, expectorant, diuretic

Dosage and routes:
Alkalosis
- *Adult and child:* IV INF 0.9-1.3 ml/min of a 2.14% sol, not to exceed 5 ml/min
Acidifier
- *Adult:* PO 4-12 g/day in divided doses
- *Child:* PO 75 mg/kg/day in divided doses
Expectorant
- *Adult:* PO 250-500 mg q2-4h as needed
Available forms: Tabs 500 mg, 1 g; inj IV 0.4, 5 mEq/ml

Side effects/adverse reactions:
CNS: Drowsiness, headache, confusion, stimulation, tremors, *twitching, hyperreflexia, tetany, EEG changes*
CV: Bradycardia, dysrhythmias, bounding pulse
GU: Glycosuria, thirst
GI: Gastric irritation, nausea, vomiting, anorexia, diarrhea
INTEG: Rash, pain at infusion site
META: Acidosis, hypokalemia, hyperchloremia, hyperglycemia
RESP: Apnea, irregular respirations, hyperventilation

Contraindications: Hypersensitivity, severe hepatic disease, severe renal disease

Precautions: Severe respiratory disease, cardiac edema, respiratory acidosis, infants, pregnancy (C), children, elderly; do not use to correct respiratory alkalosis

Pharmacokinetics: *PO:* Absorbed in 3-6 hr; metabolized in liver, excreted in urine and feces

Interactions/ incompatibilities:

- Increased toxicity: PAS
- Decreased effects of: amphetamines, tricyclic antidepressants, salicylates, sulfonylureas
- Increased risk of systemic acidosis: spironolactone
- Incompatible with chlortetracycline, codeine, dimenhydrinate, levorphanol, methadone, warfarin, alkal. sol or drugs

Lab test interferences:
Increase: Blood ammonia, AST/ ALT
Decrease: Serum magnesium, urine urobilinogen

RESPIRATORY CARE CONSIDERATIONS:
Assess/evaluate:

- Therapeutic response: Arterial blood gases for acid-base status and correction of alkalemia or increasing urinary acidity or diuresis
- Respiratory rate, rhythm, depth; notify physician of abnormalities such as hyperpnea or increasing respiratory rate and depth that may indicate acidosis
- Electrolytes and CO_2, chloride before and during treatment
- For CNS symptoms: confusion, twitching, hyperreflexia, stimulation, headache that may indicate ammonia toxicity
- For cardiac dysrhythmias

amrinone lactate
(am'ri-none)
Inocor
Func. class.: Cardiac inotropic agent
Chem. class.: Bipyrimidine derivative

Action: Positive inotropic agent with vasodilator properties; reduces preload and afterload by direct relaxation of vascular smooth muscle

Uses: Short-term management of CHF that has not responded to other medication; can be used with digitalis

Dosage and routes:
- *Adult:* IV BOL 0.75 mg/kg given over 2-3 min; start infusion of 5-10 µg/kg/min; may give another bolus ½ hr after start of therapy, not to exceed 10 mg/kg total daily dose
Available forms: Inj 5 mg/ml

Side effects/adverse reactions:
HEMA: Thrombocytopenia
CV: Dysrhythmias, hypotension, headache, chest pain
GI: Nausea, vomiting, anorexia, abdominal pain, **hepatotoxicity, ascites,** jaundice, hiccups
INTEG: Allergic reactions, burning at injection site
RESP: Pleuritis, *pulmonary densities, hypoxemia*

Contraindications: Hypersensitivity to this drug or bisulfites, severe aortic disease, severe pulmonic valvular disease, acute MI

Precautions: Lactation, pregnancy (C), children, renal disease, hepatic disease, atrial flutter/fibrillation, elderly

italic = common side effects   **bold** = life-threatening reactions

Pharmacokinetics: *IV:* Onset 2-5 min, peak 10 min, duration variable; half-life 4-6 hr, metabolized in liver, excreted in urine as drug and metabolites 60%-90%

Interactions/ incompatibilities:
- Excessive hypotension: antihypertensives
- Additive effect: cardiac glycosides
- Incompatible in furosemide or dextrose sol other than for direct dilution

RESPIRATORY CARE CONSIDERATIONS:
Assess/evaluate:
- Therapeutic response: increased cardiac output, decreased PCWP, adequate CVP, improved systemic blood pressure, decreased dyspnea, edema.
- Monitor platelet count for possible decrease and increased risk of bleeding (dose dependent).
- Monitor ECG for ventricular arrhythmias.
- Severe hypotension can result if given with the antiarrhythmic disopyramide; monitor BP.
- Assess circulatory volume of patient; drug is not a substitute for replacement of blood, plasma, or fluids.
- Assess improvement in cardiac output, and minimize airway pressures on mechanical ventilation, particularly mean airway pressure by adjusting peak flows, I:E ratios, and use of modes such as pressure support if possible, especially while patient is being stabilized.
- Monitor blood pressure with concomitant administration of beta agonist bronchodilators.

amyl nitrite
(am'il)
Amyl nitrite, Amyl Nitrite Aspirols, Amyl Nitrite Vaporole
Func. class.: Coronary vasodilator
Chem. class.: Nitrite

Action: Relaxes vascular smooth muscle; may dilate coronary blood vessels, resulting in reduced venous return, decreased cardiac output; reduces preload, afterload, which decreases left ventricular end diastolic pressure, systemic vascular resistance; converts hemoglobin to methemoglobin, which can bind cyanide

Uses: Acute angina pectoris, cyanide poisoning

Dosage and routes:
Angina
- Adult: INH 0.18-0.3 ml as needed, 1-6 inhalations from 1 cap, may repeat in 3-5 min
Cyanide poisoning
- Adult: INH 0.3 ml ampule inhaled 15 sec until preparation of sodium nitrite infusion is ready
Available forms: Inh pearls 0.18, 0.3 ml

Side effects/adverse reactions:
CV: Postural hypotension, tachycardia, cardiovascular collapse, palpitations
CNS: Headache, dizziness, weakness, syncope
GI: Nausea, vomiting, abdominal pain
INTEG: Flushing, pallor, sweating

MISC: Muscle twitching, *hemolytic anemia, methemoglobinemia*

Contraindications: Hypersensitivity to nitrites, severe anemia, increased intracranial pressure, hypertension, pregnancy (X)

Precautions: Lactation, children, drug abuse, head injury, cerebral hemorrhage, hypotension

Pharmacokinetics: *INH:* Onset 30 sec, duration 3-5 min, half-life 1-4 min, metabolized by liver, ⅓ excreted in urine,

Interactions/ incompatibilities:
■ Increased hypotension: alcohol, β-blockers, antihypertensive

RESPIRATORY CARE CONSIDERATIONS:
Assess/evaluate:
■ Therapeutic response: relief of chest pain (angina).
■ Monitor BP, pulse, and ECG if available.
■ Provide cardiopulmonary resuscitation if ventricular fibrillation or cardiac arrest occurs due to acute MI.
■ Note: alcohol or calcium channel blockers may increase risk of hypotension.
■ Evaluate for formation of methemoglobin and oxygen transport to tissues, in case of overdose or genetically abnormal hemoglobins.

Patient education:
■ Prolonged chest pain may indicate MI: seek emergency treatment.
■ Medication may explode in presence of flame.

■ Make position changes slowly to prevent orthostatic hypotension.
■ Use analgesic (preferably other than aspirin) if headache occurs.

anistreplase (APSAC)
(an-ih-strep'layz)
Eminase
Func. class.: Thrombolytic enzyme
Chem. class.: Anisolated plasminogen streptokinase activator complex

Action: Promotes thrombolysis by promoting conversion of plasminogen to plasmin

Uses: Management of acute MI; although not yet approved, anistreplase will also be used for other conditions requiring thrombolysis (i.e., PE, DVT, unclotting arteriovenous shunts).

Dosage and routes:
■ *Adult:* IV 30 U over 4-5 min as soon as possible after onset of symptoms
Available forms: Powder, lyophilized 30 U/vial

Side effects/adverse reactions:
HEMA: Decreased Hct, *GI, GU, intracranial, retroperitoneal,* surface bleeding, *thrombocytopenia*
INTEG: Rash, urticaria, phlebitis at site, itching, flushing
CNS: Headache, fever, sweating, agitation, dizziness, paresthesia, tremor, vertigo
GI: Nausea, vomiting
RESP: Altered respirations, dyspnea, *bronchospasm, lung edema*
MS: Low back pain, arthralgia

italic = common side effects   **bold** = life-threatening reactions

CV: Hypotension, dysrhythmias, conduction disorders
SYST: Anaphylaxis

Contraindications: Hypersensitivity, active internal bleeding, intraspinal or intracranial surgery, neoplasms of CNS, severe hypertension, cerebral embolism/thrombosis/hemorrhage

Precautions: Arterial emboli from left side of heart, pregnancy (B), ulcerative colitis/enteritis, renal disease, hepatic disease, hypocoagulation, COPD, subacute bacterial endocarditis, rheumatic valvular disease, intraarterial diagnostic procedure or surgery (10 days), recent major surgery

Pharmacokinetics: Half-life 105 min

Interactions/incompatibilities:
■ Increased bleeding potential: aspirin, indomethacin, phenylbutazone, anticoagulants
■ Do not mix with any other sol or drug

Lab test interferences:
Increase: PT, APTT, TT
Decrease: Fibrinogen, plasminogen

RESPIRATORY CARE CONSIDERATIONS:
Assess/evaluate:
■ Bleeding from invasive procedures, such as cutdowns, catheter insertions, or arterial punctures, is an increased risk with fibrinolytic therapy and is common.
■ Minimize arterial or venous punctures.
■ Use sites accessible to manual compression for arterial punctures.

■ Use pressure dressings for arterial puncture after prolonged manual compression.
■ Monitor for bleeding from any puncture sites.
■ Risk of fibrinolytic therapy is increased with hypertension, hemostatic defects, or treatment with anticoagulant agents.

Patient education:
Instruct patient to notify health care personnel of any swelling, hematoma, or bleeding at a puncture site.

aspirin
(as'pir-in)
Ancasal*, A.S.A., Aspergum, Aspirin*, Bayer, Bayer Children's Aspirin, Easprin, Ecotrin, Ecotrin Maximum Strength, 8-Hour Bayer Timed Release, Empirin, Entrophen*, Genprin, Maximum Bayer, Norwich Extra-Strength, Novasen*, Sal-Adult*, Sal-Infant*, St. Joseph Children's, Supasa*, Therapy Bayer, ZORprin
Func. class.: Nonnarcotic analgesic
Chem. class.: Salicylate

Action: Antiinflammatory and analgesic activity is mediated by inhibition of the prostaglandin synthetase enzyme complex. Aspirin irreversibly inhibits platelet aggregation by interfering with cyclooxygenase needed for synthesis of thromboxane A_2, a substance that causes vasoconstriction and induces platelet aggregation.

Uses: Mild to moderate pain or fever including rheumatoid arthritis, osteoarthritis, thromboembolic disorders, transient ischemic attacks in men, rheumatic fever, postmyocardial infarction, prophylaxis of myocardial infarction.

Dosage and routes:
Arthritis
- *Adult:* PO 2.6 - 5.2 g/day in divided doses q4 - 6h
- *Child:* PO 90 - 130 mg/kg/day in divided doses q4 - 6h
Pain/fever
- *Adult:* PO/REC 325 - 650 mg q4h prn, not to exceed 4 g/day
- *Child:* PO/REC 40 - 100 mg/kg/day in divided doses q4 - 6h prn
Thromboembolic disorders
- *Adult:* PO 325 - 650 mg/day or bid
Transient ischemic attacks
- *Adult:* PO 650 mg qid or 325 mg qid
Available forms: Tabs 65, 81, 325, 500, 650, 975 mg; chewable tabs 81 mg; caps 325, 500 mg; tabs controlled-release 800 mg; tabs time-release 650 mg; supp 60, 120, 125, 130, 195, 200, 300, 325, 600, 650 mg, 1.2 g; cream; gum 227.5 mg

Side effects/adverse reactions:
*HEMA: **Thrombocytopenia, agranulocytosis, leukopenia, neutropenia, hemolytic anemia,** increased pro-time, PTT, bleeding time*
*CNS: Stimulation, drowsiness, dizziness, confusion, **convulsion,** headache, flushing, hallucinations, **coma***
*GI: Nausea, vomiting, **GI bleeding,** diarrhea, heartburn, anorexia, **hepatitis***
INTEG: Rash, urticaria, bruising
EENT: Tinnitus, hearing loss

CV: Rapid pulse, pulmonary edema
RESP: Wheezing, hyperpnea
ENDO: Hypoglycemia, hyponatremia, hypokalemia

Contraindications: Hypersensitivity to salicylates, tartrazine (FDC yellow dye #5), GI bleeding, bleeding disorders, children 12 yr, children with flulike symptoms, pregnancy (D), lactation, Vit K deficiency, peptic ulcer

Precautions: Anemia, hepatic disease, renal disease, Hodgkin's disease, pre/postoperatively

Pharmacokinetics: Well absorbed PO; enteric product and rectal product may be erratic
PO: Onset 15 - 30 min, peak 1 - 2 hr, duration 4 - 6 hr
REC: Onset slow, duration 4 - 6 hr, metabolized by liver, inactive metabolites excreted by kidneys, crosses placenta, excreted in breast milk, half-life 1 - 3 ½ hr, up to 30 hrs in large doses

Interactions/incompatibilities:
- Decreased effects of aspirin: antacids, steroids, urinary alkalizers
- Increased bleeding: alcohol, heparin, valproic acid, plicamycin, cefamandole
- Increased effects of anticoagulants, insulin, methotrexate, thrombolytic agents, penicillins, phenytoin, valporic acid, oral hypoglycemics, sulfonamides
- Increased salicylate levels: urinary acidifiers
- Decreased effects of probenecid, spironolactone,

---
italic = common side effects   **bold** = life-threatening reactions

sulfinpyrazone, sulfonyla-mides
- Toxic effects: PABA, furo-semide, carbonic anhydrase inhibitors
- Decreased blood sugar levels: salicylates
- Gastric ulcer: steroids, anti-inflammatories, nonsteroidal antiinflammatories
- Ototoxicity: vancomycin

Lab test interferences:
Increase: Coagulation studies, liver function studies, serum uric acid, amylase, CO_2, urinary protein
Decrease: Serum potassium, PBI, cholesterol
Interfere: Urine catecholamines, pregnancy test, urine glucose tests (Clinistix, Tes-Tape)

RESPIRATORY CARE CONSIDERATIONS:
Assess/evaluate:
- Avoid or use with caution in subjects with asthma, nasal polyps or rhinitis; evaluate respiratory status (rate, pattern) for bronchospasm and for exacerbation of rhinitis; consider use of nonaspirin analgesic instead.
- Advise patients to avoid aspirin before undergoing bronchoscopy or other endo-scopic procedures; aspirin causes increased risk of bleed-ing during those procedures.
- Perform arterial blood sam-pling with caution in subjects on aspirin, and use adequate compression of artery to avoid hematoma.
- Salicylate overdose can cause hyperpnea (Kussmaul breathing), due to resulting metabolic acidosis.
- Monitor acid-base status, and treat metabolic acidosis

appropriately with buffering agent; ventilatory status will normalize with correction of metabolic acidosis.
- Avoid use in subjects with severe anemia or history of blood coagulation defects.

Patient education:
Advise patients, especially asthmatics, to use alternative analgesic preparations such as acetaminophen.

astemizole
(a-stem′-mi-zole)
Hismanal
Func. class.:
Antihistamine
Chem. class.: H_1-histamine antagonist

Action: Blocks the action of histamine at H_1-receptor sites on blood vessels, GI, respira-tory tract, to decrease allergic inflammatory response and in general the pharmacologic effects of histamine. There is also an anticholinergic (drying) and sedative effect.

Uses: Rhinitis, allergy symptoms

Dosage and routes:
- *Adult and child > 12 yr:* PO 10 mg qd; to reduce time to steady state may take 30 mg day 1, 20 mg day 2, followed by 10 mg daily
Available forms: Tabs 10 mg

Side effects/adverse reactions:
GU: Frequency, dysuria, urinary retention, impotence
HEMA: Hemolytic anemia, thrombocytopenia, leukopenia, agranulocytosis, pancytopenia
RESP: Thickening of bronchial secretions, dry nose, throat

GI: Nausea, diarrhea, abdominal pain, vomiting, constipation
CNS: Headache, stimulation, drowsiness, sedation, fatigue, confusion, blurred vision, tinnitus, restlessness, tremors, paradoxical excitation in children or elderly
INTEG: Rash, eczema, photosensitivity, urticaria
CV: Hypotension, palpitations, bradycardia, tachycardia, *dysrrhythmias* (rare)

Contraindications: Hypersensitivity, newborn or premature infants, lactation, severe hepatic disease

Precautions: Pregnancy (C), elderly, children, respiratory disease, narrow-angle glaucoma, prostatic hypertrophy, bladder neck obstruction, asthma, elderly

Pharmacokinetics: *PO:* Peak 1-2 hr, 97% bound to plasma proteins; half-life is biphasic 3 ½ hr, 16-23 hr

Interactions/ incompatibilities:
■ Increased CNS depression: alcohol, other CNS depressants, procarbazine
■ Increased anticholinergic effects: MAOIs
■ Decreased action of oral anticoagulants
■ Serious CV reactions: ketoconazole, itraconazole, erythromycin
■ Avoid use with antifungals, macrolide antibiotics

Lab test interferences:
False negative: Skin allergy tests

RESPIRATORY CARE CONSIDERATIONS:
Assess/evaluate:
■ Note drying of the upper airway.
■ Caution is suggested if used in asthma, although thickening of lower respiratory tract secretions has not been established.
■ Drowsiness may be a risk factor in subjects with sleep apnea; however sedative effect is less with astemizole, loratadine, and terfenadine than with other antihistamines.
■ Monitor nasal passages during long-term treatment for changes in mucus.
■ Therapeutic response: absence of running or congested nose or rashes.

Patient education:
■ Avoid hazardous activities or use caution while drug action persists.
■ Additional CNS depression may occur with concomitant use of CNS depressants (tranquilizers, sedatives, or alcohol).

atenolol
(a-ten'oh-lole)
Apo-Atenol*, Atenolol, Tenormin
Func. class.:
Antihypertensive
Chem. class.: β-1 blocker, β_1-, $_2$-blocker (high doses)

Action: Competitively blocks stimulation of β_1-adrenergic receptor within vascular smooth muscle; produces negative chronotropic activity, positive inotropic activity (decreases rate of SA node discharge, increases recovery time), slows conduction of AV

italic = common side effects   **bold** = life-threatening reactions

node, decreases heart rate, decreases O_2 consumption in myocardium; also decreases renin-aldosterone-angiotensin system at high doses, inhibits β_2-receptors in bronchial system at higher doses

Uses: Mild to moderate hypertension, prophylaxis of angina pectoris, suspected or known myocardial infarction

Dosage and routes:
- *Adult:* IV 5 mg, repeat in 10 min if initial dose is well tolerated, then start PO dose 10 min after last IV dose
- *Adult:* PO 50 mg qd, increasing q1-2 wk to 100 mg qd; may increase to 200 mg qd for angina

Available forms: Tabs 50, 100 mg

Side effects/adverse reactions:
CV: Profound hypotension, bradycardia, CHF, cold extremities, postural hypotension, 2nd or 3rd degree heart block
CNS: Insomnia, fatigue, dizziness, mental changes, memory loss, hallucinations, depression, lethargy, drowsiness, strange dreams, catatonia
GI: Nausea, diarrhea, vomiting, *mesenteric arterial thrombosis, ischemic colitis*
INTEG: Rash, fever, alopecia
HEMA: Agranulocytosis, thrombocytopenia, purpura
EENT: Sore throat, dry burning eyes
GU: Impotence
ENDO: Increased hypoglycemic response to insulin
RESP: Bronchospasm, dyspnea, wheezing

Contraindications: Hypersensitivity to β-blockers, cardiogenic shock, 2nd or 3rd degree heart block, sinus bradycardia, CHF, cardiac failure

Precautions: Major surgery, pregnancy (C), lactation, diabetes mellitus, renal disease, thyroid disease, COPD, asthma, well-compensated heart failure

Pharmacokinetics: *PO:* Peak 2-4 hr; half-life 6-7 hr, excreted unchanged in urine, protein binding 5%-15%

Interactions/ incompatibilities:
- Increased hypotension, bradycardia: reserpine, hydralazine, methyldopa, prazosin, anticholinergics, digoxin
- Decreased antihypertensive effects: indomethacin
- Increased hypoglycemic effect: insulin
- Mutual inhibition: sympathomimetics (cough, cold preparations)
- Decreased bronchodilation: theophyllines, β_2-agonists
- Paradoxical hypertension: clonidine
- Incompatible with any other drug in sol or syringe

Lab test interferences:
Interference: Glucose/insulin tolerance tests

RESPIRATORY CARE CONSIDERATIONS:
Assess/evaluate:
- Avoid use with reversible airway obstruction or bronchospastic disease such as asthma or chronic bronchitis due to potential for bronchospasm (wheezing, dyspnea, complaints of chest tightness) secondary to beta-blockade;

consider use of other classes of antihypertensive agents for these patients.
- Monitor all subjects for symptoms of increased airway resistance (wheezing, tightness in chest, difficulty breathing).
- Monitor effect on BP and pulse, especially if on positive pressure ventilatory support.
- Assess effectiveness of beta-adrenergic bronchodilator therapy for possible antagonism and effect on BP to avoid increasing BP, if used.

Patient education:
- Do not use OTC products containing α-adrenergic stimulants (nasal decongestants, OTC cold preparations) unless directed by physician
- Caution patient that orthostatic hypotension may occur.
- Report symptoms of CHF: difficulty breathing, especially on exertion or when lying down, night cough, swelling of extremities

atovaquoné
(a-tove'-a-que-one)
Mepron
Func. class.: Antiprotozoal
Chem. class.: Aromatic diamide derivative, analog of ubiquinone

Action: Interferes with DNA/RNA synthesis in protozoa

Uses: *Pneumocystis carinii* infections not sensitive to trimethoprim/sulfamethoxazole

Dosage and routes:
- *Adult:* 750 mg with food 3× a day for 21 days
Available forms: Tabs 250 mg

Side effects/adverse reactions:
CV: Hypotension
HEMA: Anemia, leukopenia
INTEG: Pruritus, urticaria, rash, oral monilia
GI: Nausea, vomiting, diarrhea, anorexia, increased AST and ALT, **acute pancreatitis,** *constipation, abdominal pain*
CNS: Dizziness, headache, anxiety
META: Hyperkalemia, hyperglycemia, hyponatremia

Contraindications: Hypersensitivity or history of developing life-threatening allergic reactions to any component of the formulation

Precautions: Blood dyscrasias, hepatic disease, diabetes mellitus, pregnancy (C), lactation, children, elderly

Pharmacokinetics: Excreted unchanged in feces (94%), highly protein bound

Interactions/incompatibilities: Use caution when administering concurrently with other highly plasma protein-bound drugs with narrow therapeutic indices

RESPIRATORY CARE CONSIDERATIONS:
Assess/evaluate:
- Monitor respiratory status to evaluate efficacy: CXR, WBC, temperature, breath sounds, respiratory rate, and pattern.
- Monitor hemoglobin and hematocrit to assess oxygen transport capability.
- Practice infection control to prevent opportunistic infection in subjects.
- Assess and screen for concomitant TB infection.

---

italic = common side effects   **bold** = life-threatening reactions

- Use isolation techniques (negative pressure booth or hood, etc.) for aerosol treatments. Nebulizers with one-way valves and expiratory filtration are preferred for concomitant aerosol drug delivery, to control risk of TB transmission to other patients or health care personnel.

atracurium besylate
(a-tra-cyoor′ee-um)
Tracrium
Func. class.: Neuromuscular blocker (nondepolarizing)
Chem. class.: Biquaternary ammonium ester

Action: Inhibits transmission of nerve impulses at the neuromuscular junction by binding with cholinergic receptor sites, antagonizing action of acetylcholine, and causing muscle weakness or paralysis, depending on dose.

Uses: Facilitation of endotracheal intubation, skeletal muscle relaxation during mechanical ventilation, surgery, or general anesthesia

Dosage and routes:
- *Adult:* IV BOL 0.4-0.5 mg/kg, then 0.08-0.10 mg/kg 20-45 min after 1st dose if needed for prolonged procedures
Available forms: Inj IV 10 mg/ml

Side effects/adverse reactions:
CV: Bradycardia, tachycardia, increased or decreased BP
RESP: Prolonged apnea, bronchospasm, cyanosis, respiratory depression
EENT: Increased secretions
INTEG: Rash, flushing, pruritus, urticaria

Contraindications: Hypersensitivity

Precautions: Pregnancy (C), cardiac disease, lactation, children <2 yr, electrolyte imbalances, dehydration, neuromuscular disease, respiratory disease

Pharmacokinetics: *IV:* Onset 2 min, duration 20-60 min; half-life 2 min, 29 min (terminal), excreted in urine, feces (metabolites), crosses placenta

Interactions/incompatibilities:
- Increased neuromuscular blockade: aminoglycosides, clindamycin, lincomycin, quinidine, local anesthetics, polymyxin antibiotics, lithium, narcotic analgesics, thiazides, enflurane, isoflurane
- Dysrhythmias: theophylline
- Do not mix with barbiturates or alkalies in solution or syringe

RESPIRATORY CARE CONSIDERATIONS:
Assess/evaluate:
- Provide airway and ventilatory support before administering drug.
- Note possible interaction with the following antibiotics, which can increase neuromuscular blockade: the aminoglycosides, the polymyxins, clindamycin, and lincomycin.
- Use with mechanical ventilation; assess patient for adequate and preferably optimal ventilator settings *before* paralyzing, if patient is "fighting" the ventilator. Provide adequately high flow rates and tidal volumes, short inspira-

tory times, and reasonable I:E ratios, check the sensitivity in assist-control mode, and provide sufficiently high rates to avoid patient fatigue. Consider paralysis if these measures fail.

■ Assess ventilator patients for pain, hypoxemia, or ventilator malfunction, if restless and anxious before instituting muscle paralysis.

■ Assess need of patient and provide for pain control and sedation during neuromuscular blockade: *neuromuscular blocking agents do not provide analgesia or sedation.*

■ Close eyelids and provide eye lubricant during prolonged paralysis.

■ Since usual signs of pain or anxiety (restlessness, tachynea, distress, thrashing) are blocked, monitor vital signs and overall patient appearance and state closely to detect problems (e.g. IV infiltration).

■ Check ventilator alarm settings for sufficient limits and sensitivity; a disconnect alarm is critical.

■ Assess reversal of drug before attempting to wean from mechanical ventilatory support.

Administer:
■ Administer by IV, not by IM, for more consistent absorption and distribution and to avoid the pain associated with IM injection of the drug.

■ Reversal: neostigmine or edrophonium, preceded by atropine to inhibit muscarinic response especially in upper airway.

atropine sulfate
(a'troe-peen)
Func. class.: Anticholinergic parasympatholytic
Chem. class.: Belladonna alkaloid

Action: Blocks acetylcholine at parasympathetic neuroeffector sites; increases cardiac output, heart rate by blocking vagal stimulation in heart; dries secretions by blocking vagus

Uses: Bradycardia, bradydysrhythmia, anticholinesterase insecticide poisoning, blocking cardiac vagal reflexes, decreasing secretions before surgery, antispasmodic with GU, biliary surgery, bronchodilator

Dosage and routes:
Bradycardia/
bradydysrhythmias
■ *Adult:* IV BOL 0.5-1 mg given q3-5 min, not to exceed 2 mg
Child: IV BOL 0.01-0.03 mg/kg up to 0.4 mg or 0.3 mg/m2; may repeat q4-6h
Insecticide poisoning
■ *Adult and child:* IM/IV 2 mg qh until muscarinic symptoms disappear, may need 6 mg qh
Presurgery
■ *Adult:* SC/IM/IV 0.4-0.6 mg before anesthesia
■ *Child:* SC 0.1-0.4 mg 30 min before surgery
Available forms: Inj 0.05, 0.1, 0.3, 0.4, 0.5, 0.8, 1 mg/ml, tabs 0.4 mg; tabs sol 0.4, 0.6 mg

Side effects/adverse reactions:
GU: Retention, hesitancy, impotence, dysuria
CNS: Headache, dizziness, involuntary movement,

---

italic = common side effects   **bold** = life-threatening reactions

confusion, psychosis, anxiety, coma, flushing, drowsiness, insomnia, weakness
GI: Dry mouth, nausea, vomiting, abdominal pain, anorexia, constipation, paralytic ileus, abdominal distention, altered taste
CV: Hypotension, paradoxical bradycardia, angina, PVCs, hypertension, tachycardia, ectopic ventricular beats
INTEG: Rash, urticaria, contact dermatitis, dry skin, flushing
EENT: Blurred vision, photophobia, glaucoma, eye pain, pupil dilation, nasal congestion
MISC: Suppression of lactation, decreased sweating

Contraindications: Hypersensitivity to belladonna alkaloids, angle-closure glaucoma, GI obstructions, myasthenia gravis, thyrotoxicosis, ulcerative colitis, prostatic hypertrophy, tachycardia/tachydysrhythmias, asthma, acute hemorrhage, hepatic disease, myocardial ischemia

Precautions: Pregnancy (C), renal disease, lactation, CHF, tachydysrhythmias, hyperthyroidism, COPD, hepatic disease, child <6 yr, hypertension, elderly, intraabdominal infections, Down syndrome, spastic paralysis, gastric ulcer

Pharmacokinetics: Well absorbed PO, IM, SC; half-life 13-40 hours, excreted by kidneys unchanged (70%-90% in 24 hr); metabolized in liver, 40%-50% crosses placenta, excreted in breast milk
IV: Peak 2-4 min, duration 4-6 hours

IM/SC: Onset 15-50 min; peak 30 min, duration 4-6 hours
PO: Onset ½ hour; peak ½-1 hour; duration 4-6 hours

Interactions/incompatibilities:
- Decreases effect of atropine; antacids
- Decreased effects of phenothiazines
- Increased anticholinergic effects of anticholinergics, tricylic antidepressants, amantadine, MAOIs, quinidine
- Incompatible with amobarbital, ampicillin, chloramphenicol, chlortetracycline, cimetidine, epinephrine, heparin, isoproterenol, levarterenol, metaraminol, methicillin, methohexital, nitrofurantoin, pentobarbital, promazine, thiopental, warfarin, $NaCo_3$ in sol or syringe

RESPIRATORY CARE CONSIDERATIONS:
Assess/evaluate:
- Therapeutic response: decreased dysrhythmias, increased heart rate, secretions, GI, GU spasms, bronchodilation.
- Consider use of other anticholinergic agents for bronchodilation, such as ipratropium bromide, which are quaternary compounds, to avoid side effects due to wide absorption and distribution throughout the body seen with atropine, which is a tertiary compound.
- Monitor heart rate for tachycardia.
- Monitor ECG if available with patient.
- Monitor respiratory status: rate, rhythm, cyanosis, wheezing, dyspnea.

*Available in Canada only

Patient education:
- That blurred vision may likely occur and reading may not be possible; this will subside.
- To avoid activities that are hazardous or require alertness if drowsiness occurs.
- That a dry mouth is likely to occur.
- To check with physician if difficulty in urination or constipation occur.

azatadine maleate
(a-za′ta-deen)
Optimine
Func. class.: Antihistamine
Chem. class.: Piperidine
H_1-receptor antagonist

Action: Blocks the action of histamine at H_1-receptor sites on blood vessels, GI, respiratory tract, to decrease allergic inflammatory response and in general the pharmacologic effects of histamine. There is also an anticholinergic (drying) and sedative effect.

Uses: Allergy symptoms, rhinitis, chronic urticaria

Dosage and routes:
- *Adult:* PO 1-2 mg bid, not to exceed 4 mg/day
Available forms: Tabs 1 mg

Side effects/adverse reactions:
CNS: Dizziness, drowsiness, poor coordination, fatigue, anxiety, euphoria, confusion, paresthesia, neuritis, sweating, chills
CV: Hypotension, palpitations, tachycardia
RESP: Increased thick secretions, wheezing, chest tightness
HEMA: **Thrombocytopenia, agranulocytosis, hemolytic anemia**

GI: Constipation, dry mouth, nausea, vomiting, anorexia, diarrhea
INTEG: Rash, urticaria, photosensitivity
GU: Retention, dysuria, frequency, impotence
EENT: Blurred vision, dilated pupils, tinnitus, nasal stuffiness, dry nose, throat, mouth

Contraindications: Hypersensitivity to H_1-receptor antagonist, acute asthma attack, lower respiratory tract disease, child <12 yr

Precautions: Increased intraocular pressure, renal disease, cardiac disease, bronchial asthma, seizure disorder, stenosed peptic ulcers, hyperthyroidism, prostatic hypertrophy, bladder neck obstruction, pregnancy (B), elderly

Pharmacokinetics:
PO: Peak 4 hr, metabolized in liver, excreted by kidneys, crosses placenta, crosses blood-brain barrier, minimally bound to plasma proteins, half-life 9-12 hr

Interactions/ incompatibilities:
- Increased CNS depression: barbiturates, narcotics, hypnotics, tricyclic antidepressants, alcohol
- Decreased effect of oral anticoagulants, heparin
- Increased effect of azatadine: MAOIs

Lab test interferences:
False negative: Skin allergy tests

RESPIRATORY CARE CONSIDERATIONS:
Assess/evaluate:
- Note drying of the upper airway.

---

italic = common side effects   **bold** = life-threatening reactions

- Caution is suggested if used in asthma, although thickening of lower respiratory tract secretions has not been established.
- Drowsiness may be a risk factor in subjects with sleep apnea.
- Monitor nasal passages during long-term treatment for changes in mucus.
- Therapeutic response: absence of running or congested nose or rashes.

Patient education:
- Avoid hazardous activities or use caution while drug action persists.
- Additional CNS depression may occur with concomitant use of CNS depressants (tranquilizers, sedatives or alcohol).

azathioprine
(ay-za-thye′oh-preen)
Imuran
Func. class.:
Immunosuppressant
Chem. class.: Purine analog

Action: Produces immunosuppression by inhibiting purine synthesis in cells

Uses: Renal transplants to prevent graft rejection, refractory rheumatoid arthritis, refractory ITP, glomerulonephritis, nephrotic syndrome, bone marrow transplant

Dosage and routes:
Prevention of rejection
- *Adult and child:* PO, IV 3 - 5 mg/kg/day, then maintenance (PO) of at least 1 - 2 mg/kg/day

Refractory rheumatoid arthritis
- *Adult:* PO 1/mg/kg/day, may increase dose after 2 mo by 0.5 mg/kg/day, not to exceed 2.5 mg/kg/day
Available forms: Tabs 50 mg; inj IV 100 mg

Side effects/adverse reactions:
GI: Nausea, vomiting, stomatitis, esophagitis, *pancreatitis, hepatotoxicity, jaundice*
HEMA: Leukopenia, thrombocytopenia, anemia, pancytopenia
INTEG: Rash
MS: Arthralgia, muscle wasting

Contraindications: Hypersensitivity, pregnancy (D)

Precautions: Severe renal disease, severe hepatic disease

Pharmacokinetics: Metabolized in liver, excreted in urine (active metabolite), crosses placenta

Interactions/ incompatibilities:
- Increased action of azathioprine: allopurinol
- Considered incompatible; do not admix with other drugs

RESPIRATORY CARE CONSIDERATIONS:
Assess/evaluate:
- Monitor for signs/ symptoms of infection, including chest radiograph.
- Use strict infection control and isolation procedures to prevent nosocomial infection while providing ventilatory support postoperatively.
- Evaluate therapeutic response of immunosuppression in autoimmune disorders.

beclomethasone dipropionate

(be-kloe-meth'a-sone)
Beclovent, Vanceril
Func. class.: Corticosteroid, synthetic
Chem. class.: Glucocorticoid

See Section III: Aerosol Agents for Oral Inhalation

beclomethasone dipropionate (nasal)

(be-kloe-meth'a-sone)
Beconase AQ Nasal, Beconase Inhalation, Vancenase AQ Nasal, Vancenase Nasal
Func. class.: Synthetic corticosteroid
Chem. class.: Beclomethasone diester

See also Section III: Aerosol Agents for Oral Inhalation

Action: Antiinflammatory, vasoconstrictive properties in nasal passages

Uses: Seasonal or perennial rhinitis

Dosage and routes:
■ *Adult and child >12 yr:*
INSTILL 1-2 sprays in each nostril bid-qid
Available forms: Aero 42 µg/spray

Side effects/adverse reactions:
EENT: Dryness, nasal irritation, burning, sneezing, secretions with blood, nasal ulcerations, *perforation of nasal septum, Candida* infection, earache, hoarseness
ENDO: Adrenal suppression
INTEG: Rash, urticaria, pruritus
CNS: Headache, paresthesia
RESP: Acute status asthmaticus

Contraindications: Hypersensitivity, systemic corticosteroid therapy

Precautions: Pregnancy (C), lactation, children <12, nasal ulcers, recurrent epistaxis respiration

Pharmacokinetics:
INSTILL: Readily absorbed; peak concentration, other data have not been determined

RESPIRATORY CARE CONSIDERATIONS:
Assess/evaluate:
■ Monitor nasal passages during long-term treatment for changes in mucus.
■ Therapeutic response: decrease in runny nose.

Patient education:
■ Review method of installation after providing written instructions from manufacturer.
■ Instruct patient to clear nasal passages before administration; use decongestant if needed; shake inhaler, invert, tilt head backward, insert nozzle into nostril, away from septum; hold other nostril closed and depress activator; inhale through nose, exhale through mouth.
■ Follow insert instructions for cleaning insufflator unit.

benazepril

(ben-a-ze'prel)
Lotensin
Func. class.: Antihypertensive
Chem. class.: Angiotensin-converting enzyme (ACE) inhibitor

Action: Selectively suppresses renin-angiotensin-aldosterone system; inhibits

ACE, prevents conversion of angiotensin I to angiotensin II; results in dilation of arterial, venous vessels

Uses: Hypertension, alone or in combination with thiazide diuretics

Dosage and routes:
- *Adult:* PO 10 mg qd initially, then 20-40 mg/day divided bid or qd
Renal impairment
- *Adult:* 5 mg qd with Ccr <30 ml/min/1.73 m^2, increase as needed to maximum of 40 mg/day
Available forms: Tabs 5, 10, 20, 40 mg

Side effects/adverse reactions:
CV: Hypotension, postural hypotension, syncope, palpitations, angina
GU: Increased BUN, creatinine, decreased libido, impotence, urinary tract infection
HEMA: Neutropenia, agranulocytosis
INTEG: Angioedema, rash, flushing, sweating
RESP: Cough, asthma, bronchitis, dyspnea, sinusitis
META: Hyperkalemia, hyponatremia
GI: Nausea, constipation, vomiting, gastritis, melena
CNS: Anxiety, hypertonia, insomnia, paresthesia, headache, dizziness, fatigue
MS: Arthralgia, arthritis, myalgia

Contraindications: Hypersensitivity to ACE inhibitors, pregnancy (D), lactation, children

Precautions: Impaired renal, liver function, dialysis patients, hypovolemia, blood dyscrasias, CHF, COPD,

asthma, elderly, bilateral renal artery stenosis

Pharmacokinetics:
PO: Peak ½-1 hr, serum protein binding 97%, half-life 10-11 hr, metabolized by liver (metabolites), excreted in urine

Interactions/ incompatibilities:
- Increased hypotension: diuretics, other antihypertensives, ganglionic blockers, adrenergic blockers
- Increased toxicity: vasodilators, hydralazine, prazosin, potassium-sparing diuretics, sympathomimetics, potassium supplements
- Decreased absorption: antacids
- Decreased antihypertensive effect: indomethacin
- Increased serum levels of digoxin, lithium
- Increased hypersensitivity: allopurinol

Lab test interferences:
False positive: Urine acetone

RESPIRATORY CARE CONSIDERATIONS:
Assess/evaluate:
- Therapeutic response: decrease in BP.
- Persistent cough and fever are common side effects of the ACE inhibitors, which should be differentiated from other possible causes, such as respiratory infection.
- Monitor for possible hypotension.
- Evaluate BP with COPD or asthmatic subjects who require beta agonists for reversible airway obstruction.
- Assess for symptoms of CHF: edema, dyspnea, wet rales, BP.

*Available in Canada only

B

benzonatate
(ben-zoe'na-tate)
Tessalon Perles
Func. class.: Antitussive,
nonnarcotic
Chem. class.: Tetracaine
derivative

Action: Inhibits cough reflex
by anesthetizing stretch receptors in respiratory system,
direct action on cough center
in medulla

Uses: Nonproductive cough

Dosage and routes:
■ *Adult and child:* PO 100 mg
tid, not to exceed 600 mg/day
■ *Child <10 yr:* PO 8 mg/kg in
3-6 divided doses
Available forms: Perles 100 mg

**Side effects/adverse
reactions:**
CNS: Dizziness, drowsiness,
headache
GI: Nausea, constipation,
upset stomach
EENT: Nasal congestion, burning eyes
CV: Increased BP, chest tightness, numbness
INTEG: Urticaria, rash, pruritus

Contraindications: Hypersensitivity

Precautions: Pregnancy (C),
lactation

Pharmacokinetics:
PO: Onset 15-20 min, duration 3-8 hr, metabolized by
liver, excreted in urine

RESPIRATORY CARE
CONSIDERATIONS:
Assess/evaluate:
■ Therapeutic response:
absence of cough.

■ Evaluate type of cough and
productivity, including assessment of breath sounds; do not
suppress a productive cough
indicative of static secretions
and bacterial infection.
■ Evaluate need for bronchial
hygiene or chest physical
therapy (percussion, postural
drainage).

Patient education:
■ To avoid driving, other hazardous activities until patient is
stabilized on this medication
■ Not to chew or break capsules; will anesthetize mouth
■ To avoid smoking, smoke-
filled rooms, perfumes, dust,
environmental pollutants,
cleaners
■ To remain well hydrated
with nondiuresing liquids
(water, juice, Gatorade,
milk—not tea, coffee).

bepridil HCl
(beh'prih-dill)
Vascor
Func. class.: Calcium
channel blocker type 4

Action: Inhibits calcium ion
influx across cell membrane
during cardiac depolarization;
produces relaxation of coronary vascular smooth muscle,
dilates coronary arteries, decreases SA/AV node conduction, dilates peripheral
arteries

Uses: Chronic stable angina,
used alone or in combination
with propranolol

Dosage and routes:
Angina
■ *Adult:* 200-450 mg qd
Available forms: Tabs, film-
coated, 200, 300, 400 mg

italic = common side effects   **bold** = life-threatening reactions

Side effects/adverse reactions:

CV: Dysrhythmia, edema, CHF, bradycardia, hypotension, palpitations, AV block
GI: Nausea, vomiting, diarrhea, gastric upset, constipation, increased liver function studies
GU: Nocturia, polyuria
CNS: Headache, fatigue, drowsiness, dizziness, anxiety, depression, weakness, insomnia, confusion, lightheadedness, nervousness

Contraindications: Sick sinus syndrome, 2nd or 3rd degree heart block, Wolff-Parkinson-White syndrome, hypotension less than 90 mm Hg systolic, cardiogenic shock, history of serious ventricular arrhythmias

Precautions: CHF, hypotension, hepatic injury, pregnancy (C), lactation, children, renal disease, idiopathic hypertropic subaortic stenosis (IHSS), concomitant β-blocker therapy

Pharmacokinetics: Peak 2-3 hr, 99% plasma protein bound, half-life 42 hr, completely metabolized in the liver and excreted in urine and feces

Interactions/incompatibilities:

■ Increased effects: β-blockers
■ Decreased effects of lithium, rifampin
■ Increased levels of digoxin

Lab test interferences:

Increase: Liver function tests, aminotransferase, CPK, LDH

RESPIRATORY CARE CONSIDERATIONS:
Assess/evaluate:
■ Therapeutic response: corrected arrhythmia, decreased anginal pain, decreased BP
■ Monitor cardiovascular status: BP, pulse, respiration, ECG
■ Watch for presence of adverse effects, especially dizziness or other signs of hypotension, bradycardia.
■ If on positive pressure ventilatory support, monitor cardiac output and/or BP, and adjust level of positive pressure to extent possible, if necessary to maintain adequate cardiac output.
■ Monitor blood pressure if beta agonists are required to treat airway obstruction.
■ Consider use of anticholinergic agent such as ipratropium bromide as an alternative to beta agonists, if bronchodilator therapy is needed; aerosol inhalation (MDI, SVN, DPI) of adrenergic bronchodilators will generally give lower systemic levels and fewer cardiovascular effects.

Patient education:
■ Note: hand tremor can occur, such as seen with beta agonist bronchodilators.
■ Change position slowly to avoid orthostatic hypotension.

beractant
(bear-ac'-tant)
Survanta
Func. Class: Exogenous surfactant
Chem. Class: Modified natural surfactant

See Section III: Aerosol Agents for Oral Inhalation

B

betamethasone/ betamethasone sodium phosphate/ betamethasone disodium phosphate/ betamethasone acetate/

(bay-ta-meth′a-sone)
Betnelan, Celestone/
Alphatrex, Betamethasone
Dipropionate, Diprosone,
Maxivate, Teladar/
Diprolene, Diprolene AF/
Betamethasone Sodium
Phosphate, Celestone Phos-
phate, Cel-U-Jec, Selestoject
Func. class.: Corticoster-
oid, synthetic
Chem. class.: Glucocorti-
coid, long-acting

Action: Decreases inflammation by suppression of migration of polymorphonuclear
leukocytes, fibroblasts, reversal of increased capillary
permeability and lysosomal
stabilization

Uses: Immunosuppression,
severe inflammation, prevention of neonatal respiratory
distress syndrome (by administration to mother)

Dosage and routes:
■ *Adult:* PO 0.6-7.2 mg qd;
IM/IV 0.6-7.2 mg qd in joint
or soft tissue (sodium phosphate)
■ *Pregnant adult:* IM 12 mg
36-48 hr, before premature
delivery, then same dose in
24 hr (betamethasone acetate)
Available forms: Tabs 0.6 mg;
syr 0.6 mg/5 ml; inj 3,
4 mg/ml

Side effects/adverse reactions:
*INTEG: Acne, poor wound healing,
ecchymosis, bruising,* petechiae
*CNS: Depression, flushing, sweat-
ing,* headache, ecchymosis,
bruising, mood changes
CV: Hypertension, **circulatory
collapse, thrombophlebitis,
embolism,** tachycardia, *necrotizing angiitis,* **CHF**
HEMA: **Thrombocytopenia**
MS: Fractures, osteoporosis,
weakness
*GI: Diarrhea, nausea, abdominal
distention,* **GI hemorrhage,** *increased appetite, pancreatitis*
EENT: Fungal infections, increased intraocular pressure,
blurred vision

Contraindications: Psychosis, hypersensitivity, idiopathic thrombocytopenia,
acute glomerulonephritis,
amebiasis, fungal infections,
nonasthmatic bronchial disease, child <2 yr, AIDS, TB

Precautions: Pregnancy (C),
diabetes mellitus, glaucoma,
osteoporosis, seizure disorders, ulcerative colitis, CHF,
myasthenia gravis, renal disease, esophagitis, peptic ulcer

Pharmacokinetics:
PO: Onset 1-2 hr, peak 1 hr,
duration 3 days
IM/IV: Onset 10 min, peak
4-8 hr, duration 1-1½ days
Metabolized in liver, excreted
in urine as steroids, crosses
placenta

Interactions/ incompatibilities:
■ Decreased action of be-
tamethasone: cholestyramine,
colestipol, barbiturates,
rifampin, ephedrine, phenytoin, theophylline

italic = common side effects   **bold** = life-threatening reactions

- Decreased effects of anticoagulants, anticonvulsants, antidiabetics, ambenonium, neostigmine, isoniazid, toxoids, vaccines, anticholinesterases, salicylates, somatrem
- Increased side effects: alcohol, salicylates, indomethacin, amphotericin B, digitalis, cyclosporine, diuretics
- Increased action of betamethasone: salicylates, estrogens, indomethacin, oral contraceptives, ketoconazole, macrolide antibiotics

Lab test interferences:
Increase: Cholesterol, sodium, blood glucose, uric acid, calcium, urine glucose
Decrease: Calcium, potassium, T4, T3, thyroid ^{131}I uptake test, urine 17-OHCS, 17-KS, PBI
False negative: Skin allergy tests

RESPIRATORY CARE CONSIDERATIONS:
Assess/evaluate:
- Monitor for side effects of increased corticosteroid level: Cushingoid symptoms (moon face, peripheral wasting, central edema).
- Monitor patients with latent tuberculosis or reactive skin tests for reactivation of the disease.
- Evaluate muscle weakness and steroid myopathy, especially in chronic lung disease patients.
- Evaluate cardiovascular system for hypertension, CHF.
- Monitor electrolytes: potassium and calcium loss can occur, with hypokalemic alkalosis.
- Infection, including pneumonia, can occur.
- Increased corticosteroid levels can mask symptoms of infection.

- If asthma is present, monitor for breakthrough symptoms (bronchospasm, wheezing) if drug is discontinued.
- Evaluate possible adrenal insufficiency when transferring from systemic to inhaled aerosol corticosteroids in asthma.
- Monitor for symptoms of adrenal insufficiency: nausea, anorexia, fatigue, dizziness, dyspnea, weakness, joint pain.

bisoprolol
(bis-o-prole'-lole)
Zebeta
Func. class.:
Antihypertensive
Chem. class.: β$_1$-blocker

Action: Preferentially and competitively blocks stimulation of β$_1$-adrenergic receptor within cardiac muscle; produces negative chronotropic and inotropic activity (decreases rate of SA node discharge, increases recovery time), slows conduction of AV node, decreases heart rate, which decreases O$_2$ consumption in myocardium; decreases renin-aldosterone-angiotensin system; inhibits β$_2$-receptors in bronchial and vascular smooth muscle at high doses

Uses: Mild to moderate hypertension

Dosage and routes:
Hypertension
- *Adult:* PO 2.5-5 mg once daily; may increase if necessary to 20 mg once daily; may need to reduce dose in presence of renal or hepatic impairment

Available forms: Tabs 5, 10 mg

Side effects/adverse reactions:

MS: Joint pain, arthralgia
MISC: Facial swelling, weight gain, decreased exercise tolerance
CV: Ventricular dysrhythmias, pro-
**found hypotension, bradycardia,
CHF,** *cold extremities, postural hypotension,* **2nd or 3rd degree heart block**
CNS: Vertigo, headache, insomnia, fatigue, dizziness, mental changes, memory loss, hallucinations, depression, lethargy, drowsiness, strange dreams, catatonia, peripheral neuropathy
GI: Nausea, diarrhea, vomiting, **mesenteric arterial thrombosis, ischemic colitis,** *flatulence, gastritis, gastric pain*
INTEG: Rash, fever, alopecia, pruritus, sweating
HEMA: **Agranulocytosis, thrombocytopenia,** *purpura, eosinophilia*
EENT: Sore throat, dry burning eyes
GU: Impotence, decreased libido
ENDO: Increased hypoglycemic response to insulin
RESP: **Bronchospasm,** *dyspnea, wheezing, cough, nasal stuffiness*

Contraindications: Hypersensitivity to β-blockers, cardiogenic shock, heart block (2nd, 3rd degree), sinus bradycardia, CHF, cardiac failure

Precautions: Major surgery, pregnancy (B), lactation, children, diabetes mellitus, renal or hepatic disease, thyroid disease, COPD, asthma, well-compensated heart failure, aortic or mitral valve disease, peripheral vascular disease, myasthenia gravis

Pharmacokinetics:
PO: Peak 2-4 hr; half-life 9-12 hr, 50% excreted unchanged in urine, protein binding 30%, metabolized in liver to inactive metabolites

Interactions/ incompatibilities:
■ Increased hypotension, bradycardia: reserpine, hydralazine, methyldopa, quinidine, prazosin
■ Decreased antihypertensive effects: indomethacin, nonsteroidal antiinflammatories, barbiturates, cholestyramine, colestipol, penicillins, salicylates
■ Increased hypoglycemic effect: insulin
■ Decreased bronchodilation: theophylline
■ Decreased hypoglycemic effect of sulfonylureas

Lab test interferences:
Increase: AST and ALT
Interference: Glucose/insulin tolerance tests

RESPIRATORY CARE CONSIDERATIONS:
Assess/evaluate:
■ Avoid use with reversible airway obstruction or bronchospastic disease such as asthma or chronic bronchitis due to potential for bronchospasm (wheezing, dyspnea, complaints of chest tightness) secondary to beta-blockade; consider use of other classes of antihypertensive agents for these patients.
■ Monitor all subjects for symptoms of increased airway resistance (wheezing, tightness in chest, difficulty breathing).
■ Monitor effect on BP and pulse, especially if on positive pressure ventilatory support.
■ Assess effectiveness of beta-adrenergic bronchodilator

---

italic = common side effects   **bold** = life-threatening reactions

therapy for possible antagonism and effect on BP to avoid increasing BP, if used.

Patient education:
- Do not use OTC products containing α-adrenergic stimulants (nasal decongestants, OTC cold preparations) unless directed by physician.
- Caution patient that orthostatic hypotension may occur.
- Report symptoms of CHF: difficulty breathing, especially on exertion or when lying down, night cough, swelling of extremities.

bitolterol mesylate
(bye-tole′-ter-ol)
Tornalate
Func. class: Beta$_2$-adrenergic bronchodilator
Chem. class: Acid ester of colterol

See section III: Aerosol Agents for Oral Inhalation

bretylium tosylate
(bre-til′ee-um)
Bretylate,* Bretylium Tosylate, Bretylol
Func. class.: Antidysrhythmic (Class III)
Chem. class.: Quaternary ammonium compound

Action: After an initial release of norepinephrine, inhibits further release by postganglionic nerve endings; prolongs action potential duration, and effective refractory period

Uses: Serious ventricular tachycardia, cardioversion, ventricular fibrillation; for short-term use only

Dosage and routes:
Severe ventricular fibrillation
- *Adult:* IV BOL 5 mg/kg, increase to 10 mg/kg repeated q15 min, up to 30 mg/kg; IV INF 1-2 mg/min or give 5-10 mg/kg over 10 min q6h (maintenance)
Ventricular dysrhythmias
- *Adult:* IV INF 500 mg diluted in 50 ml D$_5$W or NS, infuse over 10-30 min, may repeat in 1 hr, maintain with 1-2 mg/min or 5-10 mg/kg over 10-30 min q6h; IM 5-10 mg/kg undiluted; repeat in 1-2 hr if needed; maintain with same dose q6-8h
Available forms: Inj IV 50 mg/ml; 1, 2, 4 mg/ml prefilled syringes

Side effects/adverse reactions:
CNS: Syncope, dizziness, confusion, psychosis, anxiety
GI: Nausea, vomiting
CV: Hypotension, postural hypotension, bradycardia, angina, PVCs, substernal pressure, transient hypertension, precipitation of angina
RESP: Respiratory depression

Contraindications: Hypersensitivity, digitalis toxicity, aortic stenosis, pulmonary hypertension, children

Precautions: Renal disease, pregnancy (C), lactation, children

Pharmacokinetics: Well absorbed by IM/IV routes
IV: Onset 5 min; duration 6-24 hr
IM: Onset ½-2 hr, duration 6-24 hr
  Half-life 4-17 hr, excreted unchanged by kidneys (70%-80% in 24 hr)

Interactions/incompatibilities:
- Increased or decreased effects of bretylium: quinidine, procainamide, propranolol, other antidysrhythmics
- Hypotension: antihypertensives
- Toxicity: digitalis
- Incompatible with phenytoin

Lab test interferences:
Decrease: Urinary epinephrine, urinary norepinephrine, urinary VMA epinephrine

RESPIRATORY CARE CONSIDERATIONS:
Assess/evaluate:
- Monitor for initial hypertension due to catecholamine release following administration.
- Monitor for hypotension after 1-2 hours, caused by inhibition of neuronal norepinephrine release.
- Hypotension can be exacerbated by positive pressure ventilatory support: minimize mean airway pressures to extent possible.
- Monitor ECG to determine drug effectiveness, PVCs, or other dysrhythmias.

brompheniramine maleate
(brome-fen-ir'a-meen)
Bromphen, Brompheniramine, Codimal-A, Cophene-B, Dehist, Diamine T.D., Dimetane, Dimetane Extentabs, Histaject, ND Stat, Nasahist-B, Oraminic II, Veltane
Func. class.: Antihistamine
Chem. class.: Alkylamine, H_1-receptor antagonist

Action: Blocks the action of histamine at H_1-receptor sites on blood vessels, GI, respiratory tract to decrease allergic inflammatory response.

Uses: Allergy symptoms, rhinitis

Dosage and routes:
- *Adult:* PO 4-8 mg tid-qid, not to exceed 36 mg/day; TIME REL 8-12 mg bid-tid, not to exceed 36 mg/day; IM/IV/SC 5-20 mg q6-12h, not to exceed 40 mg/day
- *Child >6 yr:* PO 2 mg tid-qid, not to exceed 12 mg/day; IM/IV/SC 0.5 mg/kg/day divided tid or qid
- *Child <6 yr:* Only as directed by physician
Available forms: Tabs 4 mg; tabs, time rel 8, 12 mg; elix 2 mg/5 ml; inj IM/SC/IV 10, 100 mg/ml

Side effects/adverse reactions:
CNS: Dizziness, drowsiness, poor coordination, fatigue, anxiety, euphoria, confusion, paresthesia, neuritis
CV: Hypotension, palpitations, tachycardia
RESP: Increased thick secretions, wheezing, chest tightness
HEMA: **Thrombocytopenia, agranulocytosis, hemolytic anemia**
GI: Dry mouth, nausea, vomiting, anorexia, constipation, diarrhea
INTEG: Photosensitivity
GU: Retention, dysuria, frequency, impotence
EENT: Blurred vision, dilated pupils, tinnitus, nasal stuffiness, dry nose, throat, mouth

Contraindications: Hypersensitivity to H_1-receptor antagonists, acute asthma attack,

italic = common side effects   **bold** = life-threatening reactions

lower respiratory tract
disease, child <6 yr

Precautions: Increased
intraocular pressure, renal disease, cardiac disease, hypertension, bronchial asthma,
seizure disorder, stenosed
peptic ulcers, hyperthyroidism, prostatic hypertrophy,
bladder neck obstruction,
pregnancy (C)

Pharmacokinetics:
PO: Peak 2-5 hr, duration to
48 hr, half-life 12-34 hr, metabolized in liver, excreted by
kidneys, excreted in breast
milk.

**Interactions/
incompatibilities:**
- Increased CNS depression:
barbiturates, narcotics, hypnotics, tricyclic antidepressants, alcohol
- Decreased effect of oral anticoagulants, heparin
- Increased drying effect:
MAOIs
- Incompatible with aminophylline, insulins, pentobarbital

Lab test interferences: *False
negative:* Skin allergy tests

**RESPIRATORY CARE
CONSIDERATIONS:**
Assess/evaluate:
- Note drying of the upper
airway.
- Caution is suggested if used
in asthma, although thickening of lower respiratory tract
secretions has not been established.
- Drowsiness may be a risk
factor in subjects with sleep
apnea.
- Monitor nasal passages during long-term treatment for
changes in mucus.

- Therapeutic response: absence of running or congested
nose or rashes.

Patient education:
- Avoid hazardous activities
or use caution while drug
action persists.
- Additional CNS depression
may occur with concomitant
use of CNS depressants (tranquilizers, sedatives or alcohol).

bumetanide
(byoo-met'a-nide)
Bumex
Func. class.: Loop diuretic
Chem. class.: Sulfonamide
derivative

Action: Acts on ascending
loop of Henle by increasing
excretion of chloride, sodium

Uses: Edema in CHF, liver
disease, renal disease (nephrotic syndrome), pulmonary
edema, ascites (nephrotic
syndrome), hypertension,
anasarca

Dosage and routes:
- *Adult:* PO 0.5-2.0 mg qd;
may give 2nd or 3rd dose at
4-5 hr intervals, not to exceed
20 mg/day; may be given on
alternate days or intermittently; IV/IM 0.5-1.0 mg/day;
may give 2nd or 3rd dose at
2-3 hr intervals, not to exceed
20 mg/day
- *Child:* PO, IM, IV 0.02-0.1
mg/kg q12hr
Available forms: Tabs 0.5, 1,
2 mg; inj IV, IM 0.25 mg/ml

**Side effects/adverse
reactions:**
GU: Polyuria, **renal failure**,
glycosuria
ELECT: Hypokalemia, hypochloremic alkalosis, hypomagnesemia,

hyperuricemia, hypocalcemia, hyponatremia, hyperglycemia
CNS: Headache, fatigue, weakness, vertigo
GI: Nausea, diarrhea, dry mouth, vomiting, anorexia, cramps, upset stomach, abdominal pain, *acute pancreatitis, jaundice*
EENT: Loss of hearing, ear pain, tinnitus, blurred vision
INTEG: Rash, pruritus, purpura, *Stevens-Johnson syndrome,* sweating, photosensitivity
MS: Muscular cramps, arthritis, stiffness, tenderness
ENDO: Hyperglycemia
HEMA: Thrombocytopenia, agranulocytosis, neutropenia
CV: Chest pain, hypotension, *circulatory collapse,* ECG changes

Contraindications: Hypersensitivity to sulfonamides, anuria, hepatic coma, hypovolemia, lactation

Precautions: Dehydration, ascites, severe renal disease, pregnancy (C), hepatic cirrhosis

Pharmacokinetics:
PO: Onset ½-1 hr, duration 4 hr
IM: Onset 40 min, duration 4 hr
IV: Onset 5 min, duration 2-3 hr
Excreted by kidneys, crosses placenta, excreted by breast milk

Interactions/ incompatibilities:
■ Decreased diuretic effect: indomethacin, NSAIDs
■ Ototoxicity: cisplatin, aminoglycosides, vancomycin
■ Increased effect: antihypertensives
■ Increased toxicity: lithium, nondepolarizing skeletal muscle relaxants, digitalis

■ Decreased effects of antidiabetics
■ Incompatible with dobutamine, milrinone

RESPIRATORY CARE CONSIDERATIONS:
Assess/evaluate:
■ Monitor serum electrolytes for hyponatremia and hypokalemia, with resulting acid-base abnormalities such as metabolic alkalosis.
■ Overdose can cause reduction in blood volume and hypotension; monitor BP.
■ Hypokalemia can also cause muscular weakness, possibly complicating weaning from mechanical ventilation.
■ Monitor ECG for cardiac arrhythmias.
■ Evaluate for dehydration, especially in COPD subjects or those with excess respiratory tract secretions.
■ Monitor color, consistency of sputum.
■ Evaluate breath sounds and respiratory pattern for pulmonary congestion.
■ Evaluate chest radiograph, if used in CHF, to assess clearing of infiltrates and pulmonary edema.

caffeine
(kaf-een)
Caffedrine, Caffeine, Citrated Caffeine, Dexitac, No-Doz, Quick Pep, Tirend, Vivarin
Func. class.: Analeptic
Chem. class.: Xanthine

Action: Increases calcium permeability in sarcoplasmic reticulum; promotes accumulation of cAMP; competitively blocks adenosine receptors

italic = common side effects   **bold** = life-threatening reactions

Uses: Mild CNS stimulation in combination with analgesics, diuretics for tension and fluid retention associated with menstruation

Dosage and routes:
■ *Adult:* PO 100-200 mg q4h prn; IM 500 mg; timed rel 200-250 mg q4-6h
Available forms: Tabs 65, 100, 150, 200 mg; time rel caps 200, 250 mg; inj 250 mg/ml, time rel tabs 200 mg

Side effects/adverse reactions:
*CNS: Hyperactivity, insomnia, restlessness, talkativeness, dizzi*ness, headache, *stimulation,* irritability, aggressiveness, tremors, twitching, mild delirium, tinnitus, scintillating scotoma
HEMA: Hypoglycemia
GI: Nausea, vomiting, anorexia, gastric irritation, diarrhea
GU: Diuresis
CV: Tachycardia, extrasystole, dysrhythmias, palpitations
INTEG: Hyperesthesia

Contraindications: Hypersensitivity

Precautions: Dysrhythmias, Gilles de la Tourette's disorder, pregnancy (B), lactation, renal, psychologic disorders, depression, ulcers, diabetes mellitus

Pharmacokinetics:
PO: Onset 15 min, peak ½-1 hr, half-life 3-4 hr, metabolized by liver, less than 5% excreted unchanged by kidneys, crosses placenta, breast milk

Interactions/ incompatibilities:
■ Increased effect of caffeine: oral contraceptives, cimeti-dine, disulfiram, ciprofloxacin, endoxacin, phenyl propanolamine

Lab test interferences:
Increase: Urinary cathecholamines
False positive: Serum urate

RESPIRATORY CARE CONSIDERATIONS:
Assess/evaluate:
■ Therapeutic response: increased CNS stimulation, decreased drowsiness; respiratory stimulation in infancy
■ Monitor mental status: mood, sensorium, affect, stimulation, insomnia, irritability.
■ Monitor fluid intake, onset of diuresis, dehydration may result in elderly or children.
■ Monitor theophylline blood levels (therapeutic level is 10-20 μg/ml) if on theophylline.

Patient education:
■ Check OTC medications, current prescription medications for ephedrine, which will increase CNS stimulation; do not drink alcohol or caffeine products (tea, coffee, chocolate, colas) which will increase diuresis or add to the xanthine level (caffeine).
■ Cigarette smoking will increase metabolism of the drug, lowering blood levels.
■ Increase fluid intake if sputum becomes thicker when taking drug.
■ Use nondiuresing liquids, such as water, juice, Gatorade, milk, rather than diuretic products such as caffeinated coffee, tea, or colas.

calcium chloride/ calcium gluceptate/ calcium gluconate/ calcium lactate

Func. class.: Electrolyte replacement—calcium product
Chem. class.: Cation

Action: Cation needed for maintenance of nervous, muscular, skeletal, enzyme reactions, normal cardiac contractility, coagulation of blood; affects secretory activity of endocrine, exocrine glands

Uses: Prevention and treatment of hypocalcemia, hypermagnesemia, hypoparathyroidism, neonatal tetany, cardiac toxicity caused by hyperkalemia, lead colic, hyperphosphatemia, Vit D deficiency

Dosage and routes:
Calcium chloride
■ *Adult:* IV 500 mg-1 g q1-3 days as indicated by serum calcium levels, give at <1 ml/min; IAV 200-800 mg injected in ventricle of heart
■ *Child:* IV 25 mg/kg over several min
Calcium gluceptate
■ *Adult:* IV 5-20 ml; IM 2-5 ml
■ *Newborn:* 0.5 ml/100 ml of blood transfused
Calcium gluconate
■ *Adult:* PO 0.5-2 g bid-qid; IV 0.5-2 g at 0.5 ml/min (10% solution)
■ *Child:* PO/IV 500 mg/kg/day in divided doses
Calcium lactate
■ *Adult:* PO 325 mg-1.3 g tid with meals

■ *Child:* PO 500 mg/kg/day in divided doses
Available forms: Many; check product listings

Side effects/adverse reactions:
INTEG: Pain, burning at IV site, severe venous thrombosis, necrosis, extravasation
Hypercalcemia: Drowsiness, lethargy, muscle weakness, headache, constipation, *coma*, anorexia, nausea, vomiting, polyuria, thirst
CV: Shortened QT, heart block, hypotension, bradycardia, dysrthymias, *cardiac arrest*
GI: Vomiting, nausea, constipation

Contraindications: Hypercalcemia, digitalis toxicity, ventricular fibrillation, renal calculi

Precautions: Pregnancy (C), lactation, children, renal disease, respiratory disease, cor pulmonale, digitalized patient, respiratory failure

Interactions/ incompatibilities:
■ Increased dysrhythmias: digitalis glycosides
■ Decreased action: calcium channel blockers
■ Incompatible with amphotericin B, cephalothin, chlorpheniramine, chlortetracycline, digoxin, digitoxin, epinephrine, tetracycline, warfarin, $NaCo_3$, carbonate, phosphate, sulfate

Lab test interferences:
Increase: 11-OCHS
False decrease: Magnesium
Decrease: 17-OHCS

---

italic = common side effects   **bold** = life-threatening reactions

RESPIRATORY CARE CONSIDERATIONS:
Assess/evaluate:
- Calcium levels during treatment (8.8-10.2 mg/dl is normal level)
- ECG for decreased QT and T wave inversion: if hypercalcemia occurs, drug should be reduced or discontinued
- Cardiac status: rate, rhythm, CVP, (PWP, PAP if being monitored directly)

capreomycin sulfate
(kap-ree-oh-mye′sin)
Capastat Sulfate
Func. class.: Antitubercular
Chem. class.: S. capreolus
polypeptide antibiotic

Action: Inhibits RNA synthesis, decreases tubercle bacilli replication

Uses: Pulmonary tuberculosis as adjunct

Dosage and routes:
- *Adult:* IM 1 g qd × 2-4 mo, then 1 g 2-3 ×/wk × 18-24 mo, not to exceed 20 mg/kg/day, must be given with another antitubercular medication
Available forms: Powder for inj 1 g/10 ml vial

Side effects/adverse reactions:
INTEG: Pain, irritation, sterile abscess at injection site, rash, urticaria
CNS: Vertigo, fever, headache
EENT: Tinnitus, *deafness, ototoxicity*
GU: **Proteinuria,** decreased CrCl, increased BUN, serum Cr, *tubular necrosis,* hypokalemia, alkalosis, *hematuria, albuminuria, nephrotoxicity*

HEMA: Eosinophilia, leukocytosis, leukopenia

Contraindications: Hypersensitivity

Precautions: Renal disease, hearing impairment, allergy history, hepatic disease, pregnancy (C)

Pharmacokinetics:
IM: Peak 1-2 hr, half-life 4-6 hr, excreted in urine unchanged

Interactions/ incompatibilities:
- Increased renal toxicity: aminoglycosides, polymyxin, colistin, vancomycin
- Increased neuroblocking action: phenothiazine, tubocurarine, neostigmine

RESPIRATORY CARE CONSIDERATIONS:
Assess/evaluate:
- Monitor bacteriologic response to therapy using drug-susceptibility testing.
- Assess subject for adverse reactions to drug therapy for mycobacteria; monitor liver enzymes and evaluate hearing.
- Monitor renal function (BUN, creatinine) for nephrotoxicity.
- Respiratory care practitioners and other health care personnel should self-screen for infection with TB routinely and following exposure.
- Proper environmental and personnel protection programs should be implemented when treating subjects with TB.
- Consider the possibility of HIV infection in individuals with confirmed or suspected TB.

Patient/family education:
- That compliance with dosage schedule, duration is necessary

- Side effects, adverse reactions: hearing loss, change in urine or urinary habits

captopril
(kap'toe-pril)
Capoten
Func. class.: Antihypertensive
Chem. class.: Angiotensin-converting enzyme inhibitor

Action: Selectively suppresses renin-angiotensin-aldosterone system; inhibits ACE; prevents conversion of angiotensin I to angiotensin II; results in dilation of arterial, venous vessels

Uses: Hypertension, heart failure not responsive to conventional therapy

Dosage and routes:
Malignant hypertension
- *Adult:* PO 25 mg increasing q2h until desired response, not to exceed 450 mg/day
Hypertension
- *Initial dose:* 12.5 mg 2-3 × daily; may increase to 50 mg bid-tid at 1-2 wk intervals; usual range: 25-150 mg bid-tid; max 450 mg
CHF
- *Adult:* PO 12.5 mg 2-3 × daily given with a diuretic; may increase to 50 mg bid-tid; after 14 days, may increase to 150 mg tid if needed
Available forms: Tabs 12.5, 25, 37.5, 50, 100 mg

Side effects/adverse reactions:
CV: Hypotension, postural hypotension
GU: Impotence, dysuria, nocturia, proteinuria, *nephrotic syndrome, acute reversible renal failure*, polyuria, oliguria, frequency
HEMA: **Neutropenia**
INT: Rash, *angioedema*
RESP: **Bronchospasm**, dyspnea, cough
META: Hyperkalemia
GI: Loss of taste
CNS: Fever, chills

Contraindications: Hypersensitivity, pregnancy (C), lactation, heart block, children, K-sparing diuretics, bilateral renal artery stenosis

Precautions: Dialysis patients, hypovolemia, leukemia, scleroderma, lupus erythematosus, blood dyscrasias, CHF, diabetes mellitus, renal disease, thyroid disease, COPD, asthma

Pharmacokinetics:
PO: Peak 1 hr, duration 2-6 hr, half-life 6-7 hr, metabolized by liver (metabolites), excreted in urine, crosses placenta, excreted in breast milk

Interactions/incompatibilities:
- Increased hypotension: diuretics, other antihypertensives, ganglionic blockers, adrenergic blockers
- Do not use with potassium-sparing diuretics, sympathomimetics, potassium supplements

Lab test interferences:
False positive: Urine acetone

RESPIRATORY CARE CONSIDERATIONS:
Assess/evaluate:
- Therapeutic response: decrease in BP.
- Persistent cough and fever are common side effects of the ACE inhibitors, which should be differentiated from other

possible causes, such as respiratory infection.
- Monitor for possible hypotension.
- Evaluate BP with COPD or asthmatic subjects who require beta agonists for reversible airway obstruction.
- Assess for symptoms of CHF: edema, dyspnea, wet rales, BP.

carbidopa-levodopa
(kar-bi-doe′pa)
(lee-voe-doe′pa)
Carbidopa/Levodopa, Sinemet
Func. class.: Antiparkinson agent
Chem. class.: Catecholamine

Action: Carbidopa, used in combination with levodopa, inhibits decarboxylation of levodopa, and more levodopa is made available for transport to brain and conversion to dopamine in the brain

Uses: Parkinsonism resulting from carbon monoxide, chronic manganese intoxication, cerebral arteriosclerosis

Dosage and routes:
- *Adult:* PO 3-6 tabs of 25 mg carbidopa/250 mg levodopa qd in divided doses, not to exceed 8 tabs/day.
- *Sus. Rel:* 1 tablet bid at intervals of not less than 6 hr usual: 2-8 tabs/day at intervals of 4-8 hr
Available forms: Tabs 10/100, 25/100, 25 mg carbidopa/250 mg levodopa. Sus Rel tab: 50 mg/200 mg carbidopa/levodopa

Side effects/adverse reactions:
HEMA: Hemolytic anemia, leukopenia, agranulocytosis

CNS: Involuntary choreiform movements, hand tremors, fatigue, headache, anxiety, twitching, numbness, weakness, confusion, agitation, insomnia, nightmares, psychosis, hallucination, hypomania, severe depression, dizziness
GI: Nausea, vomiting, anorexia, abdominal distress, dry mouth, flatulence, dysphagia, bitter taste, diarrhea, constipation
INTEG: Rash, sweating, alopecia
CV: Orthostatic hypotension, tachycardia, hypertension, palpitation
EENT: Blurred vision, diplopia, dilated pupils
MISC: Urinary retention, incontinence, weight change, dark urine

Contraindications: Hypersensitivity, narrow-angle glaucoma, undiagnosed skin lesions

Precautions: Renal disease, cardiac disease, hepatic disease, respiratory disease, MI with dysrhythmias, convulsions, peptic ulcer, pregnancy (C)

Pharmacokinetics:
PO: Peak 1-3 hr, excreted in urine (metabolites)

Interactions/incompatibilities:
- Hypertensive crisis: MAOIs, furazolidone
- Decreased effects of levodopa: anticholinergics, hydantoins, methionine, papaverine, pyridoxine, tricyclics, benzodiazepines
- Increased effects of levodopa: antacids, metoclopramide

Lab test interferences:
False positive: Urine ketones
False negative: Urine glucose

C

False increase: Uric acid, urine protein
Decrease: VMA, BUN, creatinine

RESPIRATORY CARE CONSIDERATIONS:
Assess/evaluate:
- Monitor patients with severe cardiovascular or pulmonary disease carefully.
- Assess cardiovascular status (HR, BP) for hypotension or hypertension, tachycardia, palpitations, especially if on regular beta agonists in COPD or asthma.
- Assess respiratory status, including rate and breathing pattern, breath sounds, subjective comfort.
- Caution patients concerning possibility of orthostatic hypotension.

carteolol
(kar-tee′oe-lole)
Cartrol, Ocupress
Func. class.:
Antihypertensive
Chem. class.: Nonselective
β-blocker

Action: Produces fall in BP without reflex tachycardia or significant reduction in heart rate through mixture of β_1-blocking, and β_2-blocking effects; some intrinsic sympathomimetic activity reduces the decrease in cardiac output produced; elevated plasma renins are reduced

Uses: Mild to moderate hypertension

Dosage and routes:
- *Adult:* PO 2.5 mg tid initially, may gradually increase to desired response

Available forms: Tabs 2.5, 5, 10 mg

Side effects/adverse reactions:
CV: Orthostatic hypotension, *bradycardia, CHF, chest pain, ventricular dysrhythmias, AV block, peripheral vascular insufficiency,* palpitations
CNS: Dizziness, mental changes, drowsiness, fatigue, headache, catatonia, depression, anxiety, nightmares, paresthesia, lethargy, insomnia, decreased concentration
GI: Nausea, vomiting, diarrhea, dry mouth, flatulence, constipation, anorexia
INTEG: Rash, alopecia, urticaria, pruritus, fever
HEMA: Agranulocytosis, thrombocytopenic purpura (rare)
EENT: Tinnitus, visual changes, sore throat, double vision, dry burning eyes
GU: Impotence, dysuria, ejaculatory failure, urinary retention
RESP: Bronchospasm, dyspnea, wheezing, nasal stuffiness, pharyngitis
MS: Joint pain, arthralgia, muscle cramps, pain
OTHER: Facial swelling, decreased exercise tolerance, weight change, Raynaud's disease

Contraindications: Hypersensitivity to β-blockers, cardiogenic shock, heart block (2nd or 3rd degree), sinus bradycardia, CHF, bronchial asthma

Precautions: Major surgery, pregnancy (C), lactation, diabetes mellitus, renal disease, thyroid disease, COPD, well-compensated heart failure, nonallergic bronchospasm

---

italic = common side effects   **bold** = life-threatening reactions

Pharmacokinetics:
PO: Onset 1-2 hr, peak 2-4 hr, duration 8-12 hr, half-life 6-8 hr, metabolized by liver (metabolites inactive), excreted in urine, bile, crosses placenta, excreted in breast milk

Interactions/ incompatibilities:
- Increased hypotension: diuretics, other antihypertensives, halothane, nitroglycerin, prazosin
- Decreased β-blocker effects: sympathomimetics, nonsteroidal antiinflammatory agents, salicylates
- Increased hypoglycemia effect: insulin
- Increased effects of lidocaine
- Decreased bronchodilating effects of theophylline β agonists

Lab test interferences:
False increase: Urinary catecholamines
Interference: Glucose, insulin tolerance tests

RESPIRATORY CARE CONSIDERATIONS:
Assess/evaluate:
- Avoid use with reversible airway obstruction or bronchospastic disease such as asthma or chronic bronchitis due to potential for bronchospasm (wheezing, dyspnea, complaints of chest tightness) secondary to beta-blockade; consider use of other classes of antihypertensive agents for these patients.
- Monitor all subjects for symptoms of increased airway resistance (wheezing, tightness in chest, difficulty breathing).

- Monitor effect on BP as well as pulse, especially if on positive pressure ventilatory support.
- Assess effectiveness of beta-adrenergic bronchodilator therapy for possible antagonism and effect on BP to avoid increasing BP, if used.

Patient education:
- Do not use OTC products containing α-adrenergic stimulants (nasal decongestants, OTC cold preparations) unless directed by physician
- Caution patient that orthostatic hypotension may occur.
- Report symptoms of CHF: difficulty breathing, especially on exertion or when lying down, night cough, swelling of extremities

chlorothiazide
(klor-oh-thye'a-zide)
Diachlor, Diuril, Diuril Sodium
Func. class.: Diuretic
Chem. class.: Thiazide; sulfonamide derivative

Action: Acts on distal tubule by increasing excretion of water, sodium, chloride, potassium, magnesium

Uses: Edema, hypertension, diuresis

Dosage and routes:
Edema, hypertension
- *Adult:* PO/IV 500 mg-2 g qd in 2 divided doses
Diuresis
- *Child >6 mo:* PO 20 mg/kg/ day in 2 divided doses
Available forms: Tabs 250, 500 mg; oral susp 250 mg/5 ml; inj 500 mg

Side effects/adverse reactions:

CNS: Drowsiness, paresthesia, anxiety, depression, headache, *dizziness, fatigue, weakness*

CV: Irregular pulse, orthostatic hypotension, palpitations, volume depletion

EENT: Blurred vision

ELECT: *Hypokalemia,* hypercalcemia, hyponatremia, hypochloremia, hypophosphatemia, hypomagnesemia

GI: *Nausea, vomiting, anorexia,* constipation, diarrhea, cramps, pancreatitis, GI irritation, *hepatitis*

GU: *Frequency,* polyuria, *uremia,* glucosuria

HEMA: **Aplastic anemia, hemolytic anemia, leukopenia, agranulocytosis, thrombocytopenia, neutropenia**

INTEG: *Rash,* urticaria, purpura, photosensitivity, fever

META: Hyperglycemia, *hyperuricemia,* hypomagnesemia, increased creatinine, BUN

Contraindications: Hypersensitivity to thiazides or sulfonamides, anuria, renal decompensation, pregnancy (D), lactation

Precautions: Hypokalemia, renal disease, hepatic disease, gout, COPD, lupus erythematosus, diabetes mellitus, elderly

Pharmacokinetics: Not well absorbed PO

PO: Onset 2 hr, peak 4 hr, duration 6-12 hr; half-life 2 hr; crosses placenta, excreted in breast milk, excreted unchanged by the kidneys; half-life 2 hr

Interactions/ incompatibilities:

■ Incompatible in sol with amikacin, chlorpromazine, codeine, hydralazine, insulin, ionosol sol, levarterenol, levorphanol, methadone, morphine, polymyxin B, procaine, prochlorperazine, promazine, promethazine, streptomycin, tetracycline, triflupromazine, vancomycin, Vit C, Vit B with C, warfarin

■ Increased toxicity: lithium, nondepolarizing skeletal muscle relaxants, digitalis

■ Increased hypotension: other antihypertensives, alcohol

■ Decreased effects of: antidiabetics, sulfonylureas

■ Decreased absorption of thiazides: cholestyramine, colestipol

■ Decreased hypotensive response: indomethacin

■ Hypokalemia: ticarcillin, glucocorticoids, amphotericin, mezlocillin, piperacillin

■ Hyperglycemia, hyperuricemia, hypotension: diazoxide

Lab test interferences:

False negative: Phentolamine and tyramine tests

Interference: Urine steroid tests

Increase: BSP retention, Ca, amylase, parathyroid test

Decrease: PBI, PSP

RESPIRATORY CARE CONSIDERATIONS:
Assess/evaluate:

■ Monitor serum electrolytes, especially potassium, to assess hypokalemia, which will cause metabolic alkalosis.

■ Hypokalemia can also cause muscular weakness, possibly complicating weaning from mechanical ventilation.

■ Monitor ECG for cardiac arrhythmias.

■ Evaluate for dehydration, especially in COPD subjects

italic = common side effects   **bold** = life-threatening reactions

or those with excess respiratory tract secretions.
- Monitor color, consistency of sputum.
- Evaluate breath sounds and respiratory pattern for pulmonary congestion.
- Evaluate chest radiograph if used in CHF, to assess clearing of infiltrates and pulmonary edema.

chlorpheniramine maleate

(klor-fen-eer′a-meen)
Aller-Chlor, Allergy, Chlo-Amine, Chlor-100, Chlor-Pro, Chlorate, Chlorpheniramine Maleate, Chlor-Pro 10, Chlorspan-12, Chlortab-B, Chlortab-4, Chlor-Trimeton, Chlor-Trimeton Repetabs, Pedia Care Allergy Formula, Pfeiffer's Allergy, Phenetron, Telachlor, Teldrin
Func. class.: Antihistamine
Chem. class.: Alkylamine, H_1-receptor antagonist

Action: Blocks the action of histamine at H_1-receptor sites on blood vessels, GI, respiratory tract to decrease allergic inflammatory response.

Uses: Allergy symptoms, rhinitis

Dosage and routes:
- *Adult:* PO 2-4 mg tid-qid, not to exceed 36 mg/day; TIME-REL 8-12 mg bid-tid, not to exceed 36 mg/day; IM/IV/SC 5-40 mg/day
- *Child 6-12 yr:* PO 2 mg q4-6h, not to exceed 12 mg/day; SUS REL 8 mg hs or qd, SUS REL not recommended for child <6 yr

- *Child 2-5 yr:* PO 1 mg q4-6h, not to exceed 4 mg/day
Available forms: Tabs, chewable 2 mg; tabs 4 mg; tabs, time-rel 8, 12 mg, caps, time-rel 8, 12 mg; syr 2 mg/5 ml; inj IM, SC, IV 10, 100 mg/ml

Side effects/adverse reactions:
CNS: Dizziness, drowsiness, poor coordination, fatigue, anxiety, euphoria, confusion, paresthesia, neuritis
RESP: Increased thick secretions, wheezing, chest tightness
HEMA: Thrombocytopenia, agranulocytosis, hemolytic anemia
GI: Dry mouth, nausea, anorexia, diarrhea
INTEG: Photosensitivity
GU: Retention, dysuria, frequency
EENT: Blurred vision, dilated pupils, tinnitus, nasal stuffiness, dry nose, throat, mouth

Contraindications: Hypersensitivity to H_1-receptor antagonists, acute asthma attack, lower respiratory tract disease

Precautions: Increased intraocular pressure, renal disease, cardiac disease, hypertension, bronchial asthma, seizure disorder, stenosed peptic ulcers, hyperthyroidism, prostatic hypertrophy, bladder neck obstruction, pregnancy (B), elderly

Pharmacokinetics:
PO: Onset 20-60 min, duration 8-12 hr, half-life 20-24 hr, detoxified in liver, excreted by kidneys, (metabolites/free drug)

Interactions/ incompatibilities:
- Incompatible with calcium chloride, kanamycin, levarterenol, pentobarbital

*Available in Canada only

- Increased CNS depression: barbiturates, narcotics, hypnotics, tricyclic antidepressants, alcohol
- Decreased effect of: oral anticoagulants, heparin
- Increased effect of chlorpheniramine: MAOIs

Lab test interferences:
False negative: Skin allergy tests

RESPIRATORY CARE CONSIDERATIONS:
Assess/evaluate:

- Note drying of the upper airway.
- Caution is suggested if used in asthma, although thickening of lower respiratory tract secretions has not been established.
- Drowsiness may be a risk factor in subjects with sleep apnea.
- Monitor nasal passages during long-term treatment for changes in mucus.
- Therapeutic response: absence of running or congested nose or rashes.

Patient education:

- Avoid hazardous activities or use caution while drug action persists.
- Additional CNS depression may occur with concomitant use of CNS depressants (tranquilizers, sedatives or alcohol).

chlorthalidone
(klor-thal'i-done)
Chlorthalidone, Hygroton, Hylidone, Novothalidone,* Thalitone
Func. class.: Diuretic
Chem. class.: Thiazide-like; phthalimidine derivative

Action: Acts on distal tubule by increasing excretion of water, sodium, chloride, potassium, magnesium, bicarbonate

Uses: Edema, hypertension, diuresis, CHF, nephrotic syndrome

Dosage and routes:
- *Adult:* PO 25 - 100 mg/day or 100 mg every other day
- *Child:* PO 2 mg/kg 3 ×/wk
Available forms: Tabs 25, 50, 100 mg

Side effects/adverse reactions:
GU: Frequency, polyuria, *uremia*, glucosuria, impotence
CNS: Drowsiness, paresthesia, anxiety, depression, headache, *dizziness, fatigue, weakness*
GI: Nausea, vomiting, anorexia, constipation, diarrhea, cramps, pancreatitis, GI irritation, *hepatitis*
EENT: Blurred vision
INTEG: Rash, urticaria, purpura, photosensitivity, fever
META: Hyperglycemia, hyperuremia, increased creatinine, BUN, gout
HEMA: **Aplastic anemia, hemolytic anemia, leukopenia, agranulocytosis, thrombocytopenia, neutropenia**
CV: Irregular pulse, orthostatic hypotension, palpitations, volume depletion
ELECT: Hypokalemia, hypomagnesemia, hypercalcemia, hyponatremia, hypochloremia

Contraindications: Hypersensitivity to thiazides or sulfonamides, anuria, renal decompensation, lactation

Precautions: Hypokalemia, renal disease, pregnancy (C), hepatic disease, gout, diabetes mellitus, elderly

italic = common side effects   **bold** = life-threatening reactions

Pharmacokinetics:
PO: Onset 2 hr, peak 6 hr, duration 24-72 hr; half-life 40 hr, excreted unchanged by kidneys, crosses placenta, enters breast milk

Interactions/ incompatibilities:
- Increased toxicity: lithium, nondepolarizing skeletal muscle relaxants
- Decreased effects of: antidiabetics
- Decreased absorption of thiazides: cholestyramine, colestipol
- Decreased hypotensive response: indomethacin, NSAIDs
- Hyperglycemia, hyperuricemia, hypotension: diazoxide

Lab test interferences:
Increase: BSP retention, Ca, cholesterol, triglycerides, amylase
Decrease: PBI, PSP, parathyroid test

RESPIRATORY CARE CONSIDERATIONS:
Assess/evaluate:
- Monitor serum electrolytes, especially potassium, to assess hypokalemia, which will cause metabolic alkalosis.
- Hypokalemia can also cause muscular weakness, possibly complicating weaning from mechanical ventilation.
- Monitor ECG for cardiac arrhythmias.
- Evaluate for dehydration, especially in COPD subjects or those with excess respiratory tract secretions.
- Monitor color, consistency of sputum.
- Evaluate breath sounds and respiratory pattern for pulmonary congestion.

- Evaluate chest radiograph if used in CHF, to assess clearing of infiltrates and pulmonary edema.

cisatracurium besylate
(sis-a-tra-cyoor'ee-um)
Nimbex
Func. class: Nondepolarizing neuromuscular blocking agent
Chem. class: Isomer of atracurium besylate, a biquaternary ammonium ester

Action: Inhibits transmission of nerve impulses at the neuromuscular junction by binding with cholinergic receptor sites, antagonizing action of acetylcholine, and causing muscle weakness or paralysis, depending on dose.

Uses: Facilitation of endotracheal intubation, skeletal muscle relaxation during mechanical ventilation, surgery, or general anesthesia

Dosage and routes:
- *Adult:* 0.15-0.2 mg/kg given IV with a propofol/nitrous oxide/oxygen induction
- *Child (2-12 years):* 0.1 mg/kg over 5-10 seconds during either halothane or opioid anesthesia
Available forms: Inj in 5- and 10-ml vials with 2 mg/ml; 20-ml vials with 10 mg/ml

Side effects/adverse reactions:
CV: Bradycardia, hypotension
DERM: Flushing, rash
RESP: Bronchospasm

Contraindications: Hypersensitivity to cisatracurium or other bis-benzylisoquinolinium agents; hypersensitivity to benzyl alcohol, in the 10 ml vials only cisatracurium besylate

Precautions:
- Cisatracurium, as with other neuromuscular blocking agents, has no effect on consciousness or the perception of pain; block should not be induced before unconsciousness.
- Cisatracuarium is not recommended for rapid sequence endotracheal intubation because of its intermediate onset of action.
- Neuromuscular blocking agents can have a profound effect in patients with neuromuscular diseases such as myasthemia gravis; lower doses of 0.02 mg/kg are recommended, with assessment of the level of blockade using a peripheral nerve stimulator.

Pharmacokinetics: Mean half-life in healthy surgical patients ranged from 22-29 minutes.
- Cisatracurium is degraded by a Hoffmann elimination process, to form laudanosine and a monoquaternary product, which are eliminated in the kidneys
- With recommended doses of 0.15 and 0.2 mg/kg, and anesthesia induction using propofol/nitrous oxide/oxygen, blockade is sufficient for tracheal intubation in 2 and 1.5 minutes respectively.
- Infusion for up to 6 days during mechanical ventilation resulted in muscle function recovery; after infusion termination in approximately 55 minutes, compared to 178 minutes with vecuronium.

Interactions/ incompatibilities:
- Anticonvulsants, such as phenytoin or carbamazepine, decrease neuromuscular blocking action of cisatracurium.
- Isoflurane or enflurane given with nitrous oxide/ oxygen may prolong the effective duration of blocking action of cisatracurium.
- Succinylcholine: time to maximum block with cisatracurium is approximately 2 minutes faster if preceded by succinylcholine.
- Drugs such as antibiotics (aminoglycosides, tetracyclines, bacitracin, polymyxins, lincomycin, clindamycin, colistin, sodium colistimethate), magnesium salts, lithium, local anesthetics, and quinidine may enhance neuromuscular blockade with nondepolarizing agents.

RESPIRATORY CARE CONSIDERATIONS:
Assess/evaluate:
- Assess airway and ventilatory support before administering drug.
- Note possible interaction with the following antibiotics, which can increase neuromuscular blockade: the aminoglycosides, the polymyxins, clindamycin, and lincomycin.
- Use with mechanical ventilation: assess patient for adequate and preferably optimal ventilator settings *before* paralyzing; if patient is "fighting" the ventilator, provide adequately high flow rates and tidal volumes, short inspiratory times, and

---

italic = common side effects   **bold** = life-threatening reactions

reasonable I:E ratios; check the sensitivity in assist-control mode, provide sufficiently high rates to avoid patient fatigue; consider paralysis if these measures fail.
- Assess ventilator patients for pain, hypoxemia, or ventilator malfunction, if restless and anxious, before instituting muscle paralysis.
- Assess need of patient and provide for pain control and sedation during neuromuscular blockade: *neuromuscular blocking agents do not provide analgesia or sedation.*
- Close eyelids and provide eye lubricant during prolonged paralysis.
- Since usual signs of pain or anxiety (restlessness, tachypnea, distress, thrashing) are blocked, monitor vital signs closely as well as overall patient appearance and state to detect problems, such as IV infiltration.
- Check ventilator alarm settings for sufficient limits and sensitivity; a disconnect alarm is critical.
- Assess reversal of drug before attempting to wean from mechanical ventilatory support.

Administer:
- Administer by IV, not by IM, for more consistent absorption and distribution and to avoid the pain associated with IM injection of the drug.
- Reversal: neostigmine or edrophonium, preceded by atropine to inhibit muscarinic response especially in upper airway.

clemastine fumarate
(klem′as-teen)
Tavist, Tavist-|
Func. class.: Antihistamine
Chem. class.: Ethanolamine derivative, H_1-receptor antagonist

Action: Blocks the action of histamine at H_1-receptor sites on blood vessels, GI, respiratory tract, to decrease allergic inflammatory response.

Uses: Allergy symptoms, rhinitis, angioedema, urticaria

Dosage and routes:
- *Adult and child >12 yr:* PO 1.34-2.68 mg bid-tid, not to exceed 8.04 mg/day
Available forms: Tabs 1.34, 2.68 mg; syr 0.67 mg/ml

Side effects/adverse reactions:
CNS: Dizziness, drowsiness, poor coordination, fatigue, anxiety, euphoria, confusion, paresthesia, neuritis
CV: Hypotension, palpitations, tachycardia
RESP: Increased thick secretions, wheezing, chest tightness
HEMA: Thrombocytopenia, agranulocytosis, hemolytic anemia
GI: Constipation, dry mouth, nausea, vomiting, anorexia, diarrhea
INTEG: Rash, urticaria, photosensitivity
GU: Retention, dysuria, frequency
EENT: Blurred vision, dilated pupils, tinnitus, nasal stuffiness, dry nose, throat, mouth

Contraindications: Hypersensitivity to H_1-receptor antagonists, acute asthma attack, lower respiratory tract disease

Precautions: Increased intraocular pressure, renal disease, cardiac disease, hypertension, bronchial asthma, seizure disorder, stenosed peptic ulcers, hyperthyroidism, prostatic hypertrophy, bladder neck obstruction, pregnancy (B), elderly

Pharmacokinetics:
PO: Peak 5-7 hr, duration 10-12 hr or more, metabolized in liver, excreted by kidneys

Interactions/ incompatibilities:
■ Increased CNS depression: barbiturates, narcotics, hypnotics, tricyclic antidepressants, alcohol
■ Decreased effect of: oral anticoagulants, heparin
■ Increased effect of clemastine: MAOIs

Lab test interferences:
False negative: Skin allergy tests

RESPIRATORY CARE CONSIDERATIONS
Assess/evaluate:
■ Note drying of the upper airway.
■ Caution is suggested if used in asthma, although thickening of lower respiratory tract secretions has not been established.
■ Drowsiness may be a risk factor in subjects with sleep apnea.
■ Monitor nasal passages during long-term treatment for changes in mucus.
■ Therapeutic response: absence of running or congested nose or rashes.

Patient education:
■ Avoid hazardous activities or use caution while drug action persists.
■ Additional CNS depression may occur with concomitant use of CNS depressants (tranquilizers, sedatives, or alcohol).

clonidine HCl
(klon'i-deen)
Catapres, Clonidine HCl, Dixarit*
Func. class.: Antihypertensive
Chem. class.: Central α-adrenergic agonist

Action: Inhibits sympathetic vasomotor center in CNS, which reduces impulses in sympathetic nervous system; blood pressure, pulse rate, cardiac output decrease

Uses: Mild to moderate hypertension, used alone or in combination

Dosage and routes:
Hypertension
■ *Adult:* PO/TRANS 0.1 mg bid, then increase by 0.1 mg/day or 0.2 mg/day until desired response; range 0.2-0.8 mg/day in divided doses
Available forms: Tabs 0.1, 0.2, 0.3 mg; trans sys 2.5, 5, 7.5 mg delivering 0.1, 0.2, 0.3 mg/24 hr, respectively

Side effects/adverse reactions:
CNS: Drowsiness, sedation, headache, fatigue, nightmares, insomnia, mental changes, anxiety, depression, hallucinations, delirium
CV: Orthostatic hypotension, palpitations, **CHF,** ECG abnormalities
EENT: Taste change, parotid pain

ENDO: Hyperglycemia
GI: Nausea, vomiting, malaise, constipation, dry mouth
GU: Impotence, dysuria, *nocturia,* gynecomastia
INTEG: Rash, alopecia, facial pallor, pruritus, hives, edema, burning papules, excoriation (transdermal patches)
MS: Muscle, joint pain; leg cramps

Contraindications: Hypersensitivity

Precautions: MI (recent), diabetes mellitus, chronic renal failure, Raynaud's disease, thyroid disease, depression, COPD, child <12 (patches), asthma, pregnancy (C), lactation, elderly

Pharmacokinetics: Absorbed well
PO: Onset ½ to 1 hour, peak 2-4 hours, duration 8 hours, half-life 12-16 hr
TOP: Onset 3 days, duration 1 week, metabolized by liver (metabolites), excreted in urine (30% unchanged, inactive metabolites, feces), crosses blood-brain barrier, excreted in breast milk

Interactions/ incompatibilities:
- Increased CNS depression: narcotics, sedatives, hypnotics, anesthetics, alcohol
- Decreased hypotensive effects: tricyclic antidepressants, MAOIs, appetite suppressants, amphetamines
- Increased hypotensive effects: diuretics, other antihypertensive nitrates
- Increased bradycardia: β-blockers, cardiac glycosides

Lab test interferences:
Increase: Blood glucose
Decrease: VMA, catecholamines aldosterone

RESPIRATORY CARE CONSIDERATIONS
Assess/evaluate:
- Evaluate BP and pulse for efficacy of hypertension treatment and to avoid hypotension, especially if on positive pressure ventilatory support.
- Central-acting alpha-adrenergic agonists can cause drowsiness; increased sedative effect with CNS depressants such as alcohol, sedatives, tranquilizers or many analgesics (opioid). Avoid hazardous activities.
- Evaluate BP with COPD or asthmatic subjects who require beta agonists for reversible airway obstruction.
- Assess for symptoms of CHF: edema, dyspnea, wet rales, BP.
- Consider use of nonadrenergic bronchodilator such as ipratropium bromide as alternative to beta-adrenergic agents for asthmatics, COPD patients.

Patient education:
- Do not use OTC products containing α-adrenergic stimulants (nasal decongestants, OTC cold preparations) unless directed by physician.
- Caution patient that orthostatic hypotension may occur.
- Report symptoms of CHF: difficulty breathing, especially on exertion or when lying down, night cough, swelling of extremities.
- Avoid hazardous activities if drowsiness occurs.

*Available in Canada only

colfosceril palmitate
(kohl-foss'sir-ill)
Exosurf Neonatal
Func. class: Exogenous
lung surfactant
Chem. class: Synthetic
dipalmitoylphosphati-
dylcholine

See section III: Aerosol
Agents for Oral Inhalation

corticotropin (ACTH)
(kor-ti-koe-troe'pin)
ACTH, Acthar, Corticotro-
pin, ACTH-40, ACTH-80,
Duracton*, H.P. Acthar Gel
Func. class.: Pituitary
hormone
Chem. class.: Adrenocorti-
cotropic hormone

Action: Stimulates adrenal
cortex to produce, secrete cor-
ticosterone, cortisol

Uses: Testing adrenocortical
function, treatment of adrenal
insufficiency caused by administration of corticosteroids
(long term), multiple sclerosis

Dosage and routes:
Testing of adrenocortical function
■ *Adult:* IM/SC up to 80 U in
divided doses; IV 10-25 U in
500 ml D$_5$ W given over 8 hr
Inflammation
■ *Adult:* SC/IM 40 U in 4 di-
vided doses (aqueous) or 40 U
q12-24h (gel/repository form)
Available forms: Inj IM, IV, SC
25, 40 U/vial, repository inj
IM, SC 40, 80/ml

**Side effects/adverse
reactions:**
INTEG: Impaired wound healing,
rash, urticaria, hirsutism,
petechiae, ecchymoses, sweating, acne, hyperpigmentation
CNS: **Convulsions,** dizziness,
euphoria, insomnia, headache,
mood swings, behavioral
changes, depression, psychosis
GI: Nausea, vomiting, **peptic
ulcer perforation,** pancreatitis,
distention, ulcerative
esophagitis
GU: Water, sodium retention,
hypokalemia
EENT: Cataracts, glaucoma
MS: Weakness, osteoporosis,
compression fractures, muscle
atrophy, steroid myopathy,
myalgia, arthralgia
ENDO: Cushingoid symptoms,
diabetes mellitus, antibody
formation, growth retardation
in children, menstrual
irregularities

Contraindications: Hypersensitivity, scleroderma, osteoporosis, CHF, peptic ulcer
disease, hypertension, systemic fungal infections, small-
pox vaccination, recent surgery, ocular herpes simplex,
primary adrenocortical
insufficiency/hyperfunction

Precautions: Pregnancy (C),
lactation, latent TB, hepatic
disease, hypothyroiditis,
childbearing-age women,
psychiatric diagnosis,
myasthenia gravis, acute
gouty arthritis

Pharmacokinetics:
IV/IM/SC: Onset <6 hr,
duration 2-4 hr, repository
duration up to 3 days,
half-life <20 min, excreted in
urine

**Interactions/
incompatibilities:**
■ Possible ulceration: salicylates, alcohol, corticosteroids

italic = common side effects   **bold** = life-threatening reactions

- Hypokalemia: diuretics (K-depleting), amphotericin B
- Hyperglycemia: insulin or oral hypoglycemic agents
- Incompatible with aminophylline, $NaCO_3$ in sol or syringe

RESPIRATORY CARE CONSIDERATIONS
Assess/evaluate:
- Monitor for side effects of increased corticosteroid level: Cushingoid symptoms (moon face, peripheral wasting, central edema).
- Monitor patients with latent tuberculosis or reactive skin tests for reactivation of the disease.
- Evaluate muscle weakness and steroid myopathy, especially in chronic lung disease patients.
- Evaluate cardiovascular system for hypertension, CHF.
- Monitor electrolytes: potassium and calcium loss can occur with hypokalemic alkalosis.
- Infection, including pneumonia, can occur.
- Increased corticosteroid levels can mask symptoms of infection.
- If asthma is present, monitor for breakthrough symptoms (bronchospasm, wheezing) if drug is discontinued.
- Evaluate possible adrenal insufficiency when transferring from systemic to inhaled aerosol corticosteroids in asthma.
- Symptoms of adrenal insufficiency: nausea, anorexia, fatigue, dizziness, dyspnea, weakness, joint pain.

cortisone acetate
(kor'-ti-sone)
Cortone
Func. class.: Corticosteroid, synthetic
Chem. class.: Glucocorticoid, short-acting

Action: Decreases inflammation by suppression of migration of polymorphonuclear leukocytes, fibroblasts, reversal of increased capillary permeability and lysosomal stabilization

Uses: Inflammation, severe allergy, adrenal insufficiency, collagen disorders, respiratory, dermatologic disorders

Dosage and routes:
- *Adult:* PO 25-300 mg qd or q2 days, titrated to patient response
Available forms: Tabs 5, 10, 25 mg

Side effects/adverse reactions:
INTEG: Acne, poor wound healing, ecchymosis, bruising, petechiae
CNS: Depression, flushing, sweating, headache, mood changes
CV: Hypertension, circulatory collapse, thrombophlebitis, embolism, tachycardia, *necrotizing angiitis, CHF,* edema
HEMA: Thrombocytopenia
MS: Fractures, osteoporosis, weakness
GI: Diarrhea, nausea, abdominal distention, GI hemorrhage, increased appetite, *pancreatitis*
EENT: Fungal infections, increased intraocular pressure, blurred vision

Contraindications: Psychosis, hypersensitivity, idiopathic thrombocytopenia, acute glomerulonephritis, amebiasis, fungal infections, nonasthmatic bronchial disease, child <2 yr, AIDS, TB

Precautions: Pregnancy (C), diabetes mellitus, glaucoma, osteoporosis, seizure disorders, ulcerative colitis, CHF, myasthenia gravis, renal disease, esophagitis, peptic ulcer

Pharmacokinetics:
PO: Peak 2 hr, duration 1½ days
IM: Peak 20-48 hr, duration 1½ days

Interactions/ incompatibilities:
- Decreased action of cortisone: cholestyramine, colestipol, barbiturates, rifampin, ephedrine, phenytoin, theophylline
- Decreased effects of: anticoagulants, anticonvulsants, antidiabetics, ambenonium, neostigmine, isoniazid, toxoids, vaccines, anticholinesterases, salicylates, somatrem
- Increased side effects: alcohol, salicylates, indomethacin, amphotericin B, digitalis, cyclosporine, diuretics
- Increased action of cortisone: salicylates, estrogens, indomethacin, oral contraceptives, ketoconazole, macrolide antibiotics

Lab test interferences:
- *Increase:* Cholesterol, Na, blood glucose, uric acid, Ca, urine glucose
Decrease: Ca, K, T_4, T_3, thyroid ^{131}I uptake test, urine 17-OHCS, 17-KS, PBI
False negative: Skin allergy tests

RESPIRATORY CARE CONSIDERATIONS
Assess/evaluate:
- Monitor for side effects of increased corticosteroid level:

Cushingoid symptoms (moon face, peripheral wasting, central edema).
- Monitor patients with latent tuberculosis or reactive skin tests for reactivation of the disease.
- Evaluate muscle weakness and steroid myopathy, especially in chronic lung disease patients.
- Evaluate cardiovascular system for hypertension, CHF.
- Monitor electrolytes; potassium and calcium loss can occur with hypokalemic alkalosis.
- Infection, including pneumonia, can occur.
- Increased corticosteroid levels can mask symptoms of infection.
- If asthma is present, monitor for breakthrough symptoms (bronchospasm, wheezing) if drug is discontinued.
- Evaluate possible adrenal insufficiency when transferring from systemic to inhaled aerosol corticosteroids in asthma.
- Symptoms of adrenal insufficiency: nausea, anorexia, fatigue, dizziness, dyspnea, weakness, joint pain.

co-trimoxazole (sulfamethoxazole and trimethoprim)
(koe-trye-mox'a-zole)
Apo-Sulfatrim,* Bactrim, Cotrim, Comoxol, Septra, Sulfatrim, Bethaprim
Func. class.: Antibiotic
Chem. class.: Miscellaneous sulfonamide

Action: Sulfamethoxazole (SMZ) interferes with bacterial biosynthesis of proteins by competitive antagonism of PABA when adequate levels are maintained; trimethoprim (TMP) blocks synthesis of tetrahydrofolic acid; combination blocks 2 consecutive steps in bacterial synthesis of essential nucleic acids, protein

Uses: Urinary tract infections, otitis media, acute and chronic prostatitis, shigellosis, *P. carinii* pneumonia, chronic bronchitis, chancroid, traveler's diarrhea

Dosage and routes:
Urinary tract infections
- *Adult:* PO 160 mg TMP/800 mg SMZ q12h × 10-14 days
- *Child:* PO 8 mg/kg TMP/40 mg/kg SMZ qd in 2 divided doses q12h
Otitis media
- *Child:* PO 8 mg/kg TMP/40 mg/kg SMZ qd in 2 divided doses q12h × 10 days
Chronic bronchitis
- *Adult:* PO 160 mg TMP/800 mg SMZ q12h × 14 days
Pneumocystis carinii pneumonitis
- *Adult and child:* PO 20 mg/kg TMP/100 mg/kg SMZ qd in 4 divided doses q6h × 14 days; IV 15-20 mg/kg/day (based on TMP) in 3-4 divided doses for up to 14 days
- Dosage reduction necessary in moderate to severe renal impairment (CrCl 30 ml/min)
Available forms: Tabs 80 mg trimethoprim (TMP)/400 mg sulfamethoxazole (SMZ), 160 mg trimethoprim/800 mg sulfamethoxazole; susp 40 mg/200 mg/5 ml; IV inj 16 mg/80 mg/ml

Side effects/adverse reactions:
CNS: Headache, insomnia, hallucinations, depression, vertigo, fatigue, anxiety, convulsions, drug fever, chills, aseptic meningitis
CV: Allergic myocarditis
GI: Nausea, vomiting, abdominal pain, stomatitis, *hepatitis,* glossitis, pancreatitis, diarrhea, *enterocolitis,* anorexia
GU: Renal failure, toxic nephrosis; increased BUN, creatinine, crystalluria
HEMA: Leukopenia, neutropenia, thrombocytopenia, agranulocytosis, hemolytic anemia, hypoprothrombinemia, Henoch-Schönlein purpura, methemoglobinemia, eosinophilia I
INTEG: Rash, dermatitis, urticaria, *Stevens-Johnson syndrome,* erythema, photosensitivity, pain, inflammation at injection site
RESP: Cough, shortness of breath
SYST: Anaphylaxis, SLE

Contraindications: Hypersensitivity to trimethoprim or sulfonamides, pregnancy at term, megaloblastic anemia, infants <2 mo, CrCl <15 ml/min, lactation

Precautions: Pregnancy (C), renal disease, elderly, G-6-PD deficiency, impaired hepatic function, possible folate deficiency, severe allergy, bronchial asthma

Pharmacokinetics:
PO: Rapidly absorbed, peak 1-4 hr, half-life 8-13 hr, excreted in urine (metabolites and unchanged), breast milk; crosses placenta; highly bound to plasma proteins; TMP achieves high levels in prostatic tissue and fluid

Interactions/ incompatibilities:
- Increased hypoglycemic response: sulfonylurea agents
- Increased anticoagulant effects: oral anticoagulants
- Decreased hepatic clearance of: phenytoin
- Increased nephrotoxicity: cyclosporine
- Increased bone marrow depressant effects: methotrexate
- Thrombocytopenia: thiazide diuretics

Lab test interferences:
Increase: Alk phosphatase, creatinine, bilirubin
False positive: Urinary glucose test

RESPIRATORY CARE CONSIDERATIONS
Assess/evaluate:
- Caution: administer sulfonamides with caution to patients with allergies or asthma; assess for toxicity or hypersensitivity reaction and discontinue immediately.
- Hypersensitivity reaction: be prepared to support airway and provide ventilatory/ oxygenation support as needed.
- Monitor for anemia and decreased tissue oxygen transport.
- If used in patients with PCP, monitor respiratory status to evaluate efficacy: CXR, WBC, temperature, breath sounds, respiratory rate and pattern.
- Maintain sterility during procedures such as tracheal aspiration (suctioning) and asepsis with equipment to avoid infection with nonsusceptible organisms, leading to overgrowth or superinfection.

- Check indices of infection, including: WBC, temperature.
- Evaluate respiratory status, including rate, pattern, breath sounds on auscultation, dyspnea, cough, sputum production (color, consistency, amount), and chest radiograph with respiratory involvement.
- Note risk of septicemia and septic shock, with the possibility of ARDS if infections are not controlled, requiring ventilatory support.

Patient education:
- Photosensitization, leading to photoallergy or phototoxicity, may occur; take protective measures against exposure to UV or sunlight until tolerance is verified.

cromolyn sodium (disodium cromoglycate)
(kroe'moe-lin)
Intal, Intal p,* Nasalcrom, Rynacrom,* Gastrocrom
Func. class.: Antiasthmatic
Chem. class.: A bischromone

See Section III: Aerosol Agents for Oral Inhalation

cyclandelate
(sye-klan'da-late)
Cyclan, Cyclandelate, Cyclospasmol
Func. class.: Peripheral vasodilator
Chem. class.: Nonnitrate

Action: Relaxes vascular smooth muscle, dilates peripheral vascular smooth muscle by direct action

Uses: Intermittent claudication, thrombophlebitis,

Raynaud's phenomenon, ischemic cerebrovascular disease, arteriosclerosis obliterans, nocturnal leg cramps

Dosage and routes:
- *Adult:* PO 200 mg qid, not to exceed 400 mg qid; maintenance dose is 400-800 mg/day in 2-4 divided doses
Available forms: Tabs 200, 400 mg; caps 200, 400 mg

Side effects/adverse reactions:
HEMA: Increased bleeding time (rare)
CV: Tachycardia
CNS: Headache, paresthesias, dizziness, weakness
GI: Heartburn, eructation, nausea, pyrosis
INTEG: Sweating, flushing

Contraindications: Hypersensitivity

Precautions: Glaucoma, pregnancy (C), lactation, recent MI, hypertension, severe obliterative coronary artery or cerebrovascular disease

Pharmacokinetics:
PO: Onset 15 min, peak 1½ hr, duration 4 hr

RESPIRATORY CARE CONSIDERATIONS
Assess/evaluate:
- Evaluate BP and pulse for efficacy of hypertension treatment and to avoid hypotension.
- Evaluate BP with COPD or asthmatic subjects who require beta agonists for reversible airway obstruction.
- Assess for symptoms of CHF: edema, dyspnea, wet rales, BP.
- Assess BP if on mechanical ventilatory support to minimize mean airway pressures which can increase hypotensive effect through impeded venous return and decreased cardiac output; minimize inspiratory times and optimal flow patterns and avoid large tidal volumes.

Patient education:
- Do not use OTC products containing α-adrenergic stimulants (nasal decongestants, OTC cold preparations) unless directed by physician.
- Report symptoms of CHF: difficult breathing, especially on exertion or when lying down, night cough, swelling of extremities.
- It is necessary to quit smoking to prevent excessive vasoconstriction.
- Avoid hazardous activities until stabilized on medication; dizziness may occur.
- Make position changes slowly or fainting will occur.

cyclizine HCl/ cyclizine lactate
(sye'kli-zeen)
Marezine
Func. class.: Antiemetic, antihistamine, anticholinergic
Chem. class.: H₁-receptor antagonist, piperazine derivative

Action: There is reduced sensitivity of the labyrinthine apparatus. The inhibition of motion sickness and associated nausea/vomiting may be due to the anticholinergic properties of H₁-antagonists.

Uses: Motion sickness, prevention of postoperative vomiting

Dosage and routes:
Vomiting
- *Adult:* IM 50 mg ½ hr before termination of surgery, then q4-6h prn (lactate)
- *Child:* IM 3 mg/kg divided in 3 equal doses
Motion sickness
- *Adult:* PO 50 mg then q4-6h prn, not to exceed 200 mg/day (HCl)
- *Child:* PO 25 mg q4-6h prn
Available forms: Tabs 50 mg; inj 50 mg/ml

Side effects/adverse reactions:
CNS: Drowsiness, dizziness, vertigo, fatigue, restlessness, headache, insomnia, hallucinations (auditory/visual), and *convulsions* in children
GI: Nausea, anorexia
EENT: Dry mouth, blurred vision, tinnitus

Contraindications: Hypersensitivity to cyclizines, shock

Precautions: Children, narrow-angle glaucoma, urinary retention, lactation, prostatic hypertrophy, elderly, pregnancy (B)

Pharmacokinetics:
PO: Duration 4-6 hr; other pharmacokinetics not known

Interactions/ incompatibilities:
- May increase effect: alcohol, tranquilizers, narcotics

Lab test interferences:
False negative: Allergy skin testing

RESPIRATORY CARE CONSIDERATIONS
Assess/evaluate:
- Note drying of the upper airway.
- Caution is suggested if used in asthma, although thickening of lower respiratory tract secretions has not been established.
- Drowsiness may be a risk factor in subjects with sleep apnea.
- Therapeutic response: decrease or elimination in nausea, vomiting.

Patient education:
- Avoid hazardous activities or use caution while drug action persists.
- Additional CNS depression may occur with concomitant use of CNS depressants (tranquilizers, sedatives, or alcohol).

cycloserine
(sye-kloe-ser′een)
Seromycin Pulvules
Func. class.: Antitubercular
Chem. class.: S. orchidaceus, antibiotic

Action: Inhibits cell wall synthesis, analog of D-alanine

Uses: Pulmonary tuberculosis, extrapulmonary as adjunctive

Dosage and routes:
- *Adult:* PO 250 mg q12h × 14 days, then 250 mg q8h × 2 wk if there are no signs of toxicity, then 250 mg q6h if there are no signs of toxicity, not to exceed 1 g/day
- *Child:* PO 10-20 mg/kg/day (max 0.75-1 g) individual doses
Available forms: Caps 250 mg

Side effects/adverse reactions:
INTEG: Dermatitis, photosensitivity
CV: **CHF**
CNS: Headache, anxiety, drowsiness, tremors, *convulsions,* lethargy, depression, confusion, psychosis, aggression, personality changes

HEMA: Megaloblastic anemia,
Vit B_{12}, folic acid deficiency,
leukocytosis

Contraindications: Hypersensitivity, seizure disorders, renal disease, alcoholism (chronic), depression, severe anxiety, lactation, anemia

Precautions: Pregnancy (C), children

Pharmacokinetics:
PO: Peak 3 - 8 hr, excreted unchanged in urine, crosses placenta, excreted in breast milk

Interactions/ incompatibilities:
- Seizures: alcohol
- May increase CNS toxicity: isoniazid, ethionamide

Lab test interferences:
Increase: AST/ALT

RESPIRATORY CARE CONSIDERATIONS
Assess/evaluate:
- Monitor bacteriologic response to therapy using drug-susceptibility testing.
- Assess subject for adverse reactions to drug therapy for mycobacteria, such as visual acuity and color vision evaluation, liver enzymes, and hearing evaluation, if on other anti-TB drugs.
- Respiratory care practitioners and other health care personnel should self-screen for infection with TB routinely and following exposure.
- Proper environmental and personnel protection programs should be implemented when treating subjects with TB.
- Consider the possibility of HIV infection in individuals with confirmed or suspected TB.

Patient education:
- Compliance with dosage schedule, duration is necessary.
- Scheduled appointments must be kept or relapse may occur.

cyclosporine
(sye′kloe-spor-een)
Sandimmune
Func. class.:
Immunosuppressant
Chem. class.: Fungus-derived peptide

Action: Produces immunosuppression by inhibiting lymphocytes (T)

Uses: Organ transplants to prevent rejection

Dosage and routes:
- *Adult and child:* PO 15 mg/kg several hours before surgery, daily for 2 wk, reduce dosage by 2.5 mg/kg/wk to 5 - 10 mg/kg/day; IV 5 - 6 mg/kg several hours before surgery, daily, switch to PO form as soon as possible
Available forms: Oral sol 100 mg/ml; inj IV 50 mg/ml

Side effects/adverse reactions:
GI: Nausea, vomiting, diarrhea, *oral Candida, gum hyperplasia, hepatotoxicity,* pancreatitis
INTEG: Rash, acne, *hirsutism*
CNS: Tremors, headache
GU: Albuminuria, hematuria, proteinuria, renal failure

Contraindications: Hypersensitivity

Precautions: Severe renal disease, severe hepatic disease, pregnancy (C)

Pharmacokinetics: Peak 4 hr, highly protein bound, half-life (biphasic) 1.2 hr, 25 hr, metabolized in liver, excreted in feces, crosses placenta, excreted in breast milk

Interactions/ incompatibilities:
- Increased action of cyclosporine: amphotericin B, cimetidine, ketoconazole
- Decreased action of cyclosporine: phenytoin, rifampin
- Compatibility information unknown; give separately

RESPIRATORY CARE CONSIDERATIONS
Assess/evaluate:
- Monitor for signs/ symptoms of infection, including chest radiograph.
- Use strict infection control and isolation procedures to prevent nosocomial infection while providing ventilatory support postoperatively.

cyproheptadine HCl
(si-proe-hep'-ta-deen)
Cyproheptadine HCl, Periactin, Vimicon*
Func. class.: Antihistamine, H$_1$-receptor antagonist
Chem. class.: Piperidine

Action: Blocks the action of histamine at H$_1$-receptor sites on blood vessels, GI, respiratory tract to decrease allergic inflammatory response.

Uses: Allergy symptoms, rhinitis, pruritus, cold urticaria

Dosage and routes:
- *Adult:* PO 4 mg tid-qid, not to exceed 0.5 mg/kg/day
- *Child 7-14 yr:* PO 4 mg bid-tid, not to exceed 16 mg/day
- *Child 2-6 yr:* PO 2 mg bid-tid, not to exceed 12 mg/day

Available forms: Tabs 4 mg; syr 2 mg/5 ml

Side effects/adverse reactions:
CNS: Dizziness, drowsiness, poor coordination, fatigue, anxiety, euphoria, confusion, paresthesia, neuritis
CV: Hypotension, palpitations, tachycardia
RESP: Increased thick secretions, wheezing, chest tightness
GI: Constipation, dry mouth, nausea, vomiting, anorexia, diarrhea, weight gain
INTEG: Rash, urticaria, photosensitivity
GU: Retention, dysuria, frequency, increased appetite
EENT: Blurred vision, dilated pupils, tinnitus, nasal stuffiness, dry nose, throat, mouth

Contraindications: Hypersensitivity to H$_1$-receptor antagonist, acute asthma attack, lower respiratory tract disease

Precautions: Increased intraocular pressure, renal disease, cardiac disease, hypertension, bronchial asthma, seizure disorder, stenosed peptic ulcers, hyperthyroidism, prostatic hypertrophy, bladder neck obstruction, pregnancy (B), elderly

Pharmacokinetics:
PO: Duration 4-6 hr, metabolized in liver, excreted by kidneys, excreted in breast milk

Interactions/ incompatibilities:
- Increased CNS depression: barbiturates, narcotics, hypnotics, tricyclic antidepressants, alcohol
- Decreased effect of: oral anticoagulants, heparin

---

italic = common side effects   **bold** = life-threatening reactions

- Increased effect of cyproheptadine: MAOIs

Lab test interferences:
False negative: Skin allergy tests

RESPIRATORY CARE CONSIDERATIONS
Assess/evaluate:
- Note drying of the upper airway.
- Caution is suggested if used in asthma, although thickening of lower respiratory tract secretions has not been established.
- Drowsiness may be a risk factor in subjects with sleep apnea.

Patient education:
- Avoid hazardous activities or use caution while drug action persists.
- Additional CNS depression may occur with concomitant use of CNS depressants (tranquilizers, sedatives, or alcohol).

**dexamethasone/
dexamethasone
acetate/
dexamethasone
sodium phosphate**

(dex-a-meth′a-sone)
Aeroseb-Dex, Decaderm, Decaspray, Dalalone D.P., Dalalone L.A., Decadron-LA, Decaject-L.A., Dexacen LA-8, Dexamethasone Acetate, Dexasone L.A., Dexone LA, Solurex LA, Dalalone, Decadron Phosphate, Decaject, Dexacen-4, Dexamethasone Sodium Phosphate, Dexasone, Dexone, Hexadrol Phosphate, Solurex, Decadron Phosphate Respihaler
Func. class.: Corticosteroid
Chem. class.: Glucocorticoid, long-acting

See also Section III: Aerosol Agents for Oral Inhalation

Action: Decreases inflammation by suppression of migration of polymorphonuclear leukocytes, fibroblasts, reversal of increased capillary permeability and lysosomal stabilization

Uses: Inflammation, allergies, neoplasms, cerebral edema, septic shock, collagen disorders

Dosage and routes:
Inflammation
- *Adult:* PO 0.25-4 mg bid-qid
IM 4-16 mg q1-3 wk (acetate)
Shock
- *Adult:* IV 1-6 mg/kg or 40 mg q2-6h (phosphate)
Cerebral edema
- *Adult:* IV 10 mg, then 4-6 mg IM q6h × 2-4 days, then taper over 1 wk
- *Child:* PO 0.2 mg/kg/day in divided doses
Available forms: Tabs 0.25, 0.5, 0.75, 1, 1.5, 3, 4, 6 mg; inj IM acetate 8, 16 mg/ml; inj IV phosphate 4, 10 mg/ml; elix 0.5 mg/5 ml; oral sol 0.5 mg/5 ml, 0.5 mg/1 ml

Side effects/adverse reactions:
INTEG: Acne, poor wound healing, ecchymosis, petechiae
CNS: Depression, flushing, sweating, headache, mood changes
CV: Hypertension, circulatory collapse, thrombophlebitis, embolism, tachycardia, edema
HEMA: Thrombocytopenia
MS: Fractures, osteoporosis, weakness
GI: Diarrhea, nausea, abdominal distention, GI hemorrhage, increased appetite, pancreatitis

EENT: Fungal infections, increased intraocular pressure, blurred vision

Contraindications: Psychosis, hypersensitivity, idiopathic thrombocytopenia, acute glomerulonephritis, amebiasis, fungal infections, nonasthmatic bronchial disease, child <2 yr, AIDS, TB

Precautions: Pregnancy (C), diabetes mellitus, glaucoma, osteoporosis, seizure disorders, ulcerative colitis, CHF, myasthenia gravis, renal disease, peptic ulcer, esophagitis

Pharmacokinetics:
PO: Peak 1-2 h, duration 2 ⅓ days
IM: Peak 8 h, duration 6 days
   Half-life 3-4 ½ hr

Interactions/ incompatibilities:
■ Decreased action of dexamethasone: cholestyramine, colestipol, barbiturates, rifampin, ephedrine, phenytoin, theophylline, antacids
■ Decreased effects of: anticoagulants, anticonvulsants, antidiabetics, ambenonium, neostigmine, isoniazid, toxoids, vaccines, anticholinesterases, salicylates, somatrem
■ Increased side effects: alcohol, salicylates, indomethacin, amphotericin B, digitalis, cyclosporine diuretics
■ Increased action of dexamethasone: salicylates, estrogens, indomethacin, oral contraceptives, ketoconazole, macrolide antibiotics
■ Incompatible with amikacin, daunorubicin, doxorubicin, metaraminol, prochlorperazine, vancomycin

Lab test interferences:
Increase: Cholesterol, Na, blood glucose, uric acid, Ca, urine glucose
Decrease: Ca, K, T$_4$, T$_3$, thyroid ^{131}I uptake test, urine 17-OHCS, 17-KS, PBI
False negative: Skin allergy tests

RESPIRATORY CARE CONSIDERATIONS
Assess/evaluate:
■ Monitor for side effects of increased corticosteroid level: Cushingoid symptoms (moon face, peripheral wasting, central edema).
■ Monitor patients with latent tuberculosis or reactive skin tests for reactivation of the disease.
■ Evaluate muscle weakness and steroid myopathy, especially in chronic lung disease patients.
■ Evaluate cardiovascular system for hypertension, CHF.
■ Monitor electrolytes; potassium and calcium loss can occur with hypokalemic alkalosis.
■ Infection, including pneumonia, can occur.
■ Increased corticosteroid levels can mask symptoms of infection.
■ If asthma is present, monitor for breakthrough symptoms (bronchospasm, wheezing) if drug is discontinued.
■ Evaluate possible adrenal insufficiency when transferring from systemic to inhaled aerosol corticosteroids in asthma.
■ Symptoms of adrenal insufficiency: nausea, anorexia, fatigue, dizziness, dyspnea, weakness, joint pain.

---

italic = common side effects   **bold** = life-threatening reactions

dexamethasone sodium phosphate (nasal)

(dex-a-meth'a-sone)
Decadron Phosphate
Turbinaire
Func. class.: Steroid,
intranasal
Chem. class.: Glucocorticoid

Action: Long-acting synthetic adrenocorticoid with antiinflammatory activity, minimal mineralocorticoid properties

Uses: Inflammation (not within sinuses), nasal polyps, allergic conditions of nose
See also Section III: Aerosol Agents for Oral Inhalation

Dosage and routes:
■ *Adult:* Spray 1-2 sprays bid-tid, not to exceed 12/day
■ *Child 6-12 yr:* Spray 1-2 sprays bid, not to exceed 8/day
Available forms: 84 μg/ metered spray

Side effects/adverse reactions:
EENT: Nasal irritation, dryness, rebound congestion, epistaxis, sneezing, *infarction of nasal mucosa*
INTEG: Urticaria
CNS: Headache, dizziness
SYSTEMIC: CHF, convulsions, increased Na, hypertension

Contraindications: Hypersensitivity, child <12 yr, localized infection of nose, acute status asthmaticus

Precautions: Lactation, nasal trauma, pregnancy (C)

RESPIRATORY CARE CONSIDERATIONS
Assess/evaluate:
■ Therapeutic response: decreased inflammation, rhinitis.
■ Monitor nasal passages during long-term treatment for changes in mucus.

Patient education: Proper use and cleaning of spray container following manufacturer's instructions.

dexchlorpheniramine maleate

(dex-klor-fen-eer'a-meen)
Dexchlor, Dexchlorpheniramine Maleate, Poladex, Polaramine
Func. class.: Antihistamine
Chem. class.: Alkylamine derivative, H_1-receptor antagonist

Action: Blocks the action of histamine at H_1-receptor sites on blood vessels, GI, respiratory tract to decrease allergic inflammatory response.

Uses: Allergy symptoms, rhinitis, pruritus, contact dermatitis

Dosage and routes:
■ *Adult:* PO 1-2 mg tid-qid; REPEAT ACTION 4-6 mg bid-tid
■ *Child 6-11 yr:* PO 1 mg q4-6h, or TIME REL 4 mg hs
■ *Child 2-5 yr:* PO 0.5 mg q4-6h; do not use repeat action form
Available forms: Tabs 2 mg; repeat-action tab 4, 6 mg; syr 2 mg/5 ml

Side effects/adverse reactions:
CNS: Dizziness, drowsiness, poor coordination, fatigue, anxiety,

euphoria, confusion, paresthesia, neuritis
CV: Hypotension, palpitations, tachycardia
RESP: Increased thick secretions, wheezing, chest tightness
GI: Constipation, dry mouth, nausea, vomiting, anorexia, diarrhea
INTEG: Rash, urticaria, photosensitivity
GU: Retention, dysuria, frequency
EENT: Blurred vision, dilated pupils, tinnitus, nasal stuffiness, dry nose, throat, mouth

Contraindications: Hypersensitivity to H_1-receptor antagonist; acute asthma attack, lower respiratory tract disease

Precautions: Increased intraocular pressure, renal disease, cardiac disease, hypertension, bronchial asthma, seizure disorder, stenosed peptic ulcers, hyperthyroidism, prostatic hypertrophy, bladder neck obstruction, pregnancy (B), elderly

Pharmacokinetics:
PO: Onset 15 min, peak 3 hr, duration 3-6 hr, metabolized in liver, excreted by kidneys (inactive metabolites), excreted in breast milk (small amounts)

Interactions/ incompatibilities:
■ Increased CNS depression: barbiturates, narcotics, hypnotics, tricyclic antidepressants, alcohol
■ Decreased effect: oral anticoagulants, heparin
■ Increased effect of dexchlorpheniramine: MAOIs

Lab test interferences:
False negative: Skin allergy tests

RESPIRATORY CARE CONSIDERATIONS
Assess/evaluate:
■ Note drying of the upper airway.
■ Caution is suggested if used in asthma, although thickening of lower respiratory tract secretions has not been established.
■ Drowsiness may be a risk factor in subjects with sleep apnea.

Patient education:
■ Avoid hazardous activities or use caution while drug action persists.
■ Additional CNS depression may occur with concomitant use of CNS depressants (tranquilizers, sedatives, or alcohol).

dextran 40
Dextran 40, Gentran 40, LMD 10%, Rheomacrodex
Func. class.: Plasma volume expander
Chem. class.: Low molecular weight polysaccharide

Action: Similar to human albumin, which expands plasma volume by drawing fluid from interstitial space to intravascular space

Uses: Expand plasma volume, prophylaxis of embolism, thrombosis

Dosage and routes:
Shock
■ *Adult:* IV INF 500 ml over 15-30 min, total dose in 24 hr not to exceed 20 ml/kg; then subsequent doses given

slowly; if given >24 hr, not to exceed 10 ml/kg/day; not to exceed therapy >5 days
Thrombosis/embolism
- *Adult:* IV INF 500-1000 ml, then 500 ml/day × 3 days, then 500 ml q2-3 days × 2 wk if needed
Available forms: 10% dextran 40/5% dextrose, 10% dextran 40/0.9% sodium chloride

Side effects/adverse reactions:
HEMA: Decreased hematocrit, platelet function, increased bleeding/coagulation times
INTEG: Rash, urticaria, pruritus, angioedema, chills, fever, flushing
RESP: Wheezing, dyspnea, *bronchospasm, pulmonary edema*
CV: Hypotension, *cardiac arrest*
GU: Osmotic nephrosis; renal failure, stasis, hyponatremia
GI: Nausea, vomiting, increased AST, ALT
SYST: Anaphylaxis

Contraindications: Hypersensitivity, renal failure, CHF (severe), extreme dehydration

Precautions: Active hemorrhage, pregnancy (C)

Pharmacokinetics:
IV: Expands blood volume 1-2 × amount infused; excreted in urine and feces

Interactions/ incompatibilities
- Incompatible with chlortetracycline, phytonadione, promethazine
- Incompatible with any drug in dextran sol

Lab test interferences:
False increase: Blood glucose, urinary protein, bilirubin, total protein

Interference: Rh test, blood typing/crossmatching

RESPIRATORY CARE CONSIDERATIONS
Assess/evaluate:
- Evaluate therapeutic response of increased circulatory volume and improvement of blood pressure.
- Monitor subject for allergic reactions causing wheezing, dyspnea, or bronchospasm.
- Monitor breath sounds for wheezing or rales suggestive of pulmonary edema indicating volume overload.
- Monitor BP for decreases suggesting high output failure. Ventilatory parameters should be monitored and adjusted if possible to prevent or minimize high thoracic pressures causing impeded venous return and decreased cardiac output if hypotension occurs.
- Note alteration (decrease) of hematocrit and hemoglobin laboratory values following administration.
- Note possible adverse effects.

dextran 70/75
Dextran 70, Dextran 75, Gentran 75, Macrodex
Func. class.: Plasma volume expander
Chem. class.: High molecular weight polysaccharide

Action: Similar to human albumin, which expands plasma volume by drawing fluid from interstitial space to intravascular space

Uses: Expand plasma volume in hypovolemic shock or impending shock

Dosage and routes:
- *Adult:* IV INF 500-1000 ml not to exceed 20-40 ml/min, not to exceed 10 ml/kg/24 hr if therapy >24 hr
Available forms: 70/75 dextran in 0.9% NaCl, D$_5$%

Side effects/adverse reactions:
HEMA: Decreased hematocrit, platelet function, increased bleeding/coagulation times
INTEG: Rash, urticaria, pruritus, angioedema, chills, fever, flushing
RESP: Wheezing, dyspnea, *bronchospasm, pulmonary edema*
CV: Hypotension, *cardiac arrest*
GU: Osmotic nephrosis, renal failure, stasis, hypernatremia
GI: Nausea, vomiting, increased AST, ALT
SYST: Anaphylaxis

Contraindications: Hypersensitivity, renal failure, CHF (severe), extreme dehydration

Precautions: Active hemorrhage, pregnancy (C)

Pharmacokinetics:
IV: Expands blood volume 1-2 × amount infused; excreted in urine and feces

Lab test interferences:
False increase: Blood glucose, urinary protein, bilirubin, total protein
Interferences: Rh test, blood typing/crossmatching

RESPIRATORY CARE CONSIDERATIONS
Assess/evaluate:
- Evaluate therapeutic response of increased circulatory volume and improvement of blood pressure.
- Monitor subject for allergic reactions causing wheezing, dyspnea, or bronchospasm.
- Monitor breath sounds for wheezing or rales suggestive of pulmonary edema indicating volume overload.
- Monitor BP for decreases suggesting high output failure. Ventilatory parameters should be monitored and adjusted if possible to prevent or minimize high thoracic pressures causing impeded venous return and decreased cardiac output if hypotension occurs.
- Note alteration (decrease) of hematocrit and hemoglobin laboratory values following administration.
- Note possible adverse effects.

dextromethorphan hydrobromide
(dex-troe-meth-or'fan)
Benylin DM, Children's Hold, Delsym, Dextromethorphan, Hold DM, Pertussin, Pertussin ES, Robitussin Cough Calmers, Robitussin Pediatric, St. Joseph Cough Suppressant, Sucrets Cough Control, Suppress, Trocal, Vicks Formula 44
Func. class.: Antitussive, nonnarcotic
Chem. class.: Levorphanol derivative

Action: Dextromethorphan is a nonnarcotic antitussive, which is the d-isomer of the codeine analog of levorphanol. Although it lacks analgesic and addictive properties, the drug depresses the cough center in the medulla.

Uses: Nonproductive cough

Dosage and routes:
- *Adult:* PO 10-20 mg q4h, or 30 mg q6-8h, not to exceed 120 mg/day; CON-REL LIQ 60 mg bid, not to exceed 120 mg/day
- *Child 6-12 yr:* PO 5-10 mg q4h; CON-REL LIQ 30 mg bid, not to exceed 60 mg/day
- *Child 2-6 yr:* PO 2.5-5 mg q4h, or 7.5 mg q6-8h, not to exceed 30 mg/day

Available forms: Loz 5 mg; sol 5, 7.5, 10, 15 mg/5 ml

Side effects/adverse reactions:
CNS: Dizziness
GI: Nausea

Contraindications: Hypersensitivity, asthma/emphysema, productive cough

Precautions: Nausea/vomiting, increased temperature, persistent headache, pregnancy (C)

Pharmacokinetics:
PO: Onset 15-30 min, duration 3-6 hr

Interactions/incompatibilities:
- Do not give with MAOIs or within 2 wk of MAOIs, penicillins, salicylates, tetracyclines, phenobarbital, iodines (high doses)

RESPIRATORY CARE CONSIDERATIONS
Assess/evaluate:
- Monitor cough: type, frequency, character including sputum.
- Avoid suppressing a productive cough when respiratory infection is present.

Patient education:
- Increased nondiuretic fluids can help liquefy secretions; humidify (cool humidifier) patient's room.
- Avoid hazardous activities if drowsiness occurs.
- Avoid smoking, smoke-filled rooms, perfumes, dust, environmental pollutants, cleaners that increase cough.

diazoxide
(dye-az-ox'ide)
Diazoxide Injection, Hyperstat
Func. class.: Antihypertensive
Chem. class.: Vasodilator

Action: Vasodilates arteriolar smooth muscle by direct relaxation; reduces blood pressure with concomitant increases in heart rate, cardiac output

Uses: Hypertensive crisis when urgent decrease of diastolic pressure required; increase blood glucose levels in hyperinsulinism

Dosage and routes:
- *Adult:* IV BOL 1-3 mg/kg rapidly up to a max of 150 mg in a single injection; dose may be repeated at 5-15 min intervals until desired response is achieved; give IV in 30 sec or less
- *Child:* IV BOL 1-2 mg/kg rapidly; administration same as adult, not to exceed 150 mg

Available forms: Inj IV 15 mg/ml

Side effects/adverse reactions:
CV: Hypotension, T-wave changes, angina pectoris, palpitations, *supraventricular tachycardia, edema,* rebound hypertension
CNS: Headache, sleepiness, euphoria, anxiety, extrapyrami-

dal symptoms, confusion, tinnitus, blurred vision, dizziness, weakness

GI: Nausea, vomiting, dry mouth

INTEG: Rash

HEMA: Decreased hemoglobin, hematocrit, *thrombocytopenia*

GU: Breast tenderness; increased BUN, fluid, electrolyte imbalances; Na, water retention

ENDO: Hyperglycemia in diabetics, transient hyperglycemia in nondiabetics

Contraindications: Hypersensitivity to thiazides, sulfonamides, hypertension associated with aortic coarctation or AV shunt, pheochromocytoma, dissecting aortic aneurysm

Precautions: Tachycardia, fluid, electrolyte imbalances, pregnancy (B), lactation, impaired cerebral or cardiac circulation, children

Pharmacokinetics:
IV: Onset 1-2 min, peak 5 min, duration 3-12 hr, half-life 20-36 hr, excreted slowly in urine, crosses blood-brain barrier, placenta

Interactions/ incompatibilities:
- Increased effects: thiazide diuretics, antihypertensives, coumadin, guanethidine, sympathomimetics
- Do not mix with any drug in syringe or solution
- Increased effects of: warfarin, other coumarins
- Hyperglycemia/ hyperuricemia: thiazides, diuretics
- Decreased pharmacologic effects of both: sulfonylureas

RESPIRATORY CARE CONSIDERATIONS
Assess/evaluate:
- Evaluate BP and pulse for efficacy of hypertension treatment and to avoid hypotension.
- Evaluate BP with COPD or asthmatic subjects who require beta agonists for reversible airway obstruction.
- Assess for symptoms of CHF: edema, dyspnea, wet rales, BP.
- Assess BP if on mechanical ventilatory support to minimize mean airway pressures which can increase hypotensive effect through impeded venous return and decreased cardiac output; minimize inspiratory times and optimize flow patterns and avoid large tidal volumes.

Patient education:
- Do not use OTC products containing α-adrenergic stimulants (nasal decongestants, OTC cold preparations) unless directed by physician.
- Report symptoms of CHF: difficult breathing, especially on exertion or when lying down, night cough, swelling of extremities.
- Stop smoking to prevent excessive vasoconstriction.
- Avoid hazardous activities until stabilized on medication; dizziness may occur.
- Make position changes slowly or fainting will occur.

didanosine (ddI, dideoxyinosine)
(dye-dan'-o-seen)
Videx, ddI, Dideoxyinosine
Func. class.: Antiviral
Chem. class.: Synthetic purine nucleoside of deoxyadenosine

---

italic = common side effects   **bold** = life-threatening reactions

Action: Didanosine, or ddI, is a nucleoside analog which inhibits viral replication. Didanosine is converted in a cell to dideoxyadenosine triphosphate (ddATP); this active metabolite lacks the 3'-hydroxyl group needed for DNA chain extension and also interferes with reverse transcriptase.

Uses: Advanced HIV infections in adults and children who have been unable to use zidovudine or who have not responded to treatment

Dosage and routes:
- *Adult:* PO >75 kg, 300 mg bid tabs, or 375 mg bid buffered powder
50 - 74 kg, 200 mg bid tabs, or 250 mg bid buffered powder
35 - 49 kg, 125 mg bid tabs, or 167 mg bid buffered powder
- *Child:* PO 1.1 - 1.4 m$_2$, 100 mg bid tabs, or 125 mg bid pedi powder
0.8 - 1 m$_2$, 75 mg bid tabs, or 94 mg bid pedi powder
0.5 - 0.7 m$_2$, 50 mg bid tabs, or 62 mg bid pedi powder
< 0.4 m^2, 25 mg bid tabs, or 31 mg bid pedi powder
Available forms: Tabs, buffered, chewable/dispersible 25, 50, 100, 150 mg; powder for oral sol, buffered 100, 167, 250, 375 mg; powder for oral sol, pedi 2, 4 g

Side effects/adverse reactions:
GI: Pancreatitis, diarrhea, nausea, vomiting, abdominal pain, constipation, stomatitis, dyspepsia, liver abnormalities, flatulence, taste perversion, dry mouth, oral thrush, melena, increased ALT, AST, Alk phosphatase, amylase

GU: Increased bilirubin, uric acid
CNS: Peripheral neuropathy, seizures, confusion, anxiety, hypertonia, abnormal thinking, asthenia, insomnia, *CNS depression,* pain, dizziness, chills, fever
RESP: Cough, pneumonia, dyspnea, asthma, epistaxis, hypoventilation, sinusitis
INTEG: Rash, pruritus, alopecia, ecchymosis, hemorrhage, petechiae, sweating
MS: Myalgia, arthritis, myopathy, muscular atrophy
CV: Hypertension, vasodilation, dysrhythmia, syncope, CHF, palpitation
EENT: Ear pain, otitis, photophobia, visual impairment
HEMA: Leukopenia, granulocytopenia, thrombocytopenia, anemia

Contraindications: Hypersensitivity

Precautions: Renal, hepatic disease, pregnancy (B), lactation, children, Na-restricted diets, elevated amylase, preexistent peripheral neuropathy

Pharmacokinetics:
PO: Elimination half-life 1.62 hr, extensive metabolism is thought to occur; administration within 5 min of food will decrease absorption

Interactions/ incompatibilities:
- Decreased absorption: ketoconazole, dapsone, food
- Do not administer with tetracyclines
- Decreased concentrations of: fluoroquinolone antibiotics

RESPIRATORY CARE CONSIDERATIONS
Assess/evaluate:
- Practice infection control to prevent opportunistic infection in subjects.
- Monitor subject for respiratory infections, especially *P. carinii* pneumonia (PCP).
- If subject is HIV positive, assess and screen for concomitant TB infection.
- Use isolation techniques (negative pressure booth or hood, etc.) for aerosol treatments. Nebulizers with one-way valves and expiratory filtration are preferred for aerosol drug delivery.

digitoxin
(di-ji-tox'in)
Digitaline*, Digitoxin
Func. class.: Antidysrhythmic, cardiac glycoside cardiotonic
Chem. class.: Digitalis preparation

Action: Acts by increased influx of calcium ions from extracellular to intracellular cytoplasm, increasing force of contraction and cardiac output; decreases conduction velocity through AV node; prolongs effective refractory period

Uses: CHF, atrial fibrillation, atrial flutter, atrial tachycardia, rapid digitalization in these disorders

Dosage and routes:
- *Adult and child >12 yr:* 1.2-1.6 initially; give in divided doses over 24 hr; 150 µg qd
- *Neonates:* 22 µg/kg; 2 wk-1 yr: 45 µg/kg; 1-2 yr: 40 µg/kg; 2-12 yr: 30 µg/kg

- *Maintenance dose:* 10% initial dose
Available forms: Powder, tabs 50, 100, 150, 200 µg

Side effects/adverse reactions:
CNS: Headache, drowsiness, apathy, confusion, disorientation, fatigue, depression, hallucinations
CV: **Dysrhythmias, hypotension, bradycardia,** AV block
GI: Nausea, vomiting, anorexia, abdominal pain, diarrhea
EENT: Blurred vision, yellow-green halos, photophobia, diplopia
MS: Muscular weakness

Contraindications: Hypersensitivity to digitalis, ventricular fibrillation, ventricular tachycardia, carotid sinus syndrome, 2nd or 3rd degree heart block

Precautions: Hepatic disease, acute MI, AV block, hypokalemia, hypomagnesemia, sinus node disease, lactation, severe respiratory disease, hypothyroidism, elderly, pregnancy (C)

Pharmacokinetics:
PO: Onset ½-2 hr, peak 4-12 hr, duration 2-3 wk, half-life 4-20 days, metabolized in liver, excreted in urine

Interactions/ incompatibilities:
- Hypokalemia: thiazides
- Increased blood levels: spironolactone
- Decreased effects: hydantoins, aminoglutethimide, rifampin, phenylbutazone, barbiturates, cholestyramine, colestipol
- Toxicity: adrenergics, diuretics, succinylcholine, quinidine, thioamines

---

italic = common side effects   **bold** = life-threatening reactions

- Decreased level of digitoxin: thyroid agents

Lab test interferences:
Increase: CPK

RESPIRATORY CARE CONSIDERATIONS
Assess/evaluate:
- Monitor patient for cardiac arrhythmias, due to both direct effects of the glycosides and to coronary vasoconstriction.
- Monitor serum electrolytes: hypokalemia, hypercalcemia, hypomagnesemia can predispose to digitalis toxicity.
- Assess cardiac output (BP, pulse volume, reduced heart rate) for efficacy of treatment.

digoxin
(di-jox'in)
Digoxin, Lanoxicaps, Lanoxin
Func. class.: Antidysrhythmic, cardiac glycoside
Chem. class.: Digitalis preparation

Action: Inhibits the sodium-potassium ATPase, which makes more calcium available for contractile proteins, resulting in increased cardiac output

Uses: CHF, atrial fibrillation, atrial flutter, atrial tachycardia, rapid digitalization in these disorders

Dosage and routes:
- *Adult:* IV 0.5 mg given over >5 min, then PO 0.125-0.5 mg qd in divided doses q4-6hr as needed
- *Elderly:* PO 0.125 mg qd maintenance
- *Child >2 yr:* PO 0.02-0.04 mg/kg divided q8h over 24 hr; maintenance 0.006-0.012 mg/kg qd in divided doses q12hr; IV loading dose 0.015-0.035 mg/kg over >5 min
- *Child 1 mo-2 yr:* IV 0.03-0.05 mg/kg in divided doses over >5 min q48h; change to PO as soon as possible; PO 0.035-0.060 mg/kg divided in 3 doses over 24 hr; maintenance 0.01-0.02 mg/kg in divided doses q12h
- *Neonates:* IV loading dose 0.02-0.03 mg/kg over >5 min in divided doses q4-8h; change to PO as soon as possible; PO loading dose 0.035 mg/kg divided q8h over 24h; maintenance 0.01 mg/kg in divided doses q12hr
- *Premature infants:* IV 0.015-0.025 mg/kg divided in 3 doses over 24 hr, given over >5 min; maintenance 0.003-0.009 mg/kg in divided doses q12h
Available forms: Caps 50, 100, 200 μg; elix 50 μg/ml; tabs 125, 250, 500 μg; inj 100, 250 μg/ml

Side effects/adverse reactions:
CNS: Headache, drowsiness, apathy, confusion, disorientation, fatigue, depression, hallucinations
CV: **Dysrhythmias, hypotension,** bradycardia, *AV block*
EENT: Blurred vision, yellow-green halos, photophobia, diplopia
GI: Nausea, vomiting, anorexia, abdominal pain, diarrhea

Contraindications: Hypersensitivity to digitalis, ventricular fibrillation, ventricular tachycardia, carotid sinus syndrome, 2nd or 3rd degree heart block

Precautions: Renal disease, acute MI, AV block, severe respiratory disease, hypothyroidism, elderly, pregnancy (C), sinus nodal disease, lactation, hypokalemia

Pharmacokinetics:
PO: Onset ½-2 hr, peak 6-8 hrs, duration 3-4 days
IV: Onset 5-30 min, peak 1-5 hr, duration variable, half-life 1.5, days excreted in urine

Interactions/ incompatibilities:
■ Hypokalemia: diuretics, amphotericin B, carbenicillin, ticarcillin, corticosteroids, piperacillin
■ Decreased digoxin level: thyroid agents
■ Increased blood levels: propantheline bromide, spirono-lactone quinidine, verapamil, aminoglycosides PO, amiodarone, anticholinergics, quinine
■ Increased bradycardia: β-adrenergic blockers, antidysrythmics
■ Toxicity: adrenergics, amphotericin, corticosteroids, diuretics, glucose, insulin, reserpine, succinylcholine, quinidine, thioamines
■ Incompatible with acids, alkalies, Ca salts

Lab test interferences:
Increase: CPK

RESPIRATORY CARE CONSIDERATIONS
Assess/evaluate:
■ Monitor patient for cardiac arrhythmias, due to both direct effects of the glycosides, and to coronary vasoconstriction.
■ Monitor serum electrolytes: hypokalemia, hypercalcemia, hypomagnesemia can predispose to digitalis toxicity.
■ Assess cardiac output (BP, pulse volume, reduced heart rate) for efficacy of treatment.

D

digoxin immune FAB (ovine)
Digibind
Func. class.: Antidote—digoxin specific
Chem. class.: Antidigitoxin antibodies

Action: Antibody fragments bind to free digoxin to reverse digoxin toxicity by not allowing digoxin to bind to sites of action

Uses: Life-threatening digoxin or digitoxin toxicity

Dosage and routes:
Digoxin toxicity
■ *Adult:* IV dose (mg) = Dose ingested (mg) $\times$ 0.8 $\times$ 66.7; if ingested amount is unknown, give 800 mg IV.
If digoxin liquid caps or digitoxin used, do not multiply ingested dose by 0.8
Available forms: Inj 40 mg/vial (binds 0.6 mg digoxin or digitoxin)

Side effects/adverse reactions:
CV: **CHF,** ventricular rate increase, **atrial fibrillation,** low cardiac output
RESP: **Impaired respiratory function, rapid respiratory rate**
META: Hypokalemia
INTEG: Hypersensitivity, allergic reactions

Contraindications: Mild digoxin toxicity

Precautions: Children, lactation, cardiac disease, renal disease, pregnancy (C)

---

italic = common side effects   **bold** = life-threatening reactions

Pharmacokinetics:
IV: Peaks after completion of infusion, onset 30 min (variable); not known if crosses placenta, breast milk; half-life biphasic 14-20 hr; prolonged in renal disease; excreted by kidneys

**Interactions/
incompatibilities**
▪ Considered incompatible with all drugs in syringe or sol

Lab test interferences:
Interfere: Immunoassay digoxin

RESPIRATORY CARE CONSIDERATIONS
Assess/evaluate:
▪ Monitor patient for cardiac arrhythmias, due to both direct effects of the glycosides and to coronary vasoconstriction.
▪ Monitor serum electrolytes: hypokalemia, hypercalcemia, hypomagnesemia can predispose to digitalis toxicity.

diltiazem HCl
(dil-tye'a-zem)
Cardizem, Cardizem SR, Cardizem CD, Diltiazem, DilacorXR
Func. class.: Calcium channel blocker
Chem. class.: Benzothiazepine

Action: Inhibits calcium ion influx across cell membrane during cardiac depolarization; produces relaxation of coronary vascular smooth muscle, dilates coronary arteries, slows SA/AV node conduction times, dilates peripheral arteries

Uses: Oral: angina pectoris due to coronary insufficiency, hypertension. Parenteral: atrial fibrillation, flutter, paroxysmal supraventricular tachycardia

Dosage and routes:
▪ *Adult:* PO 30 mg qid, increasing dose gradually to 180-360 mg/day in divided doses or 60-120 mg bid; may increase to 240-360 mg/day
▪ *Adult IV:* 0.25 mg/kg over BOL 2 min initially, then 0.35 mg/kg may be given after 15 min; if no response, may give Cont Inf 5-15 mg/hr for up to 24 hrs
▪ *Adult:* PO (Cardizem CD) qd
Available forms: Tabs 30, 60, 90, 120 mg, sus rel 60, 90, 120, 150 mg; Inj (IV) 5 mg/ml (5, 10 ml)

Side effects/adverse reactions:
CV: Dysrhythmia, edema, CHF, bradycardia, hypotension, palpitations, heart block, peripheral edema, angina
GI: Nausea, vomiting, diarrhea, gastric upset, constipation, increased liver function studies
GU: Nocturia, polyuria, *acute renal failure*
INTEG: Rash, pruritus, flushing, photosensitivity
CNS: Headache, fatigue, drowsiness, dizziness, depression, weakness, insomnia, tremor, paresthesia

Contraindications: Sick sinus syndrome, 2nd or 3rd degree heart block, hypotension less than 90 mm Hg systolic, acute MI, pulmonary congestion

Precautions: CHF, hypotension, hepatic injury, pregnancy (C), lactation, children, renal disease

Pharmacokinetics: Onset 30-60 min, peak 2-3 hr, immediate rel, 6-11 sus rel, half-life 3 ½-9 hr; metabolized by liver; excreted in urine (96% as metabolites)

Interactions/ incompatibilities:
■ Increased effects of: β-blockers, digitalis, lithium, carbamazepine, cyclosporine
■ Increased effects of diltiazem: cimetidine

RESPIRATORY CARE CONSIDERATIONS
Assess/evaluate:
■ Therapeutic response: corrected arrhythmia, decreased anginal pain, decreased BP.
■ Monitor cardiovascular status: BP, pulse, respiration, ECG.
■ Check for presence of adverse effects, especially dizziness or other signs of hypotension bradycardia.
■ If on positive pressure ventilatory support, monitor cardiac output and/or BP, and adjust level of positive pressure to extent possible, if necessary to maintain adequate cardiac output.
■ Monitor blood pressure if beta agonists are required to treat airway obstruction.
■ Consider use of anticholinergic agent such as ipratropium bromide as an alternative to beta agonists, if bronchodilator therapy is needed; aerosol inhalation (MDI, SVN, DPI) of adrenergic bronchodilators will generally give lower systemic levels and fewer cardiovascular effects.

Patient education:
■ Note: hand tremor can occur, such as seen with beta agonist bronchodilators.
■ Change position slowly to avoid orthostatic hypotension.

dimenhydrinate
(dye-men-hye'dri-nate)
Calm-X, Dimenhydrinate, Dinate, Dommanate, Dramamine, Dramanate, Dramocen, Dramoject, Dymenate, Gravol*, Hydrate, Marmine, Nauseal*, Nauseatol*, Nico-Vert, Novodimenate*, Travamine*, Triptone Caplets, Vertab
Func. class.: Antiemetic, antihistamine, anticholinergic
Chem. class.: H_1-receptor antagonist, ethanolamine derivative

Action: Dimenhydrinate is a combination of diphenhydramine, an antihistamine, and chlorotheophylline. Dimenhydrinate acts by depressing the hyperstimulated labyrinthine function. The antiemetic effect is believed to be due the antihistamine action. The inhibition of motion sickness and associated nausea/vomiting may be due to the anticholinergic properties of H_1 antagonists.

Uses: Motion sickness, nausea, vomiting

Dosage and routes:
■ *Adult:* PO 50-100 mg q4h; REC 100 mg qd or bid; IM/IV 50 mg as needed
■ *Child:* IM/PO 5 mg/kg divided in 4 equal doses
Available forms: Tabs 50 mg; inj 500 mg/ml; liq 12.5 mg/4 ml; supp 50, 100 mg

Side effects/adverse reactions:
CNS: Drowsiness, restlessness, headache, dizziness,

italic = common side effects   **bold** = life-threatening reactions

insomnia, confusion, nervousness, tingling, vertigo; hallucinations and *convulsions* in young children
GI: Nausea, anorexia, diarrhea, vomiting, constipation
CV: Hypertension, hypotension, palpitation
INTEG: Rash, urticaria, fever, chills, flushing
EENT: Dry mouth, blurred vision, diplopia, nasal congestion, photosensitivity

Contraindications: Hypersensitivity to narcotics, shock

Precautions: Children, cardiac dysrhythmias, elderly, asthma, pregnancy (B), prostatic hypertrophy, bladder-neck obstruction, narrow-angle glaucoma, stenosing peptic ulcer, pyloroduodenal obstruction

Pharmacokinetics:
IM/PO: Duration 4-6 hr

Interactions/ incompatibilities:
■ Incompatible with aminophylline, ammonium chloride, amobarbital, butorphanol, chlordiazepoxide, chlorpromazine, diphenhydramine, glycopyrrolate, heparin, hydrocortisone, hydroxyzine, midazolam, pentobarbital, phenobarbital, phenytoin, prednisolone, prochlorperazine, promazine, promethazine, tetracyclines, trifluoperzine, thiopental
■ Increased effect: alcohol, other CNS depressants
■ May mask ototoxic symptoms associated with aminoglycosides

Lab test interferences:
False negative: Allergy skin testing

RESPIRATORY CARE CONSIDERATIONS
Assess/evaluate:
■ Note drying of the upper airway.
■ Caution is suggested if used in asthma, although thickening of lower respiratory tract secretions has not been established.
■ Drowsiness may be a risk factor in subjects with sleep apnea.

Patient education:
■ Avoid hazardous activities or use caution while drug action persists.
■ Additional CNS depression may occur with concomitant use of CNS depressants (tranquilers, sedatives, or alcohol).

diphenhydramine HCl
(dye-fen-hye′dra-meen)
Allermax, Banophen, Belix, Bena-D 10, Bena-D 50, Benadryl, Benadryl 25, Benadryl Kapseals, Benahist 10, Benahist 50, Ben-Allergin-50, Benoject, Benoject-10, Benoject-50, Benylin Cough, Bydramine, Compoz, Dermamycin, Diahist, Diphenacen-50, Diphen Cough, Diphenhist, Diphenhydramine HCl, Dormarex 2, Dormin, Dyrexin, Genahist, Hydramine, Hydramyn, Hyrexin-50, Nidryl, Nordryl, Nordryl Cough, Nytol, Phendry, Scot-Tussin Allergy, Silphen Cough, Sleep-Eze 3, Sleepinal, Sominex 2, Sominex Caplets, Tusstat, Twilite, Uni-Bent Cough, Wehdryl
Func. class.: Antihistamine
Chem. class.: Ethanolamine derivative, H_1-receptor antagonist

D

Action: Blocks the action of histamine at H_1-receptor sites on blood vessels, GI, respiratory tract to decrease allergic inflammatory response and in general the pharmacologic effects of histamine. There is also an anticholinergic (drying) and sedative effect. There is reduced sensitivity of the labyrinthine apparatus. The inhibition of motion sickness and associated nausea/vomiting may be due to the anticholinergic property.

Uses: Allergy symptoms, rhinitis, motion sickness, antiparkinsonism, nighttime sedation, infant colic, nonproductive cough

Dosage and routes:
- *Adult:* PO 25-50 mg q4-6h, not to exceed 400 mg/day; IM/IV 10-50 mg, not to exceed 400 mg/day
- *Child >12 kg:* PO/IM/IV 5 mg/kg/day in 4 divided doses, not to exceed 300 mg/day

Available forms: Caps 25, 50 mg; tabs 50 mg; elix 12.5 mg/5 ml; syr 12.5 mg/5 ml; inj IM, IV 10, 50 mg/ml

Side effects/adverse reactions:
CNS: Dizziness, drowsiness, poor coordination, fatigue, anxiety, euphoria, confusion, paresthesia, neuritis
RESP: Increased thick secretions, wheezing, chest tightness
*HEMA: **Thrombocytopenia, agranulocytosis, hemolytic anemia***
GI: Dry mouth, nausea, anorexia, diarrhea
INTEG: Photosensitivity
GU: Retention, dysuria, frequency

EENT: Blurred vision, dilated pupils, tinnitus, nasal stuffiness, dry nose, throat, mouth

Contraindications: Hypersensitivity to H_1-receptor antagonist, acute asthma attack, lower respiratory tract disease

Precautions: Increased intraocular pressure, renal disease, cardiac disease, hypertension, bronchial asthma, seizure disorder, stenosed peptic ulcers, hyperthyroidism, prostatic hypertrophy, bladder neck obstruction, pregnancy (C)

Pharmacokinetics:
PO: Peak 1-3 hr, duration 4-7 hr
IM: Onset ½ hr, peak 1-4 hr, duration 4-7 hr
IV: Onset immediate, duration 4-7 hr
   Metabolized in liver, excreted by kidneys, crosses placenta, excreted in breast milk, half-life 2-7 hr

Interactions/incompatibilities:
- Incompatible with: amobarbital, amphotericin B, cephalothin, dexamethasone, furosemide, methylprednisolone, pentobarbital, phenytoin, secobarbital
- Increased CNS depression: barbiturates, narcotics, hypnotics, tricyclic antidepressants, alcohol
- Decreased effect of: oral anticoagulants, heparin
- Increased effect of diphenhydramine: MAOIs

Lab test interferences:
False negative: Skin allergy tests

---

italic = common side effects   **bold** = life-threatening reactions

RESPIRATORY CARE CONSIDERATIONS

Assess/evaluate:

- Note drying of the upper airway.
- Caution is suggested if used in asthma, although thickening of lower respiratory tract secretions has not been established.
- Drowsiness may be a risk factor in subjects with sleep apnea.

Patient Education:

- Avoid hazardous activities or use caution while drug action persists.
- Additional CNS depression may occur with concomitant use of CNS depressants (tranquilizers, sedatives, or alcohol).

dipyridamole

(dye-peer-id′a-mole)
Dipyridamole, Persantine, Persantine IV, Pyridamole
Func. class.: Coronary vasodilator, antiplatelet
Chem. class.: Nonnitrate

Action: Platelet adhesion inhibitor and coronary vasodilator, possibly through inhibition of adenosine uptake.

Uses: As adjunctive therapy with coumarin anticoagulants to prevent postoperative thromboembolic formation with cardiac valve replacement; evaluation of coronary artery disease with patients who cannot exercise during performance of a thallium scan.

Dosage and routes:
TIA

- *Adult:* PO 50 mg tid, 1 hr ac, not to exceed 400 mg qd
Inhibition of platelet adhesion

- *Adult:* PO 50-75 mg qid in combination with aspirin or warfarin
Available forms: Tabs 25, 50, 75 mg, IV

Side effects/adverse reactions:
CV: Postural hypotension
CNS: Headache, dizziness, weakness, fainting, syncope
GI: Nausea, vomiting, anorexia, diarrhea
INTEG: Rash, flushing

Contraindications: Hypersensitivity, hypotension

Precautions: Pregnancy (C)

Pharmacokinetics:
PO: Peak 2-2 ½ hr, duration 6 hr therapeutic response may take several months; metabolized in liver, excreted in bile, undergoes enterohepatic recirculation

Interactions/ incompatibilities:

- Incompatibility not known
- Additive antiplatelet effects: ASA, NSAID
- Increased bleeding: Coumadin

RESPIRATORY CARE CONSIDERATIONS

Assess/evaluate:

- Monitor BP, pulse during treatment until stable; take BP lying, standing; orthostatic hypotension is common.
- Monitor cardiac status and reports of chest pain; avoid stressors that aggravate.
- Therapeutic response: decreased chest pain (angina), decreased platelet adhesion.
- Note risk of bleeding with platelet inhibition; assess puncture site during arterial blood sampling, apply adequate pressure.

D

disopyramide

(dye-soe-peer'a-mide)

Disopyramide, Norpace, Norpace CR

Func. class.: Antidysrhythmic (Class IA)

Chem. class.: Nonnitrate

Action: Prolongs action, potential duration, and effective refractory period; reduces disparity in refractory between normal and infarcted myocardium

Uses: PVCs, ventricular tachycardia, supraventricular tachycardia, atrial flutter, fibrillation

Dosage and routes:
▪ *Adult:* PO 100-200 mg q6h, in renal dysfunction 100 mg q6h; SUS REL CAPS 200 mg q12h
▪ *Child 12-18 yr:* PO 6-15 mg/kg/day, in divided doses q6h
▪ *Child 4-12 yr:* PO 10-15 mg/kg/day in divided doses q6h
▪ *Child 1-4 yr:* PO 10-20 mg/kg/day in divided doses q6h
▪ *Child <1 yr:* PO 10-30 mg/kg/day, in divided doses q6h
Available forms: Caps 100, 150 mg (as phosphate), caps rel 100, 150 mg

Side effects/adverse reactions:
GU: Retention, hesitancy, impotence, urinary frequency, urgency
CNS: Headache, dizziness, psychosis, fatigue, depression, paresthesias, anxiety, insomnia
GI: Dry mouth, constipation, nausea, anorexia, flatulence, diarrhea, vomiting
CV: Hypotension, bradycardia, angina, PVCs, tachycardia, increases QRS, QT segments, *cardiac arrest,* edema, weight gain, AV block, *CHF,* syncope, chest pain
META: Hypoglycemia
INTEG: Rash, pruritus, urticaria
MS: Weakness, pain in extremities
EENT: Blurred vision, dry nose, throat, eyes, narrow-angle glaucoma
HEMA: **Thrombocytopenia, agranulocytosis,** anemia (rare), decreased hemoglobin, hematocrit

Contraindications: Hypersensitivity, 2nd or 3rd degree heart block, cardiogenic shock, CHF (uncompensated), sick sinus syndrome, QT prolongation

Precautions: Pregnancy (C), lactation, diabetes mellitus, renal disease, children, hepatic disease, myasthenia gravis, narrow-angle glaucoma, cardiomyopathy, conduction abnormalities

Pharmacokinetics:
PO: Peak 30 min-3 hr, duration 6-12 hr, half-life 4-10 hr, metabolized in liver, excreted in feces, urine, breast milk crosses placenta

Interactions/incompatibilities:
▪ Increased effects of disopyramide: quinidine, procainamide, propranolol, lidocaine, atenolol, other antidysrhythmics
▪ Do not administer within 48 hr of verapamil
▪ Increased side effects of disopyramide: anticholinergics
▪ Decreased effects of disopyramide: phenytoin, rifampin

Lab test interferences:
Increase: Liver enzymes, lipids, BUN, creatinine
Decrease: Hgb/Hct, blood glucose

italic = common side effects   **bold** = life-threatening reactions

RESPIRATORY CARE CONSIDERATIONS
Assess/evaluate:
- ECG; check for increased QT, widening QRS; if either occurs, drug should be discontinued.
- Monitor for dehydration or hypovolemia, I&O ratio, electrolytes (Na, K, Cl).
- Assess BP for hypotension or hypertension, pulse rate.
- Monitor respiratory rate and pattern (labored, dyspnea).
- Provide resuscitation support in the event of cardiac arrest.
- Evaluate therapeutic response: decreased dysrhythmias.

Patient education:
- Avoid alcohol or severe hypotension may occur; avoid OTC drugs or serious drug interactions may occur.
- Make position change slowly to prevent orthostatic hypotension and fainting.
- Avoid hazardous activities if dizziness or blurred vision occurs.

dobutamine HCl
(doe-byoo′ta-meen)
Dobutrex
Func. class.: Adrenergic direct-acting β_1-agonist
Chem. class.: Catecholamine

Action: Causes increased contractility, increased coronary blood flow and heart rate by acting on β_1-receptors in heart

Uses: Cardiac surgery, refractory heart failure

Dosage and routes:
- *Adult:* IV INF 2.5 - 10 µg/kg/min; may increase to 40 µg/kg/min if needed

Available forms: Inj 250 mg vial IV

Side effects/adverse reactions:
CNS: Anxiety, headache, dizziness
CV: Palpitations, tachycardia, hypertension, PVCs, angina
GI: Heartburn, nausea, vomiting
MS: Muscle cramps (leg)

Contraindications: Hypersensitivity, idiopathic hypertrophic subaortic stenosis

Precautions: Pregnancy (C), lactation, children, hypertension

Pharmacokinetics:
IV: Onset 1 - 5 min, peak 10 min, half-life 2 min, metabolized in liver (inactive metabolites), excreted in urine

Interactions/incompatibilities:
- Dysrhythmias: general anesthetics
- Decreased action of dobutamine: other β-blockers
- Increased BP: oxytocics
- Increased pressor effect and dysrhythmias: tricyclic antidepressant, MAOIs
- Incompatible with $NaHCO_3$, acyclovir, aminophylline, bretylium, bumetamide, CaCl, calcium gluconate, cefamandole, cefazolin, cephalothin, diazepam, digoxin, furosemide, heparin, hydrocortisone, insulins, $MgSO_4$, penicillin, phenytoin, potassium phosphate, sodium ethacrynate

RESPIRATORY CARE CONSIDERATIONS
Assess/evaluate:
- Therapeutic response: increased cardiac output, decreased PCWP, adequate CVP,

improved systemic blood pressure, decreased dyspnea, edema.
- Monitor ECG for tachycardia and BP for hypertension.
- Assess circulatory volume of patient; dobutamine is not a substitute for replacement of blood, plasma, or fluids.
- Monitor for allergic reactions including anaphylaxis due to sulfite ingredient in product.
- Assess improvement in cardiac output and minimize airway pressures on mechanical ventilation, particularly mean airway pressure by adjusting peak flows, I:E ratios, and use of modes such as pressure support if possible, especially while patient is being stabilized.
- Monitor BP with concomitant administration of beta-agonist bronchodilators.

dopamine HCl
(doe′pa-meen)
Dopamine HCl, Intropin, Revimine*
Func. class.: Agonist
Chem. class.: Catecholamine

Action: An endogenous catecholamine and a precursor of norepinephrine; dopamine exerts its pharmacological effects by acting on alpha and beta$_1$-receptors. Stimulation of beta$_1$-receptors produces a positive inotropic effect and causes increased cardiac output. Alpha effects causing vasoconstriction are minimal at low and intermediate dosages. When low doses are administered, renal and mesenteric vasodilation are presumably due to dopaminergic stimulation. At higher doses, peripheral resistance increases, and renal blood flow decreases, due to vasoconstriction mediated by alpha stimulation.

Uses: Shock increase perfusion (low doses) hypotension

Dosage and routes:
- *Adult:* IV INF 2-5 µg/kg/min, not to exceed 50 µg/kg/min, titrate to patient's response
Available forms: Inj 0.8, 1.6, 40, 80, 160 mg/ml

Side effects/adverse reactions:
CNS: Headache
CV: Palpitations, tachycardia, hypertension, ectopic beats, angina, wide QRS complex, peripheral vasoconstriction
GI: Nausea, vomiting, diarrhea
INTEG: Necrosis, tissue sloughing with extravasation, gangrene
RESP: Dyspnea

Contraindications: Hypersensitivity, ventricular fibrillation, tachydysrhythmias, pheochromocytoma

Precautions: Pregnancy (C), lactation, arterial embolism, peripheral vascular disease

Pharmacokinetics:
IV: Onset 5 min, duration <10 min, metabolized in liver, excreted in urine (metabolites)

Interactions/incompatibilities:
- Incompatible with acyclovir, amphotericin B, cephalothin, gentamicin, sodium bicarbonate, alkaline sol
- Do not use within 2 wk of MAOIs, phenytoin, barbiturates, or hypertensive crisis may result

- Dysrhythmias: general anesthetics
- Decreased action of dopamine: other β-blockers
- Increased BP: oxytocics
- Increased pressor effect: tricyclic antidepressants, MAOIs
- Additive effect: diuretics

RESPIRATORY CARE CONSIDERATIONS
Assess/evaluate:
- Assess for hypovolemia and correct prior to administration of dopamine.
- Monitor urine flow, cardiac output, and BP during treatment.
- Monitor for allergic reactions especially in asthmatics, including anaphylaxis due to sulfite ingredient in product.
- Assess improvement in cardiac output or BP, and minimize airway pressures on mechanical ventilation, particularly mean airway pressure by adjusting peak flows, I:E ratios, and use of modes such as pressure support if possible, especially while patient is being stabilized.
- Monitor BP with concomitant administration of beta agonist bronchodilators.

Dornase alfa, DNase (recombinant human deoxyribonuclease I)
Pulmozyme
Func. class.: Cystic fibrosis agent (orphan drug)
Chem. class.: Recombinant human enzyme

See Section III: Aerosol Agents for Oral Inhalation

doxacurium chloride
(dox′a-cure-ee-um)
Nuromax
Func. class.: Neuromuscular blocker (nondepolarizing)
Chem. class.: Isoquinolone derivative

Action: Inhibits transmission of nerve impulses at the neuromuscular junction by binding with cholinergic receptor sites, antagonizing action of acetylcholine, and causing muscle weakness or paralysis, depending on dose.

Uses: Facilitation of endotracheal intubation, skeletal muscle relaxation during mechanical ventilation, surgery, or general anesthesia

Dosage and routes:
- *Adult:* IV 0.05 mg/kg; 0.08 mg/kg is used for prolonged neuromuscular blockade; maintenance 0.025 mg/kg
Available forms: Inj 1 mg/ml

Side effects/adverse reactions:
CV: Decreased BP, ventricular fibrillation, myocardial infarction, cardiovascular accident
RESP: Prolonged apnea, bronchospasm, wheezing, respiratory depression
EENT: Diplopia
MS: Weakness, prolonged skeletal muscle relaxation, *paralysis*
INTEG: Rash, urticaria

Contraindications: Hypersensitivity

Precautions: Pregnancy (C), renal, hepatic disease, lactation, children <3 mo, fluid and electrolyte imbalances, neuromuscular disease, respiratory disease, obesity, elderly, severe burns

D

Pharmacokinetics: Not metabolized; excretion of unchanged drug in urine and bile

**Interactions/
incompatibilities:**
▪ Increased neuromuscular blockade: Aminoglycosides, quinidine, local anesthetics, polymyxin antibiotics, enflurane, isoflurane, tetracyclines, halothane, Mg, colistin, procainamide, bacitracin, lincomycin, clindamycin, lithium
▪ Longer onset and shorter duration of doxacurium: phenytoin, carbamazepine

**RESPIRATORY CARE
CONSIDERATIONS
Assess/evaluate:**
▪ Provide airway and ventilatory support before administering drug.
▪ Note possible interaction with the following antibiotics, which can increase neuromuscular blockade: the aminoglycosides, the polymyxins, clindamycin, and lincomycin.
▪ Use with mechanical ventilation, assess patient for adequate and preferably optimal ventilator settings *before* paralyzing. If patient is "fighting" the ventilator, provide adequately high flow rates and tidal volumes, short inspiratory times, and reasonable I:E ratios, check the sensitivity in assist-control mode, provide sufficiently high rates to avoid patient fatigue; consider paralysis if these measures fail.
▪ Assess ventilator patients for pain, hypoxemia, or ventilator malfunction, if restless and anxious, before instituting muscle paralysis.
▪ Assess need of patient and provide for pain control and

sedation during neuromuscular blockade: *neuromuscular blocking agents do not provide analgesia or sedation.*
▪ Close eyelids and provide eye lubricant during prolonged paralysis.
▪ Since usual signs of pain or anxiety (restlessness, tachynea, distress, thrashing) are blocked, monitor vital signs closely and overall patient appearance and state to detect problems (e.g., IV infiltration).
▪ Check ventilator alarm settings for sufficient limits and sensitivity; a disconnect alarm is critical.
▪ Assess reversal of drug before attempting to wean from mechanical ventilatory support.

Administer:
▪ Administer by IV, not by IM, for more consistent absorption and distribution and to avoid the pain associated with IM injection of the drug.
▪ Reversal: neostigmine or edrophonium, preceded by atropine to inhibit muscarinic response especially in upper airway.

doxapram HCl
(dox'a-pram)
Dopram
Func. class.: Analeptic
Chem. class.: Synthetic compound

Action: Respiratory stimulation through activation of peripheral carotid chemoreceptor; with higher doses medullary respiratory centers are stimulated

Uses: Chronic obstructive pulmonary disease (COPD), postanesthesia respiratory stimulation, acute hypercapnia, drug-induced CNS depression

Dosage and routes:
Postanesthesia
- *Adult:* IV inj 0.5-1 mg/kg, not to exceed 1.5 mg/kg total as a single injection; IV inf 250 mg in 250 ml sol, not to exceed 4 mg/kg; run at 1-3 mg/min

Drug-induced CNS depression
- Priming IV dose of 2 mg/kg, repeated in 5 min; repeat q1-2h till patient awakes; IV inf priming dose 2 mg/kg at 1-3 mg/min, not to exceed 3 g/d

COPD
- *Adult:* IV inf 1-2 mg/min, not to exceed 3 mg/min for no longer than 2 hr

Available forms: Inj IV 20 mg/ml

Side effects/adverse reactions:
*CNS: **Convulsions** (clonus/generalized), headache, restlessness, dizziness, confusion, paresthesias, flushing, sweating, bilateral Babinski's sign, rigidity, depression*
GI: Nausea, vomiting, diarrhea, hiccups
GU: Retention, incontinence
CV: Chest pain, hypertension, change in heart rate, lowered T waves, tachycardia, arrhythmias
INTEG: Pruritus, irritation at injection site
EENT: Pupil dilation, sneezing
*RESP: **Laryngospasm, bronchospasm**, rebound hypoventilation, dyspnea, cough, tachypnea, hiccoughs*

Contraindications:
Hypersensitivity, seizure disorders, severe hypertension, severe bronchial asthma, severe dyspnea, severe cardiac disorders, pneumothorax, pulmonary embolism, severe respiratory disease, newborns

Precautions:
Bronchial asthma, pheochromocytoma, severe tachycardia, dysrhythmias, pregnancy (B), hypertension, lactation, children

Pharmacokinetics:
IV: Onset 20-40 sec, peak 1-2 min, duration 5-10 min, half-life 2½-4 hr metabolized by liver, excreted by kidneys (metabolites)

Interactions/incompatibilities:
- Synergistic pressor effect: MAOIs, sympathomimetics
- Cardiac dysrhythmias: halothane, cyclopropane, enflurane
- Incompatible with aminophylline, carbenicillin, cefaperazone, cefotaxime, cefotetan, cefuroxime, dexamethasone, diazepam, digoxin, dobutamine, furosemide, hydrocortisone, ketamine, methylprednisolone, minocycline, pentobarbital, phenobarbital, secobarbital, thiopental, ticarcillin

RESPIRATORY CARE CONSIDERATIONS
Assess/evaluate:
- Assess effect on respiratory rate and depth.
- Monitor for possible respiratory failure and need for ventilatory support: arterial blood gases, respiratory pattern.
- Monitor for pressor effect, increased BP.
- Doxapram HCl can cause increased release of catecholamines; monitor for hypertension if on beta agonists.

- Doxapram HCl can reverse respiratory depression.
- Note: it will not reverse analgesia; monitor patients for symptoms of pain.
- Monitor for possible respiratory effects: cough, dyspnea, increased WOB, need for ventilatory support, laryngospasm, bronchospasm.
- Convulsive seizures can result from OD, requiring short-acting barbiturates, O_2, resuscitation.

doxazosin mesylate
Cardura
Func. class.: Peripheral α_1-adrenergic blocker
Chem. class.: Quinazoline

Action: Peripheral blood vessels are dilated, peripheral resistance lowered; reduction in blood pressure results from α-adrenergic receptors being blocked

Uses: Hypertension

Dosage and routes:
- *Adult:* PO 1 mg qd, increasing up to 16 mg qd if required; usual range 4-16 mg/day
Available forms: Tabs 1, 2, 4, 8 mg

Side effects/adverse reactions:
CV: Palpitations, orthostatic hypotension, tachycardia, edema, dysrhythmias, chest pain
CNS: Dizziness, headache, drowsiness, anxiety, depression, vertigo, weakness, fatigue, asthenia
GI: Nausea, vomiting, diarrhea, constipation, abdominal pain
GU: Incontinence, polyuria
EENT: Epistaxis, tinnitus, dry mouth, red sclera, pharyngitis, rhinitis

Contraindications: Hypersensitivity to quinazolines

Precautions: Pregnancy (C), children, lactation, hepatic disease

Pharmacokinetics:
PO: Onset 2 hr, peak 2-6 hr, duration 6-12 hr, half-life 22 hr, metabolized in liver, excreted via bile/feces (<63%) and in urine (9%), extensively protein bound (98%)

Interaction/ incompatibilities:
- Increased hypotensive effects: β-blockers, verapamil
- Decreased hypotensive effects: indomethacin

RESPIRATORY CARE CONSIDERATIONS
Assess/evaluate:
- Monitor for "first dose" effect: marked hypotension (especially postural), syncope with loss of consciousness with first few doses.
- Monitor effect on BP and pulse, especially if on positive pressure ventilatory support.
- Assess effectiveness of beta-adrenergic bronchodilator therapy for possible antagonistic effect on BP to avoid increasing BP, or decreasing BP due to beta receptor stimulation of vascular smooth muscle in the presence of blocked alpha receptors.
- Consider use of nonadrenergic bronchodilator such as ipratropium bromide as alternative to beta-adrenergic agents for asthmatics or COPD patients.
- Note: since alpha receptors are blocked, other adrenergic agents that stimulate both types of sympathetic receptors

or beta receptors, such as epinephrine, may cause exaggerated response of tachycardia and hypotension.

■ Treatment of overdose with epinephrine can cause worsening of hypotension, as outlined previously; use leg elevation, discontinue the drug, support circulation.

Patient education:

■ Do not use OTC products containing α-adrenergic stimulants (nasal decongestants, OTC cold preparations) or other sympathomimetics unless directed by physician.

■ Report symptoms of CHF: difficulty breathing, especially on exertion or when lying down, night cough, swelling of extremities.

dyphylline

(dye'fi-lin)

Dilor, Dyflex-200, Dyflex-400, Dylline, Dyphylline, Lufyllin, Lufyllin-400, Neothylline, Protophylline*

Func. class.: Bronchodilator
Chem. class.: Xanthine, a theophylline derivative (dihydroxypropyl theophylline)

Action: Relaxes smooth muscle of respiratory system by unknown mechanism, possibly adenosine receptor antagonism

Uses: Bronchial asthma, bronchospasm in chronic bronchitis, COPD

Dosage and routes:

■ *Adult:* PO 200-800 mg q6h; IM 250-500 mg q6h injected slowly

■ *Child >6 yr:* PO 4-7 mg/kg/day in 4 divided doses
Available forms: Tabs 200, 400 mg; elix 100, 160 mg/15 ml; inj IM 250 mg/ml

Side effects/adverse reactions:

CNS: Anxiety, restlessness, insomnia, dizziness, **convulsions,** *headache, lightheadedness, muscle twitching*
CV: Palpitations, sinus tachycardia, hypotension, flushing, dysrhythmias
GI: Nausea, vomiting, anorexia, dyspepsia, epigastric pain
INTEG: Flushing, urticaria
RESP: Tachypnea
OTHER: Fever, dehydration, **albuminuria,** *hyperglycemia*

Contraindications: Hypersensitivity to xanthines, tachydysrhythmias

Precautions: Elderly, CHF, cor pulmonale, hepatic disease, active peptic ulcer disease, diabetes mellitus, hyperthyroidism, hypertension, children, renal disease, pregnancy (C), glaucoma

Pharmacokinetics: Peak 1 hr, half-life 2 hr, excreted in urine unchanged

Interactions/incompatibilities:

■ Do not mix in syringe with other drugs
■ Increased action of dyphylline: cimetidine, propranolol, erythromycin, troleandomycin
■ May increase effects of: anticoagulants
■ Cardiotoxicity: β-blockers
■ Increased metabolism: barbiturates, phenytoin
■ Decreased elimination of dyphylline: uricosurics

*Available in Canada only

RESPIRATORY CARE CONSIDERATIONS

Assess/evaluate:

- Note: Dyphylline is about one-tenth as potent as theophylline; equivalent dosage with theophylline not known.
- Therapeutic response: decreased dyspnea, respiratory rate and pattern respiratory stimulation in infancy.
- Monitor fluid intake for the onset of diuresis; dehydration may result in elderly or children.
- Monitor respiratory rate, rhythm, depth; auscultate lung fields bilaterally; notify physician of abnormalities.
- Allergic reactions: rash, urticaria; if these occur, drug should be discontinued.
- Assess side effects reported, and evaluate dose.

Patient education:

- Take doses as prescribed; do not skip dose.
- Check OTC medications, current prescription medications for ephedrine; dyphylline will increase CNS stimulation. Do not drink alcohol or caffeine products (tea, coffee, chocolate, colas) which will increase diuresis or add to the xanthine level (caffeine).
- Avoid hazardous activities; dizziness may occur.
- If GI upset occurs, take drug with 8 oz water; avoid food, since absorption may be decreased.
- Notify physician of toxicity: insomnia, anxiety, nausea, vomiting, rapid pulse, convulsions.
- Cigarette smoking will increase metabolism of the drug, lowering blood levels.

- Increase fluid intake if sputum becomes thicker when taking drug.
- Use nondiuresing liquids, such as water, juice, Gatorade, milk rather than diuretic products such as caffeinated coffee, tea or colas.

E

edrophonium chloride

(ed-roe-foe′nee-um)

Enlon, Reversol, Tensilon

Func. class.: Cholinergics, anticholinesterase

Chem. class.: Quaternary ammonium compound

Action: An indirect-acting cholinergic that inhibits cholinesterase enzyme, preventing the destruction of acetylcholine; this increases concentration at sites where acetylcholine is released and facilitates neuromuscular transmission.

Uses: To diagnose myasthenia gravis; curare antagonist; differentiation of myasthenic crisis from cholinergic crisis

Dosage and routes:

Tensilon test

- *Adult:* IV 1-2 mg over 15-30 sec, then 8 mg if no response; IM: 10 mg; if cholinergic reaction occurs, retest after ½ hr with 2 mg IM
- *Child >34 kg:* IV 2 mg; if no response in 45 sec, then 1 mg q45 sec, not to exceed 10 mg
- *Child <34 kg:* IV 1 mg; if no response in 45 sec, then 1 mg q45 sec, not to exceed 5 mg
- *Infant:* IV 0.5 mg

Curare antagonist

- *Adult:* IV 10 mg over 30-45 sec, may repeat, not to exceed 40 mg

---

italic = common side effects   **bold** = life-threatening reactions

Differentiation of myasthenic crisis from cholinergic crisis
■ *Adult:* IV 1 mg, if no response in 1 min, may repeat
Available forms: Inj IV 10 mg/ml

Side effects/adverse reactions:
INTEG: Rash, urticaria
CNS: Dizziness, headache, sweating, weakness, *convulsions*, incoordination, *paralysis*, drowsiness, *loss of consciousness*
GI: Nausea, diarrhea, vomiting, cramps, increased salivary and gastric secretions, dysphagia, increased peristalsis
CV: Tachycardia, dysrhythmias, bradycardia, hypotension, AV block, ECG changes, *cardiac arrest*, syncope
GU: Frequency, incontinence, urgency
RESP: Respiratory depression, bronchospasm, constriction, laryngospasm, respiratory arrest, dyspnea
EENT: Miosis, blurred vision, lacrimation, visual changes

Contraindications: Obstruction of intestine, renal system, hypersensitivity

Precautions: Seizure disorders, bronchial asthma, coronary occlusion, hyperthyroidism, dysrhythmias, peptic ulcer, megacolon, poor GI motility, pregnancy (C), bradycardia, hypotension

Pharmacokinetics:
IV: Onset 30-60 sec, duration 6-24 min
IM: Onset 2-10 min, duration 12-45 min

Interactions/ incompatibilities:
■ Decreased action of edrophonium: procainamide, quinidine, aminoglycosides, anesthetics, mecamylamine, polymyxin, Mg, corticosteroids, antidysrythmics
■ Bradycardia: digitalis
■ Considered incompatible with any drug in syringe or sol

RESPIRATORY CARE CONSIDERATIONS

Assess/evaluate:
■ Therapeutic response: reversal of neuromuscular blockade, or improved muscle function, especially diaphragmatic contractile force as evidenced by tidal volume, vital capacity, grip strength.
■ In reversing neuromuscular blockade, maintain airway and ventilatory support until complete recovery of adequate ventilation is seen in spontaneous respiratory rate and pattern.
■ Monitor for exacerbation of asthma or airway resistance in COPD subject, due to parasympathetic induced bronchoconstriction.
■ Assess respiratory rate and pattern, breath sounds for wheezing.
■ Assess subjective response of patient for difficulty in breathing, tightness in chest.
■ Assess pulse for bradycardia and BP for decrease.
■ Note: use of a cholinergic agent can intensify and prolong a depolarizing blockade induced by succinylcholine, due to the inactivation of acetylcholine needed for neuromuscular transmission.

enalapril maleate/enalaprilat

(en-al-a'prel)

Vasotec, Vasotec IV

Func. class.: Antihypertensive

Chem. class.: Angiotensin-converting enzyme inhibitor

Action: Selectively suppresses renin-angiotensin-aldosterone system; inhibits ACE; prevents conversion of angiotensin I to angiotensin II, dilation of arterial, venous vessels

Uses: Hypertension, CHF

Dosage and routes:
- *Adult:* PO 5 mg/day, may increase or decrease to desired response range 10-40 mg/day

Hypertension
- *Adult:* IV 1.25 mg q6h over 5 min

Patients on diuretics
- *Adult:* IV 0.625 mg over 5 min, may give additional doses of 1.25 mg q6h

Renal impairment
- *Adult:* IV 1.25 mg q6h with CrCl <3 mg/dl or 0.625 mg if CrCl >3 mg/dl

Available forms: Tabs 2.5, 5, 10, 20 mg, inj 1.25 mg/ml

Side effects/adverse reactions:

CV: Hypotension, chest pain, tachycardia, dysrhythmias

CNS: Insomnia, dizziness, paresthesias, headache, fatigue, anxiety

GI: Nausea, vomiting, colitis, cramps, diarrhea, constipation, flatulence, dry mouth, loss of taste

INTEG: Rash, purpura, alopecia, hyperhidrosis

HEMA: **Agranulocytosis, neutropenia**

EENT: Tinnitus, visual changes, sore throat, double vision, dry burning eyes

GU: **Proteinuria, renal failure,** increased frequency of polyuria or oliguria

RESP: Dyspnea, cough, rales, angioedema

META: Hyperkalemia

Contraindications: Pregnancy (C), lactation

Precautions: Renal disease, hyperkalemia

Pharmacokinetics:
PO: Peak 4-6 hr, half-life 1½ hr metabolized by liver to active metabolite, excreted in urine *IV:* Onset 5-15 min, peak up to 4 hr

Interactions/incompatibilities:
- Hypersensitivity: allopurinol
- Severe hypotension: diuretics, other antihypertensives
- Decreased effects of enalapril: aspirin, antacids
- Increased K levels: salt substitutes, K-sparing diuretics, K supplements
- May increase effects of: ergots, neuromuscular blocking agents, antihypertensives, hypoglycemics, barbiturates, reserpine, levodopa
- Effects may be increased by phenothiazines, diuretics, phenytoin, quinidine, nifedipine

Lab test interferences:
Interference: Glucose/insulin tolerance tests

RESPIRATORY CARE CONSIDERATIONS

Assess/evaluate:
- Therapeutic response: decrease in BP.

- Persistent cough and fever are common side effects of the ACE inhibitors, which should be differentiated from other possible causes, such as respiratory infection.
- Monitor for possible hypotension.
- Evaluate BP with COPD or asthmatic subjects who require beta agonists for reversible airway obstruction.
- Assess for symptoms of CHF: edema, dyspnea, wet rales, BP.

enoxaparin sodium

(in-ox′a-par-in)
Lovenox
Func. class.: Anticoagulant
Chem. class.: Unfractionated porcine heparin

Action: Prevents conversion of fibrinogen to fibrin and prothrombin to thrombin by enhancing inhibitory effects of antithrombin III; produces higher ratio of anti-factor Xa to anti-factor IIa

Uses: Prevention of deep vein thrombosis, pulmonary emboli in hip and knee replacement

Dosage and routes:
- *Adult:* SC 30 mg bid immediately after surgery; continue to administer until deep vein thrombosis no longer a threat (7-14 days)
Available forms: Inj 30 mg/ 0.3 ml

Side effects/adverse reactions:
CNS: Fever, confusion
GI: Nausea
GU: Edema, peripheral edema
HEMA: Hypochromic anemia
INTEG: Ecchymosis

Contraindications: Hypersensitivity to this drug, heparin, or pork; hemophilia, leukemia with bleeding, peptic ulcer disease, thrombocytopenic purpura

Precautions: Alcoholism, elderly, pregnancy (C), hepatic disease (severe), renal disease (severe), blood dyscrasias, severe hypertension, subacute bacterial endocarditis, acute nephritis, lactation, children

Pharmacokinetics:
SC: Maximum antithrombin activity (3-5 hr), elimination half-life 4½ hr

Interactions/ incompatibilities:
- Increased action of enoxaprin: oral anticoagulants, salicylates
- Do not mix with other drugs or infusion fluids

RESPIRATORY CARE CONSIDERATIONS
Assess/evaluate:
- Avoid or minimize arterial punctures for blood gas analysis.
- Use sites accessible to manual compression for arterial punctures.
- Use pressure dressings for arterial puncture after prolonged manual compression.
- Monitor for bleeding from any puncture sites.
- Risk of fibrinolytic therapy is increased with hypertension, hemostatic defects.
- Assess possibility of bleeding with unexplained fall in hematocrit or BP.

*Available in Canada only

Patient education:
■ Instruct patient to notify health care personnel of any swelling, hematoma, or bleeding at a puncture site.

ephedrine sulfate (nasal)
(e-fed′rin)
Vatronol Nose Drops
Func. class.: Nasal decongestant
Chem. class.: Indirect/direct sympathomimetic amine

Action: Stimulates alpha- and beta-adrenergic receptors; increases diameter of nasal passages by alpha-mediated vasoconstriction.

Uses: Nasal congestion associated with colds, hay fever, sinusitis, other allergic conditions, adjunct in middle ear infections

Dosage and routes:
■ *Adult and child:* Instill 3-4 gtts q4h or small amount of gel in each nostril q4h
Available forms: Sol 0.5% sulfate, gel 0.6% HCl

Side effects/adverse reactions:
GI: Nausea, vomiting, anorexia
EENT: Irritation, burning, sneezing, stinging, dryness, rebound congestion
INTEG: Contact dermatitis
CNS: Anxiety, restlessness, tremors, weakness, insomnia, dizziness, fever, headache

Contraindications: Hypersensitivity to sympathomimetic amines

Precautions: Child <6 yr, elderly, diabetes, cardiovascular disease, hypertension, hyperthyroidism, increased ICP, prostatic hypertrophy, pregnancy (C)

Interactions/ incompatibilities:
■ Hypertension: MAOIs, β-adrenergic blockers
■ Hypotension: methyldopa, mecamylamine, reserpine

RESPIRATORY CARE CONSIDERATIONS
Assess/evaluate:
■ Therapeutic response: decreased nasal congestion.
■ Assess subject's BP if using beta agonist bronchodilator simultaneously, for possible increases.
■ Monitor BP for possible increases and hypertension with repeated use of drug.

Patient education:
■ Environmental humidification may help to decrease nasal congestion, dryness.
■ Warn patient that rebound nasal congestion can occur.
■ Use for short-term symptoms only; prolonged rhinitis should be evaluated by physician, ENT specialist, or allergist.

ephedrine sulfate
(e-fed′rin)
Ephedrine, Ephedrine sulfate, Neorespin
Func. class.: Adrenergic, mixed direct and indirect effects
Chem. class.: Phenylisopropylamine

Action: Causes increased contractility and heart rate by acting on β-receptors in the heart; also acts on α-receptors, causing vasoconstriction in blood vessels

Uses: Shock, increased perfusion, hypotension, bronchodilation

Dosage and routes:
- *Adult:* IM/SC 25-50 mg, not to exceed 150 mg/24 hr IV 10-25 mg, not to exceed 150 mg/24 hr
- *Child:* SC/IV 3 mg/kg/day in divided doses q4-6h
Bronchodilator
- *Adult:* PO 12.5-50 mg bid-qid, not to exceed 400 mg/day
- *Child:* PO 2-3 mg/kg/day in 4-6 divided doses
Available forms: Inj 25, 50 mg/ml, IM, SC, IV; caps 25, 50 mg; syr 11, 20 mg/5 ml

Side effects/adverse reactions:
CNS: Tremors, anxiety, insomnia, headache, dizziness, confusion, hallucinations, *convulsions, CNS depression*
GU: Dysuria, urinary retention
CV: Palpitations, tachycardia, hypertension, chest pain, *dysrhythmias*
GI: Anorexia, nausea, vomiting
RESP: Dyspnea

Contraindications: Hypersensitivity to sympathomimetics, narrow-angle glaucoma

Precautions: Pregnancy (C), cardiac disorders, hyperthyroidism, diabetes mellitus, prostatic hypertrophy

Pharmacokinetics:
PO: Onset 15-60 min, duration 2-4 hr
IV: Onset 5 min, duration 2 hr
Metabolized in liver; excreted in urine (unchanged); crosses blood-brain barrier, placenta, breast milk

Interactions/ incompatibilities:
- Do not use with MAOIs or tricyclic antidepressants; hypertensive crisis may occur
- Decreased effect of ephedrine: methyldopa, urinary acidifiers, rauwolfia alkaloids
- Increased effect of this drug: urinary alkalizers
- Dysrhythmia: halothane, anesthetics, digitalis
- Decreased effect of: guanethidine
- Incompatible with alkaline sol, hydrocortisone, pentobarbital, phenobarbital, secobarbital, thiopental

RESPIRATORY CARE CONSIDERATIONS
Assess/evaluate:
- Note: less optimal than other bronchodilating agents, if used for airway obstruction due to lack of adrenergic receptor selectivity.
- Assess effectiveness of drug therapy based on the indication(s): presence of reversible airflow due to primary bronchospasm or other obstruction secondary to an inflammatory response and/or secretions, improvement of blood pressure with hypotension.
- Monitor expiratory flow rates using office or bedside peak flow meters or laboratory reports of pulmonary function, especially before and after bronchodilator studies, to assess reversibility of airflow obstruction.
- Assess breathing rate and pattern.
- Assess breath sounds by auscultation before and after treatment.

---

*Available in Canada only

- Assess pulse before and after treatment.
- Assess patient's subjective reaction to treatment for any change in breathing effort or pattern.
- Monitor BP and pulse rate if subject is on other beta-adrenergic agents or tricyclic antidepressants.

Patient education:
- Instruct asthmatic patients in use and interpretation of disposable peak flow meters to assess severity of asthmatic episodes.

epinephrine/ epinephrine bitartrate/ epinephrine HCl

(ep-i-nef′rin)

Adrenalin Chloride, Adrenalin Chloride Solution, Asthma Haler, Asthma Nefrin, Bronitin Mist, Bronkaid Mist, Epinephrine, Epinephrine HCl, Epinephrine Pediatric, Medihaler-Epi, Micro-Nefrin, Nephron Inhalant, Primatene Mist, S-2 Inhalant, Sus-Phrine, Vaponefrin
Func. class.: Adrenergic
Chem. class.: Catecholamine

See also Section III: Aerosol Agents for Oral Inhalation

Action: Stimulates alpha-, beta$_1$-, beta$_2$-adrenergic receptors; β_1 and β_2 agonist causes increased levels of cyclic AMP producing bronchodilation, cardiac, and CNS stimulation; large doses cause vasoconstriction; small doses can cause vasodilation via β_2-vascular receptors

Uses: Acute asthmatic attacks, hemostasis, bronchospasm, anaphylaxis, allergic reactions, cardiac arrest

Dosage and routes:
- *Adult:* IM/SC 0.1-0.5 ml of 1:1000 sol, may repeat q10-15 min IV 0.1-0.25 ml of 1:1000 sol
- *Child:* SC 0.01 ml of 1:1000/kg, may repeat q20min to 4 hr; INH 0.005 ml/kg of 1:200 solution, may repeat q8-12h
Asthma
- *Adult and child:* MDI 1-2 puffs prn or as ordered; SVN 0.25-0.5 ml of 1:100 or 2.25% racemic q15min or as ordered.
Hemostasis
- *Adult:* TOP 1:50,000-1:1000 applied as needed to stop bleeding
Cardiac arrest
- *Adult:* IC, IV, endotracheal 0.1-1 mg repeat q5min PRN
- *Child:* IC, IV, endotracheal 5-10 μg q5min, may use 0.1 μ/kg/min IV inf after inital dose
Available forms: Aerosol 0.16 mg/spray, 0.2 mg/spray, 0.25 mg/spray, inj 1:1000 (1 mg/ml), 1:200 (5 mg/ml), 0.01 mg/ml (1:100,000), 0.1 mg/ml (1:10,000), 0.5 mg/ml (1:2,000); IM, IV, SC; sol for nebulization 1:100, 1.25% 2.25% (base)

Side effects/adverse reactions:
GU: Urinary retention
CNS: Tremors, anxiety, insomnia, headache, dizziness, confusion, hallucinations, *cerebral hemorrhage*
CV: Palpitations, tachycardia, hypertension, *dysrhythmias,* increased T wave
GI: Anorexia, nausea, vomiting
RESP: Dyspnea

---

italic = common side effects   **bold** = life-threatening reactions

Contraindications: Hypersensitivity to sympathomimetics, narrow-angle glaucoma

Precautions: Pregnancy (C), cardiac disorders, hyperthyroidism, diabetes mellitus, prostatic hypertrophy

Pharmacokinetics:
SC: Onset 3-5 min, duration 20 min
PO, INH: Onset 1 min

Interactions/ incompatibilities:
- Do not use with MAOIs or tricyclic antidepressants; hypertensive crisis may occur
- Decreased effect of epinephrine: methyldopa, urinary acidifiers, rauwolfia alkaloids and β-blockers
- Increased effect of epinephrine: urinary alkalizers
- Incompatible with any other drug in syringe; unstable in sol with aminophylline, cephapirin, mephentermine, $NaCO_3$, warfarin

RESPIRATORY CARE CONSIDERATIONS
Assess/evaluate:
- Assess effectiveness of drug therapy based on the indication(s) for the aerosol agent: presence of reversible airflow due to primary bronchospasm or other obstruction secondary to an inflammatory response and/or secretions, either acute or chronic; control of bleeding if used for hemostasis during bronchoscopy.
- Monitor flow rates using office or bedside peak flow meters or laboratory reports of pulmonary function, especially before and after bronchodilator studies, to assess reversibility of airflow obstruction.

- Assess breathing rate and pattern.
- Assess breath sounds by auscultation before and after treatment.
- Assess pulse before and after treatment.
- Assess patient's subjective reaction to treatment, for any change in breathing effort or pattern.
- Assess arterial blood gases or pulse oximeter saturation, as needed, for acute states with asthma or COPD to monitor changes in ventilation and gas exchange (oxygenation).
- Note effect of beta agonists on blood glucose (increase) and K^+ (decrease) laboratory values, if these are available.
- Monitor BP and pulse rate if subject is on other adrenergic agents or tricyclic antidepressants.
- Long-term: monitor pulmonary function studies of lung volumes, capacities, and flows.

Patient education:
- Caution patient that the duration of action is very short (1-2 hours), and symptoms of airflow obstruction may return.
- Epinephrine does not inhibit late phase reaction in asthma; symptoms may return and worsen several hours later.
- Instruct asthmatic patients in use and interpretation of disposable peak flow meters to assess severity of asthmatic episodes.
- Instruct patients in use, assembly, and especially cleaning of aerosol inhalation devices.

- Note: death has been associated with excessive use of inhaled adrenergic agents in severe acute asthma crises; individuals using such drugs should be instructed to contact a physician or an emergency room if there is no response to the usual dose of the inhaled agent.

epinephrine HCl (nasal)

(ep-i-nef′rin)
Adrenalin Chloride
Func. class.: Nasal decongestant
Chem. class.: Sympathomimetic amine

Action: Increases diameter of nasal passage by action on alpha-adrenergic receptors, causing vasoconstriction.

Uses: Nasal congestion, superficial bleeding

Dosage and routes:
- *Adult and child >6 yr:* TOP apply to affected area with sterile swab
Available forms: Sol 0.1%

Side effects/adverse reactions:
GI: Nausea, vomiting, anorexia
EENT: Irritation, burning, sneezing, stinging, dryness, rebound congestion
INTEG: Contact dermatitis
CNS: Anxiety, restlessness, tremors, weakness, insomnia, dizziness, fever, headache

Contraindications: Hypersensitivity to sympathomimetic amines

Precautions: Child <6 yr, elderly, diabetes, cardiovascular disease, hypertension,

hyperthyroidism, increased ICP, prostatic hypertrophy, pregnancy (C)

Interactions/ incompatibilities:
- Hypertension: MAOIs, β-adrenergic blockers
- Hypotension: methyldopa, mecamylamine, reserpine

RESPIRATORY CARE CONSIDERATIONS
Assess/evaluate:
- Therapeutic response: decrease in runny nose, opening of nasal passages.
- Assess subject's BP if using beta agonist bronchodilator simultaneously, for possible increases.

Patient education:
- Discuss method of installation after providing written instructions from manufacturer.
- Clear nasal passages before administration; use decongestant if needed; shake inhaler, invert, tilt head backward, insert nozzle into nostril, away from septum; hold other nostril closed and depress activator, inhale through nose, exhale through mouth.
- Follow insert instructions for cleaning insufflator unit.
- Avoid prolonged use; rebound congestion can occur.

erythrityl tetranitrate

Cardilate
Func. class.: Vasodilator, coronary
Chem. class.: Nitrate

Action: Decreases preload, afterload, which is responsible for decreasing left ventricular end diastolic pressure, systemic vascular resistance; improves exercise tolerance

Uses: Chronic stable angina pectoris, prophylaxis of angina pain, pulmonary arteriolar dilation

Dosage and routes:
■ *Adult:* PO 10-30 mg tid; SL 5-15 mg before stressful activity
Available forms: Chew tabs 10 mg; tabs PO, SL 5, 10 mg

Side effects/adverse reactions:
CV: Postural hypotension, tachycardia, *collapse,* syncope, edema
GI: Nausea, vomiting
INTEG: Pallor, sweating, rash
CNS: Headache, flushing, dizziness, weakness, fainting
MISC: Twitching, hemolytic anemia, *methemoglobinemia*

Contraindications: Hypersensitivity to this drug or nitrites, severe anemia, increased intracranial pressure, cerebral hemorrhage, acute MI, head trauma

Precautions: Postural hypotension, pregnancy (C), lactation, children, hypertropic cardiomyopathy, glaucoma

Pharmacokinetics:
PO: Onset 30 min, peak 1-1½ hr, duration 6 hr
SL: Onset 5-10 min, peak 30-45 min, duration 3 hr metabolized by liver, excreted in urine

Interactions/ incompatibilities:
■ Increased effects: β-blockers, diuretics, antihypertensives, alcohol products

Lab test interferences:
Decrease: Cholesterol

RESPIRATORY CARE CONSIDERATIONS
Assess/evaluate:
■ Therapeutic response: relief of chest pain (angina).
■ Monitor BP, pulse, and ECG if available.
■ Provide cardiopulmonary resuscitation if ventricular fibrillation or cardiac arrest occurs due to acute MI.
■ Note: alcohol or calcium channel blockers may increase risk of hypotension.
■ Evaluate for formation of methemoglobin and oxygen transport to tissues in case of overdose or genetically abnormal hemoglobins.
■ Note possible respiratory adverse effects: bronchitis, pneumonia, URI. Monitor respiratory status (rate, pattern, auscultation, patient report of breathing).

Patient education:
■ Prolonged chest pain may indicate MI; seek emergency treatment.
■ Make position changes slowly to prevent orthostatic hypotension.
■ Use of aspirin may increase serum levels and effect of nitrates.

erythropoietin recombinant
(er-ith-row-poe'-ee-tin)
r-HuEPO, eprex*
Func. class.: Hormone
Chem. class.: Amino acid polypeptide

Action: Erythropoietin is one factor controlling rate of red cell production; drug is developed by recombinant DNA technology

*Available in Canada only

Uses: Anemia caused by reduced endogenous erythropoietin production, primarily end-stage renal disease; to correct hemostatic defect in uremia

Dosage and routes:
- *Adult:* IV 5-500 U/kg 3 ×/wk

Side effects/adverse reactions:
CV: Hypertension, hypertensive encephalopathy
CNS: Seizures, coldness, sweating
MS: Bone pain

Contraindications: Hypersensitivity

Pharmacokinetics:
IV: Metabolized in body, extent of metabolism unknown, onset of increased reticulocyte count 1-2 wk

RESPIRATORY CARE CONSIDERATIONS
Assess/evaluate:
- Assess efficacy of therapy: improvement in red cell count. Assess hemoglobin and hematocrit.
- Evaluate oxygen transport ability, based on hemoglobin and cardiac output.
- Assess patient symptoms of fatigue, dyspnea resulting from poor oxygen transport.

esmolol HCl
(ess'moe-lol)
Brevibloc
Func. class.: Beta$_1$-selective adrenergic blocker
Chem. class.: Modified catecholamine structure

Action: Competitively blocks stimulation of β$_1$-adrenergic receptors in the myocardium; produces negative chronotropic, inotropic activity (decreases rate of SA node discharge, increases recovery time), slows conduction of AV node, decreases heart rate, decreases O$_2$ consumption in myocardium; also decreases renin-aldosterone-angiotensin system at high doses; inhibits β$_2$-receptors in bronchial system slightly

Uses: Supraventricular tachycardia, noncompensatory tachycardia, hypertensive crisis

Dosage and routes:
- *Adult:* IV loading dose—500 μg/kg/min over 1 min; maintenance—50 μg/kg/min for 4 min; may repeat q5min, increasing maintenance inf by 50 μg/kg/min (max of 200 μg/kg/min), titrate to patient response
Available forms: Inj IV 10 mg, conc 250 mg/ml

Side effects/adverse reactions:
INTEG: Induration, inflammation at site, discoloration, edema, erythema, burning pallor, flushing, rash, pruritus, dry skin, alopecia
CNS: Confusion, lightheadedness, paresthesia, somnolence, fever, dizziness, fatigue, headache, depression, anxiety
GI: Nausea, vomiting, anorexia, gastric pain, flatulence, constipation, heartburn, bloating
CV: Hypotension, bradycardia, chest pain, peripheral ischemia, shortness of breath, CHF, conduction disturbances
GU: Urinary retention, impotence, dysuria
RESP: Bronchospasm, dyspnea, cough, wheeziness, nasal stuffiness

italic = common side effects   **bold** = life-threatening reactions

Contraindications: 2nd or 3rd degree heart block, cardiogenic shock, CHF, cardiac failure, hypersensitivity

Precautions: Hypotension, pregnancy (C), peripheral vascular disease, diabetes, hypoglycemia, thyrotoxicosis, renal disease, lactation

Pharmacokinetics: Onset very rapid, duration short, half-life 9 min, metabolized by hydrolysis of the ester linkage, excreted via kidneys

Interactions/ incompatibilities:
- Increased digoxin levels: digoxin
- Increased esmolol levels: morphine
- Reversal of esmolol effects: isoproterenol, norepinephrine, dopamine, dobutamine
- Increased effects of both drugs: disopyramide
- Increased effects of: lidocaine
- Incompatible with $NaCO_3$, furosemide; do not mix with any drug before full dilution

Lab test interferences:
Interference: Glucose/insulin tolerance test

RESPIRATORY CARE CONSIDERATIONS
Assess/evaluate:
- Avoid use with reversible airway obstruction or bronchospastic disease such as asthma or chronic bronchitis due to potential for bronchospasm (wheezing, dyspnea, complaints of chest tightness) secondary to beta blockade; consider use of other classes of antihypertensive agents for these patients.
- Monitor all subjects for symptoms of increased airway resistance (wheezing, tightness in chest, difficulty breathing).
- Monitor effect on BP and pulse, especially if on positive pressure ventilatory support.
- Assess effectiveness of beta-adrenergic bronchodilator therapy, if used, for possible antagonism and effect on BP to avoid increasing BP.
- Consider use of nonadrenergic bronchodilator such as ipratropium bromide as alternative to beta-adrenergic agents for patients to avoid positive inotropic effect.

Patient education:
- Do not use OTC products containing α-adrenergic stimulants (nasal decongestants, OTC cold preparations) unless directed by physician.
- Caution patient that orthostatic hypotension may occur.
- Report symptoms of CHF: difficulty breathing, especially on exertion or when lying down, night cough, swelling of extremities.

ethacrynate sodium/ ethacrynic acid
(eth-a-kri′nate)
Edecrin, Edecrin Sodium
Func. class.: Loop diuretic
Chem. class.: Ketone derivative

Action: Acts on loop of Henle by increasing excretion of chloride, sodium

Uses: Pulmonary edema, edema in CHF, liver disease, nephrotic syndrome, ascites

Dosage and routes:
- *Adult:* PO 50-200 mg/day; may give up to 200 mg bid
- *Child:* PO 25 mg, increased by 25 mg/day until desired effect occurs

Pulmonary edema
- *Adult:* IV 50 mg given over several minutes or 0.5-1 mg/kg

Available forms: Tabs 25, 50 mg; powder for inj 50 mg

Side effects/adverse reactions:

GU: Polyuria, *renal failure,* glycosuria

ELECT: Hypokalemia, hypochloremic alkalosis, hypomagnesemia, hyperuricemia, hypocalcemia, hyponatremia, decreased glucose tolerance

CNS: Headache, fatigue, weakness, vertigo

GI: Nausea, *severe diarrhea,* dry mouth, vomiting, anorexia, cramps, upset stomach, abdominal pain, *acute pancreatitis,* jaundice, *GI bleeding;* abdominal distention

EENT: Loss of hearing, ear pain, tinnitus, blurred vision

INTEG: Rash, pruritus, purpura, *Stevens-Johnson syndrome,* sweating, photosensitivity

MS: Cramps, arthritis, stiffness

ENDO: Hyperglycemia

HEMA: Thrombocytopenia, agranulocytosis, leukopenia, neutropenia

CV: Chest pain, hypotension, *circulatory collapse,* ECG changes

Contraindications: Hypersensitivity to sulfonamides, anuria, hypovolemia, lactation, electrolyte depletion, infants

Precautions: Dehydration, ascites, severe renal disease, pregnancy (D), hypoproteinemia

Pharmacokinetics:
PO: Onset ½ hr, peak 2 hr, duration 6-8 hr
IV: Onset 5 min, peak 15-30 min, duration 2 hr
Excreted by kidneys, crosses placenta, half-life 30-70 min

Interactions/ incompatibilities:
- Increased hypotension: antihypertensives
- Decreased diuretic effect: indomethacin, NSAIDs
- Increased ototoxicity: cisplatin, aminoglycosides, rancomycin
- Increased toxicity: lithium, nondepolarizing skeletal muscle relaxants, digitalis
- Increased anticoagulant activity: warfarin
- Incompatible with hydralazine, procainamide, reserpine, tolazine, triflupromazine, blood, blood products

RESPIRATORY CARE CONSIDERATIONS
Assess/evaluate:
- Monitor serum electrolytes for hyponatremia and hypokalemia, with resulting acid-base abnormalities such as metabolic alkalosis.
- Overdose can cause reduction in blood volume and hypotension.
- Hypokalemia can also cause muscular weakness, possibly complicating weaning from mechanical ventilation.
- Monitor ECG for cardiac arrhythmias.
- Evaluate for dehydration, especially in COPD subjects or those with excess respiratory tract secretions.
- Monitor color, consistency of sputum.

---

italic = common side effects   **bold** = life-threatening reactions

- Evaluate breath sounds and respiratory pattern for pulmonary congestion.
- Evaluate chest radiograph if used in CHF, to assess clearing of infiltrates and pulmonary edema.

ethambutol HCI

(e-tham'byoo-tole)
Etibi,* Myambutol
Func. class.: Antitubercular
Chem. class.: Diisopropylethylene diamide derivative

Action: Inhibits RNA synthesis, decreases tubercle bacilli replication

Uses: Pulmonary tuberculosis, as an adjunct

Dosage and routes:
- *Adult and child >13 yr:* PO 15 mg/kg/day as a single dose
Retreatment
- *Adult and child >13 yr:* PO 25 mg/kg/day as single dose × 2 mo with at least 1 other drug, then decrease to 15 mg/kg/day as single dose
Available forms: Tabs 100, 400 mg

Side effects/adverse reactions:
GI: Abdominal distress, anorexia, nausea, vomiting
INTEG: Dermatitis, pruritis
CNS: Headache, confusion, fever, malaise, dizziness, disorientation, hallucinations
EENT: Blurred vision, optic neuritis, photophobia, decreased visual acuity
META: Elevated uric acid, acute gout, liver function impairment
MISC: Thrombocytopenia, joint pain, bloody sputum

Contraindications: Hypersensitivity, optic neuritis, child <13 yr

Precautions: Pregnancy (D), renal disease, diabetic retinopathy, cataracts, ocular defects, hepatic and hematopoietic disorders

Pharmacokinetics:
PO: Peak 2 - 4 hr, half-life 3 hr metabolized in liver excreted in urine (unchanged drug/inactive metabolites, unchanged drug in feces)

Interactions/incompatibilities:
- Increased renal toxicity: aminoglycosides, cisplatin
- Delayed absorption of ethambutol: aluminum salts

RESPIRATORY CARE CONSIDERATIONS
Assess/evaluate:
- Monitor bacteriologic response to therapy using drug-susceptibility testing.
- Assess subject for adverse reactions to drug therapy for mycobacteria, such as visual acuity and color vision evaluation, liver enzymes, and hearing evaluation if on multiple drug therapies.
- Respiratory care practitioners and other health care personnel should self-screen for infection with TB routinely and following exposure.
- Proper environmental and personnel protection programs should be implemented when treating subjects with TB.
- Consider the possibility of HIV infection in individuals with confirmed or suspected TB.

Patient education:
- Compliance with dosage schedule, duration is necessary.

*Available in Canada only

- Scheduled appointments must be kept or relapse may occur.

ethionamide
(e-thye-on-am-ide)
Trecator-SC
Func. class.: Antitubercular
Chem. class.: Thiomine derivative

Action: Bacteriostatic against *M. tuberculosis*

Uses: Pulmonary, extrapulmonary TB when other antitubercular drugs have failed

Dosage and routes:
- *Adult:* PO 500 mg-1 g qd in divided doses, with another antitubercular drug and pyridoxine
- *Child:* PO 15-20 mg/kg/day in 3-4 doses, not to exceed 1g
Available forms: Tabs 250 mg

Side effects/adverse reactions:
INTEG: Dermatitis, alopecia, acne
CV: Severe postural hypotension
CNS: Headache, drowsiness, tremors, *convulsions,* depression, psychosis, dizziness, peripheral neuritis
GI: Anorexia, nausea, vomiting, diarrhea, metallic taste
EENT: Blurred vision, optic neuritis
HEMA: Thrombocytopenia, purpura
MISC: Gynecomastia, impotence, menorrhagia, difficulty managing diabetes mellitus

Contraindications: Hypersensitivity, severe hepatic disease

Precautions: Pregnancy (D), renal disease, diabetic retin-opathy, cataracts, ocular defects, child <13 yr

Pharmacokinetics:
PO: Peak 3 hr, duration 9 hr, half-life 3 hr metabolized in liver excreted in urine (unchanged drug/inactive) crosses placenta

Interactions/ incompatibilities:
- Increased neurotoxicity: cycloserine, ethyl alcohol
- Increased adverse reactions: TB test agents, anti-TB drugs

RESPIRATORY CARE CONSIDERATIONS
Assess/evaluate:
- Monitor bacteriologic response to therapy using drug-susceptibility testing.
- Assess subject for adverse reactions to drug therapy for mycobacteria, such as liver enzymes, and GI disturbance.
- Respiratory care practitioners and other health care personnel should self-screen for infection with TB routinely and following exposure.
- Proper environmental and personnel protection programs should be implemented when treating subjects with TB.
- Consider the possibility of HIV infection in individuals with confirmed or suspected TB.

ethylnorepinephrine HCl
(eth-il-nor-ep-i-nef'rin)
Bronkephrine
Func. class.: Adrenergic
Chem. class.: Catecholamine

Action: α-stimulation with vasoconstriction, pressor response, nasal decongestion;

nonselective beta-adrenergic stimulation can cause tachycardia, vasodilation, and bronchial dilation, although this is less than with epinephrine due to drug's greater preference for alpha receptors compared to beta receptors.

Uses: Bronchospasm (more selective beta$_2$-adrenergic agents are preferred today)

Dosage and routes:
- *Adult:* IM/SC 0.5-1 ml
- *Child:* IM/SC 0.1-0.5 ml
Available forms: Inj 2 mg/ml IM, SC

Side effects/adverse reactions:
CNS: Tremors, anxiety, insomnia, headache, dizziness, confusion
CV: Palpitations, tachycardia, hypertension, chest pain, *dysrhythmias*
GI: Anorexia, nausea, vomiting

Contraindications: Hypersensitivity to sympathomimetics, narrow-angle glaucoma

Precautions: Pregnancy (C), cardiac disorders, hyperthyroidism, diabetes mellitus, prostatic hypertrophy

Pharmacokinetics:
IM/SC: Onset 6-12 min, duration 1-2 hr

Interactions/ incompatibilities:
- Do not use with MAOIs or tricyclic antidepressants; hypertensive crisis may occur
- Decreased effect of ethylnorepinephrine when used with methyldopa, urinary acidifiers, rauwolfia alkaloids
- Increased effect of ethylnorepinephrine when used with urinary alkalizers

RESPIRATORY CARE CONSIDERATIONS
Assess/evaluate:
- Assess effectiveness of drug therapy based on the indication(s) for the aerosol agent: presence of reversible airflow due to primary bronchospasm or other obstruction secondary to an inflammatory response and/or secretions, either acute or chronic.
- Monitor flow rates using office or bedside peak flow meters or laboratory reports of pulmonary function, especially before and after bronchodilator studies, to assess reversibility of airflow obstruction.
- Assess breathing rate and pattern.
- Assess breath sounds by auscultation before and after treatment.
- Assess pulse before and after treatment.
- Assess patient's subjective reaction to treatment for any change in breathing effort or pattern.
- Assess arterial blood gases or pulse oximeter saturation, as needed, for acute states with asthma or COPD to monitor changes in ventilation and gas exchange (oxygenation).
- Monitor BP and pulse rate if subject is on other adrenergic agents or tricyclic antidepressants.

Patient education:
- Instruct asthmatic patients in use and interpretation of disposable peak flow meters to assess severity of asthmatic episodes.

*Available in Canada only

■ Caution patient that adrenergic catecholamines are relatively short-acting (1-2 hours); symptoms may return.
■ Advise patient that adrenergic agonists do not protect against the late-phase reaction in asthma; symptoms may return or increase following use of adrenergic bronchodilator alone.
■ Note: death has been associated with excessive use of inhaled adrenergic agents in severe acute asthma crises; individuals using such drugs should be instructed to contact a physician or an emergency room if there is no response to the usual dose of the inhaled agent.

factor IX complex (human)
AlphaNine, Konyne HT, Proplex T, Proplex SX-T, Profilnine Heat-Treated
Func. class.: Hemostatic
Chem. class.: Factors II, VII, IX, X

Action: Causes an increase in blood levels of clotting factors II, VII, IX, X

Uses: Hemophilia B (Christmas disease), factor IX deficiency, anticoagulant reversal, control of bleeding in patients with factor VIII inhibitors

Dosage and routes:
■ *Adult and child:* IV 1 U/kg × desired % increase
Available forms: Inj IV (number of units noted on label)

Side effects/adverse reactions:
GI: Nausea, vomiting, abdominal cramps, jaundice, *viral hepatitis*

INTEG: Rash, flushing, *urticaria*
CNS: Headache, dizziness, malaise, paresthesia, *lethargy, chills, fever, flushing*
HEMA: **Thrombosis, hemolysis, AIDS, DIC**
CV: Hypotension, tachycardia, MI, **venous thrombosis, pulmonary embolism**
RESP: **Bronchospasm**

Contraindications: Hypersensitivity, hepatic disease, DIC, elective surgery, mild factor IX deficiency

Precautions: Neonates/infants, pregnancy (C)

Pharmacokinetics:
IV: Half-life factor VII—3-6 hr, factor IX—24-36 hr; rapidly cleared from plasma

Interactions/ incompatiblilities:
■ Incompatible with protein products
■ Increased risk of thrombosis: aminocaproic acid; do not administer

RESPIRATORY CARE CONSIDERATIONS
Assess/evaluate:
■ Avoid or minimize arterial punctures for blood gas analysis.
■ Use sites accessible to manual compression for arterial punctures.
■ Use pressure dressings for arterial puncture after prolonged manual compression.
■ Monitor for bleeding from any puncture sites.
■ Assess possibility of bleeding with unexplained fall in hematocrit or BP.
■ Check laboratory studies to assess bleeding times and improvement (PT, PTT).

italic = common side effects   **bold** = life-threatening reactions

Patient education:
■ Instruct patient to notify health care personnel of any swelling, hematoma, or bleeding at a puncture site.

felodipine
(fell-od'a-pine)
Plendil
Func. class.: Calcium-channel blocker
Chem. class.: Dihydropyridine

Action: Inhibits calcium ion influx across cell membrane, resulting in dilation of peripheral arteries

Uses: Essential hypertension, alone or with other antihypertensives

Dosage and routes:
■ *Adult:* PO 5 mg qd initially, usual range 5-10 mg qd; do not exceed 20 mg qd; do not adjust dosage at intervals of <2 wk
Available forms: Ext rel tabs 5, 10 mg

Side effects/adverse reactions:
CV: Dysrhythmia, edema, CHF, hypotension, palpitations, *MI, pulmonary edema,* tachycardia, syncope, AV block, angina
GI: Nausea, vomiting, diarrhea, gastric upset, constipation, increased liver function studies, dry mouth
GU: Nocturia, polyuria
INTEG: Rash, pruritus
MISC: Flushing, sexual difficulties, cough, nasal congestion, shortness of breath, wheezing, epistaxis, respiratory infection, chest pain
CNS: Headache, fatigue, drowsiness, dizziness, anxiety, depression, nervousness, insomnia, lightheadedness, paresthesia, tinnitus, psychosis, somnolence
HEMA: Anemia

Contraindications: Hypersensitivity, sick sinus syndrome, 2nd or 3rd degree heart block

Precautions: CHF, hypotension <90 mm Hg systolic, hepatic injury, pregnancy (C), lactation, children, renal disease, elderly

Pharmacokinetics: Peak plasma levels 2½-5 hr; highly protein bound, >99% metabolized in liver, 0.5% excreted unchanged in urine, elimination half-life 11-16 hr

Interactions/ incompatibilities:
■ Increased effects of: β-blockers, antihypertensives, digitalis
■ Increased felodipine level: cimetidine, ranitidine

RESPIRATORY CARE CONSIDERATIONS
Assess/evaluate:
■ Therapeutic response: corrected arrhythmia, decreased anginal pain, decreased BP.
■ Monitor cardiovascular status: BP, pulse, respiration, ECG.
■ Check for presence of adverse effects, especially dizziness or other signs of hypotension; bradycardia.
■ If on positive pressure ventilatory support, monitor cardiac output and/or BP and adjust level of positive pressure to extent possible, if necessary to maintain adequate cardiac output.

■ Monitor blood pressure if beta agonists are required to treat airway obstruction.

■ Consider use of anticholinergic agent such as ipratropium bromide as an alternative to beta agonists, if bronchodilator therapy is needed; aerosol inhalation (MDI, SVN, DPI) of adrenergic bronchodilators will generally give lower systemic levels and fewer cardiovascular effects.

Patient education:

■ Note: hand tremor can occur, such as seen with beta agonist bronchodilators.

■ Change position slowly to avoid orthostatic hypotension.

flecainide acetate

(fle-kay′nide)
Tambocor
Func. class.: Antidysrhythmic (Class IC)
Chem. class.: A benzamide

Action: Decreases conduction in all parts of the heart, with greatest effect on His-Purkinje system, which stabilizes cardiac membrane

Uses: Life-threatening ventricular dysrhythmias, sustained ventricular tachycardia

Dosage and routes:

■ *Adult:* PO 100 mg q12h; may increase q4d by 50 mg q12h to desired response, not to exceed 400 mg/day

Available forms: Tabs 50, 100, 150 mg

Side effects/adverse reactions:

CNS: Headache, dizziness, involuntary movement, confusion, psychosis, restlessness, irrita-

bility, paresthesias, ataxia, flushing, somnolence, depression, anxiety, malaise

EENT: Tinnitus, *blurred vision,* hearing loss

GI: Nausea, vomiting, anorexia, constipation, abdominal pain, flatulence, change in taste

CV: Hypotension, bradycardia, angina, PVCs, *heart block, cardiovascular collapse, arrest, dysrhythmias, CHF, fatal ventricular tachycardia*

RESP: Dyspnea, *respiratory depression*

INTEG: Rash, urticaria, edema, swelling

HEMA: Leukopenia, thrombocytopenia

GU: Impotence, decreased libido, polyuria, urinary retention

Contraindications: Hypersensitivity, severe heart block, cardiogenic shock, nonsustained ventricular dysrhythmias, frequent PVCs, non-life-threatening dysrhythmias

Precautions: Pregnancy (C), lactation, children, renal disease, liver disease, CHF, respiratory depression, myasthenia gravis

Pharmacokinetics:

PO: Peak 3 hr, half-life 12-27 hr, metabolized by liver, excreted unchanged by kidneys (10%) excreted in breast milk

Interactions/ incompatibilities:

■ Increased levels of both drugs: propranolol

■ Increased level of flecainide: amiodarone, cimetidine

■ Increased negative inotropic effects: disopyramide, verapamil

■ Increased digoxin level: digoxin

italic = common side effects   **bold** = life-threatening reactions

Lab test interferences:
Increase: CPK

RESPIRATORY CARE CONSIDERATIONS:
Assess/evaluate:
- Monitor ECG; in case of increased QT or widening QRS, drug should be discontinued.
- For dehydration or hypovolemia monitor I&O ratio, electrolytes (Na, K, Cl).
- Monitor pulse and BP for hypotension, hypertension.
- Monitor respiratory rate and pattern (labored, dyspnea).
- Provide resuscitation support in the event of cardiac arrest, life-threatening arrhythmias.
- Evaluate therapeutic response: decreased dysrhythmias.

Patient education:
- Make position change slowly to prevent orthostatic hypotension and fainting.
- Avoid hazardous activities if dizziness or blurred vision occurs.

---

flumazenil
(floo-maz′een-ill)
Mazicon, Romazicon
Func. class.: Benzodiazepine receptor antagonist
Chem. class.: Imidazobenzodiazepine derivative

Action: Antagonizes the actions of benzodiazepines on the CNS, competitively inhibits the activity at the benzodiazepine recognition site on the GABA/benzodiazepine receptor complex

Uses: Reversal of the sedative effects of benzodiazepines

Dosage and routes:
Reversal of conscious sedation or in general anesthesia
- *Adult:* IV 0.2 mg (2 ml) given over 15 sec; wait 45 sec, then give 0.2 mg (2 ml) if consciousness does not occur; may be repeated at 60-sec intervals as needed, up to 4 additional times (max total dose 1 mg); dose is to be individualized
Management of suspected benzodiazepine overdose
- *Adult:* IV 0.2 mg (2 ml) given over 30 sec; wait 30 sec, then give 0.3 mg (3 ml) over 30 sec if consciousness does not occur; further doses of 0.5 mg (5 ml) can be given over 30 sec at intervals of 1 min up to cumulative dose of 3 mg
Available forms: Inj 0.1 mg/ml

Side effects/adverse reactions:
EENT: Abnormal vision, blurred vision, tinnitus
CV: Hypertension, palpitations, cutaneous vasodilation, dysrhythmias, bradycardia, tachycardia, chest pain
GI: Nausea, vomiting, hiccups
CNS: Dizziness, agitation, emotional lability, confusion, *convulsions*, somnolence
SYST: Headache, injection site pain, increased sweating, fatigue, rigors

Contraindications: Hypersensitivity to this drug or benzodiazepines, serious cyclic antidepressant overdose, patients given benzodiazepine for control of life-threatening condition

Precautions: Pregnancy (C), lactation, children, elderly, renal disease, seizure disorders, head injury, labor and delivery, hepatic disease, hypoventilation, panic disorder, drug and alcohol dependency, ambulatory patients

Pharmacokinetics: Terminal half-life 41-79 min; metabolized in liver

Interactions/ incompatibilities:
▪ Toxicity: mixed drug overdosage
▪ Ingestion of food during IV INF: Increased flumazenil clearance

RESPIRATORY CARE CONSIDERATIONS:
Assess/evaluate:
▪ Therapeutic response: decreased sedation. Monitor respiratory rate and depth, sensorium, alertness.
▪ Provide airway and ventilatory support as necessary until reversal is sufficient.
▪ Check airway and IV access before administration.
▪ GI symptoms: nausea, vomiting; place in side-lying position to prevent aspiration.
▪ Allergic reactions: flushing, rash, urticaria, pruritus.

Patient education:
▪ Do not engage in hazardous activities for 18-24 hr after discharge.
▪ Do not take any alcohol or nonprescription drugs for 18-24 hr.

flunisolide
(floo-niss'oh-lide)
AeroBid
Func. class.: Corticosteroid
Chem. class.: Glucocorticoid

See Section III: Aerosol Agents for Oral Inhalation

flunisolide
(floo-niss'oh-lide)
Nasalide
Func. class.: Corticosteroid
Chem. class.: Glucocorticoid

See also Section III: Aerosol Agents for Oral Inhalation

Action: Decreases inflammation by suppression of migration of polymorphonuclear leukocytes, fibroblasts, reversal of increased capillary permeability and lysosomal stabilization; does not depress hypothalamus

Uses: Rhinitis, allergies, nasal polyps

Dosage and routes:
▪ *Adults:* SPRAY 2 puffs in each nostril bid, not to exceed 8 sprays in each nostril daily.
▪ *Children:* 1 SPRAY in each nostril 3 times daily, or 2 sprays in each nostril 2 times a day. Maximum daily dose is 4 sprays in each nostril.
Available forms: Nasal sol 25 µg/metered dose (Nasalide)

Side effects/adverse reactions:
CNS: Headache, nervousness, restlessness
EENT: Hoarseness, *Candida* infection of oral cavity, sore throat
GI: Nausea, vomiting, dry mouth

Contraindications: Hypersensitivity, child <6 yr

Precautions: Nonasthmatic bronchial disease; bacterial, fungal, viral infections of mouth, throat, lungs; respiratory TB; untreated fungal, bacterial, or viral infections; pregnancy (C); glaucoma

italic = common side effects   **bold** = life-threatening reactions

Pharmacokinetics:
INH: Duration 12 hr

RESPIRATORY CARE CONSIDERATIONS:
Assess/evaluate:
■ Monitor nasal passages during long-term treatment for changes in mucus.
■ Therapeutic response: decrease in runny nose.

Patient education:
■ Discuss method of installation after providing written instructions from manufacturer.
■ Clear nasal passages before administration; use decongestant if needed; shake inhaler, invert, tilt head backward, insert nozzle into nostril, away from septum; hold other nostril closed and depress activator, inhale through nose, exhale through mouth.
■ Follow insert instructions for cleaning insufflator unit.

fosinopril
(foss-in-o'pril)
Monopril
Func. class.:
Antihypertensive
Chem. class.: Angiotension-converting enzyme (ACE) inhibitor

Action: Selectively suppresses renin-angiotensin-aldosterone system; inhibits ACE; prevents conversion of angiotensin I to angiotensin II; results in dilation of arterial, venous vessels

Uses: Hypertension, alone or in combination with thiazide diuretics

Dosage and routes:
■ *Adult:* PO 10 mg qd initially, then 20-40 mg/day divided bid or qd
Available forms: Tabs 10, 20 mg

Side effects/adverse reactions:
CV: Hypotension, chest pain, palpitations, angina, orthostatic hypotension
GU: Proteinuria increased BUN, creatinine, decreased libido
HEMA: Decreased Hct, Hgb, *eosinophilia, leukopenia, neutropenia*
INTEG: Angioedema, rash, flushing, sweating, photosensitivity, pruritus
RESP: Cough, sinusitis, dyspnea, *bronchospasm*
META: Hyperkalemia
GI: Nausea, constipation, vomiting, diarrhea
CNS: Insomnia, paresthesia, headache, dizziness, fatigue, memory disturbance, tremor, mood change
MS: Arthralgia, myalgia

Contraindications: Hypersensitivity to ACE inhibitors, pregnancy (D), lactation, children

Precautions: Impaired liver function, hypovolemia, blood dyscrasias, CHF, COPD, asthma, elderly

Pharmacokinetics:
PO: Peak 3 hr, serum protein binding 97%, half-life 12 hr, metabolized by liver (metabolites excreted in urine, feces)

Interactions/incompatibilities:
■ Increased hypotension: diuretics, other antihypertensives, ganglionic blockers, adrenergic blockers

■ Increased toxicity: vasodilators, hydralazine, prazosin, K-sparing diuretics, sympathomimetics
■ Decreased absorption: antacids
■ Decreased antihypertensive effect: indomethacin
■ Increased serum levels of: digoxin, lithium
■ Increased hypersensitivity: allopurinol

Lab test interferences:
False positive: Urine acetone

RESPIRATORY CARE CONSIDERATIONS
Assess/evaluate:
■ Therapeutic response: decrease in BP.
■ Persistent cough and fever are common side effects of the ACE inhibitors, which should be differentiated from other possible causes, such as respiratory infection.
■ Monitor for possible hypotension.
■ Evaluate BP with COPD or asthmatic subjects who require beta agonists for reversible airway obstruction.
■ Assess for symptoms of CHF: edema, dyspnea, wet rales, BP.

furosemide
(fur-oh′se-mide)
Fumide, Furomide M.D., Furosemide, Lasix, Luramide, Novosemide,* Uritol*
Func. class.: Loop diuretic
Chem. class.: Sulfonamide derivative

Action: Furosemide inhibits the reabsorption of sodium and chloride in the proximal and distal tubules, and loop of Henle.

Uses: Pulmonary edema, edema in CHF, liver disease, nephrotic syndrome, ascites, hypertension

Dosage and routes:
■ *Adult:* PO 20-80 mg/day in AM; may give another dose in 6 hr up to 600 mg/day; IM/IV 20-40 mg, increased by 20 mg q2h until desired response
■ *Child:* PO/IM/IV 2 mg/kg; may increase by 1-2 mg/kg/ q6-8h up to 6 mg/kg
Pulmonary edema
■ *Adult:* IV 40 mg given over several minutes, repeated in 1 hr; increase to 80 mg if needed
Available forms: Tabs 20, 40, 80 mg; oral sol 10 mg/ml; inj IM, IV 10 mg/ml

Side effects/adverse reactions:
CNS: Headache, fatigue, weakness, vertigo, paresthesias
CV: Orthostatic hypotension, chest pain, ECG changes, *circulatory collapse*
EENT: **Loss of hearing,** ear pain, tinnitus, blurred vision
ELECT: Hypokalemia, hypochloremic alkalosis, hypomagnesemia, hyperuricemia, hypocalcemia, hyponatremia, metabolic alkalosis
ENDO: Hyperglycemia
GI: Nausea, diarrhea, dry mouth, vomiting, anorexia, cramps, oral, gastric irritations, pancreatitis
GU: Polyuria, **renal failure,** glycosuria
HEMA: **Thrombocytopenia, agranulocytosis, leukopenia, neutropenia, anemia**
INTEG: Rash, pruritus, purpura, **Stevens-Johnson syndrome,** sweating, photosensitivity, urticaria

---

italic = common side effects   **bold** = life-threatening reactions

MS: Cramps, stiffness

Contraindications: Hypersensitivity to sulfonamides, anuria, hypovolemia, infants, lactation, electrolyte depletion

Precautions: Diabetes mellitus, dehydration, severe renal disease, pregnancy (C)

Pharmacokinetics:
PO: Onset 1 hr, peak 1-2 hr, duration 6-8 hr, absorbed 70%
IV: Onset 5 min, peak ½ hr, duration 2 hr (metabolized by the liver 30%)
Excreted in urine, some as unchanged drug, feces; crosses placenta; excreted in breast milk; half-life ½-1 hour

Interactions/ incompatibilities:
■ Increased toxicity: lithium, nondepolarizing skeletal muscle relaxants, digitalis
■ Increased action of: antihypertensives, oral anticoagulants, nitrates
■ Increased ototoxicity: aminoglycosides, cisplatin, vancomycin
■ Decreased antihypertensive effect of furosemide: indomethacin, metolazone
■ Incompatible in sol with acidic sol, Vit C, corticosteroids, diphenhydramine, dobutamine, esmolol, epinephrine, gentamicin, levarterenol, meperidine, milrione, netilmicin, reserpine, spironolactone, tetracyclines; incompatible with any drug in syringe

Lab test interferences:
Interference: GTT

RESPIRATORY CARE CONSIDERATIONS
Assess/evaluate:
■ Monitor serum electrolytes for hyponatremia and hypokalemia, with resulting acid-base abnormalities such as metabolic alkalosis.
■ Overdose can cause reduction in blood volume and hypotension.
■ Hypokalemia can also cause muscular weakness, possibly complicating weaning from mechanical ventilation.
■ Monitor ECG for cardiac arrhythmias.
■ Evaluate for dehydration, especially in COPD subjects or those with excess respiratory tract secretions.
■ Monitor color, consistency of sputum.
■ Evaluate breath sounds and respiratory pattern for pulmonary congestion.
■ Evaluate chest radiograph, if used in CHF, to assess clearing of infiltrates and pulmonary edema.

gallamine triethiodide
(gal'a-meen)
Flaxedil
Func. class.: Neuromuscular blocker (nondepolarizing)

Action: Inhibits transmission of nerve impulses at the neuromuscular junction, by binding with cholinergic receptor sites, antagonizing action of acetylcholine, and causing muscle weakness or paralysis, depending on dose.

Uses: Facilitation of endotracheal intubation, skeletal muscle relaxation during mechanical ventilation, surgery, or general anesthesia

Dosage and routes:
■ *Adult and child >1 mo:* IV 1 mg/kg, not to exceed 100 mg, then 0.5-1 mg/kg q30-40 min
■ *Child <1 mo, >5 kg:* IV 0.25-0.75 mg/kg, then 0.01-0.05 mg/kg q30-40 min
Available forms: Inj IV 20 mg/ml

Side effects/adverse reactions:
CV: Bradycardia, tachycardia, increased, decreased BP
RESP: Prolonged apnea, bronchospasm, cyanosis, respiratory depression
EENT: Increased secretions
INTEG: Rash, flushing, pruritus, urticaria
CNS: Malignant hyperthermia
GI: Decreased motility

Contraindications: Hypersensitivity to iodides

Precautions: Pregnancy (C), thyroid disease, collagen disease, cardiac disease, lactation, children <2 yr, electrolyte imbalances, dehydration, neuromuscular disease (myasthenia gravis), respiratory disease, renal disease

Pharmacokinetics:
IV: Onset 2 min, duration 20-60 min; half-life 2 min, 29 min (terminal); excreted in urine, feces (metabolites); crosses placenta

Interactions/ incompatibilities:
■ Increased neuromuscular blockade: aminoglycosides, clindamycin, lincomycin, quinidine, local anesthetics, polymyxin antibiotics, lithium, narcotic analgesics, thiazides, enflurane, isoflurane; when used with cyclopropane, may provoke ventricular dysrhythmias
■ Dysrhythmias: theophylline
■ Incompatible with anesthetics, barbiturates in sol; incompatible with any other drug in syringe

RESPIRATORY CARE CONSIDERATIONS
Assess/evaluate:
■ Provide airway and ventilatory support before administering drug.
■ Note possible interaction with the following antibiotics, which can increase neuromuscular blockade: the aminoglycosides, the polymyxins, clindamycin, and lincomycin.
■ Use with mechanical ventilation: assess patient for adequate and preferably optimal ventilator settings *before* paralyzing; if patient is "fighting" the ventilator, provide adequately high flow rates and tidal volumes, short inspiratory times, and reasonable I:E ratios, check the sensitivity in assist-control mode, and provide sufficiently high rates to avoid patient fatigue. Consider paralysis if these measures fail.
■ Assess ventilator patients for pain, hypoxemia, or ventilator malfunction, if restless and anxious, before instituting muscle paralysis.
■ Assess need of patient and provide for pain control and

italic = common side effects   **bold** = life-threatening reactions

sedation during neuromuscular blockade *neuromuscular blocking agents do not provide analgesia or sedation.*

- Close eyelids and provide eye lubricant during prolonged paralysis.
- Since usual signs of pain or anxiety (restlessness, tachynea, distress, thrashing) are blocked, monitor vital signs closely, and overall patient appearance and state to detect problems (e.g., IV infiltration).
- Check ventilator alarm settings for sufficient limits and sensitivity; a disconnect alarm is critical.
- Assess reversal of drug before attempting to wean from mechanical ventilatory support.

Administer:
- Administer by IV, not by IM, for more consistent absorption and distribution and to avoid the pain associated with IM injection of the drug.
- Reversal: neostigmine or edrophonium, preceded by atropine to inhibit muscarinic response especially in upper airway.

glycopyrrolate
(glye-koe-pye′roe-late)
Glycopyrrolate, Robinul, Robinul Forte
Func. class.: Cholinergic blocker
Chem. class.: Quaternary ammonium compound

Action: Blocks acetylcholine receptor sites in autonomic nervous system, which controls secretions, free acids in stomach

Uses: Decreased secretions before surgery or reversal of neuromuscular blockade; peptic ulcer disease, irritable bowel syndrome, anticholinergic bronchodilator as alternative to atropine

Dosage and routes:
Preoperatively
- *Adult:* IM 0.002 mg/lb ½-1 hr before surgery
Child 2-12 yr: IM 0.002-0.004 mg/lb
- *Child <2 yr:* IM 0.004 mg/lb
Reversal of neuromuscular blockage
- *Adult:* IV 0.2 mg for each 1 mg of neostigmine or 5 mg IV of pyridostigmine simultaneously
GI disorders
- *Adult:* PO 1-2 mg bid-tid; IM/IV 0.1-0.2 mg tid-qid, titrated to patient response
Available forms: Tabs 1, 2 mg; inj 0.2 mg/ml

Side effects/adverse reactions:
INTEG: Urticaria, allergic reactions
MISC: Suppression of lactation, nasal congestion, decreased sweating
CNS: Confusion, anxiety, restlessness, irritability, delusions, hallucinations, headache, sedation, depression, incoherence, dizziness, lethargy, flushing, weakness
EENT: Blurred vision, photophobia, dilated pupils, difficulty swallowing, increased intraocular pressure, mydriasis, cycloplegia

CV: Palpitations, tachycardia, postural hypotension, paradoxical bradycardia
GI: Dryness of mouth, constipation, nausea, vomiting, abdominal distress, paralytic ileus, altered taste perception
GU: Hesitancy, retention, impotence

Contraindications: Hypersensitivity, narrow-angle glaucoma, myasthenia gravis, GI/GU obstruction, child <3 yr, tachycardia, myocardial ischemia, hepatic disease, ulcerative colitis, toxic megacolon

Precautions: Pregnancy (C), elderly, lactation, prostatic hypertrophy, renal disease, CHF, pulmonary disease, hyperthyroidism

Pharmacokinetics:
PO: Peak 1 hr, duration 6 hr
IM: Peak 30-45 min, duration 7 hr
IV: Peak 10-15 min, duration 4 hr
Excreted in urine, bile, feces (unchanged)

Interactions/ incompatibilities:
▪ Increased anticholinergic effect: alcohol, antihistamines, phenothiazines, amantadine, tricyclics
▪ Incompatible with alkaline sol, dexamethasone, dimenhydrinate, methohexital, methylprednisolone, pentazocine, phenothiazines, secobarbital, thiopental, diazepam, chloramphenicol, pentobarbital, sodium bicarbonate, in syringe or sol

RESPIRATORY CARE CONSIDERATIONS:
Assess/evaluate:
▪ Note: glycopyrrolate has been used in the past as an anticholinergic bronchodilator as an alternative to aerosolized atropine to avoid the unwanted systemic distribution and side effects of atropine.
▪ Therapeutic response: decreased secretions, GI, GU spasms, bronchodilation.
▪ Consider use of other anticholinergic agents for bronchodilation, such as ipratropium bromide, which are also quaternary compounds and which are FDA approved for aerosol administration.
▪ Use of glycopyrrolate by inhaled aerosol (SVN) requires clear and specific written physician order, since it is not FDA approved for use as a bronchodilator or by the aerosol route.
▪ Monitor heart rate for tachycardia.
▪ Monitor ECG if available with patient.
▪ Monitor respiratory status: rate, rhythm, cyanosis, wheezing, dyspnea.

Patient education:
▪ Blurred vision may occur, and reading may not be possible; this will subside.
▪ Avoid activities that are hazardous or require alertness if drowsiness occurs.
▪ A dry mouth is likely to occur.
▪ If difficulty in urination or constipation occur, check with physician.

italic = common side effects   **bold** = life-threatening reactions

guaifenesin

(gwye-fen'e-sin)
Amonidrin, Anti-tuss,
Balminil,* Breonesin, Fenesin,
Gee-Gee, Genatuss, GG-Cen,
Glyate, Glycotuss, Glytuss,
Guaifenesin, Guiatuss,
Halotussin, Humibid, Humibid
L.A., Hytuss, Hytuss 2X,
Malotuss, Mytussin, Naldecon
Senior EX, Resyl,* Robitussin,
Scot-Tussin Expectorant,
Sinumist-SR, Uni-Tussin
Func. class.: Expectorant

Action: Acts as an expectorant by stimulating a gastric mucosal reflex to increase the production of mucus in the respiratory tract

Uses: Dry, nonproductive cough, or to aid mucociliary clearance of respiratory tract secretions

Dosage and routes:
■ *Adult:* PO 100-400 mg q4-6h, not to exceed 1.2 g/day
■ *Child:* PO 12 mg/kg/day in 6 divided doses
Available forms: Tabs 100, 200 mg; caps 200 mg; syr 100 mg/5 ml

Side effects/adverse reactions:
CNS: Drowsiness
GI: Nausea, anorexia, vomiting

Contraindications: Hypersensitivity, persistent cough

Precautions: Pregnancy (C)

Lab test interferences: May cause color interference with certain laboratory determination of 5-hydroxy indoleacetic

acid (5-HIAA) and vanillylmandelic acid (VMA).

RESPIRATORY CARE CONSIDERATIONS
Assess/evaluate:
■ Therapeutic response: improved clearance of secretions, productive cough, and decrease in dry irritated cough.
■ Monitor color, consistency, and amount of sputum produced.
■ Assess changes in respiratory infection: WBC, breath sounds, chest radiograph, patient report of breathing, temperature.
■ Assess patient's adequacy of cough and level of consciousness to determine need for mechanical suctioning of airway.
■ Assess patient's ability to clear and expectorate secretions; consider adjunct bronchial hygiene such as postural drainage, percussion, PEP therapy, or autogenic drainage.

guanabenz acetate

(gwan'a-benz)
Wytensin
Func. class.:
Antihypertensive
Chem. class.: Central α_2-adrenergic agonist

Action: Stimulates central α_2-adrenergic receptors, resulting in decreased sympathetic outflow from brain

Uses: Hypertension

Dosage and routes:
■ *Adult:* PO 4 mg bid, increasing in increments of 4-8 mg/day q1-2wk, not to exceed 32 mg bid
Available forms: Tabs 4, 8, 16 mg

Side effects/adverse reactions:
*CV: **Severe rebound hypertension**, chest pain, dysrhythmias, palpitations*
CNS: Drowsiness, dizziness, sedation, headache, depression, weakness
EENT: Dry mouth, nasal congestion, blurred vision
GI: Nausea, diarrhea, constipation
GU: Impotence

Contraindications: Hypersensitivity to guanabenz

Precautions: Pregnancy (C), lactation, children <12 yr, severe coronary insufficiency, recent myocardial infarction, cerebrovascular disease, severe hepatic or renal failure

Pharmacokinetics:
PO: Peak 2-4 hr, half-life 6 hr, excreted in urine

Interactions/ incompatibilities:
■ Increased sedation: CNS depressants

RESPIRATORY CARE CONSIDERATIONS:
Assess/evaluate:
■ Evaluate BP and pulse for efficacy of hypertension treatment and to avoid hypotension, especially if on positive pressure ventilatory support.
■ Central-acting alpha-adrenergic agonists can cause drowsiness; increased sedative effect with CNS depressants such as alcohol, sedatives, tranquilizers, or many analgesics (opioid). Avoid hazardous activities.
■ Evaluate BP with COPD or asthmatic subjects who require beta agonists for reversible airway obstruction.
■ Assess for symptoms of CHF: edema, dyspnea, wet rales, BP.
■ Consider use of nonadrenergic bronchodilator such as ipratropium bromide as alternative to beta-adrenergic agents for asthmatics, COPD patients.

Patient education:
■ Do not use OTC products containing α-adrenergic stimulants (nasal decongestants, OTC cold preparations) unless directed by physician
■ Caution patient that orthostatic hypotension may occur.
■ Report symptoms of CHF: difficulty breathing, especially on exertion or when lying down, night cough, swelling of extremities
■ Avoid hazardous activities if drowsiness occurs.

guanadrel sulfate
(gwahn'a-drel)
Hylorel
Func. class.: Antihypertensive
Chem. class.: Adrenergic blocker, peripheral guanethidine derivative

Action: Inhibits sympathetic vasoconstriction by inhibiting release of norepinephrine, depletes norepinephrine stores in adrenergic nerve endings

Uses: Hypertension

Dosage and routes:
■ *Adult:* PO 5 mg bid, adjusted to desired response; may need 20-75 mg/day in divided doses
Available forms: Tabs 10, 25 mg

Side effects/adverse reactions:

CV: Orthostatic hypotension, bradycardia, CHF, palpitations, chest pain, tachycardia, dysrhythmias

CNS: Drowsiness, fatigue, weakness, feeling of faintness, insomnia, dizziness, mental changes, memory loss, hallucinations, *depression,* anxiety, *confusion, paresthesias, headache*

GI: Nausea, cramps, diarrhea, constipation, dry mouth, anorexia, indigestion

INTEG: Rash, purpura, alopecia

EENT: Nasal stuffiness, tinnitus, visual changes, sore throat, double vision, dry burning eyes

GU: Ejaculation failure, impotence, dysuria, nocturia, frequency

RESP: Bronchospasm, dyspnea, cough, rales, SOB

MS: Leg cramps, aching, pain, inflammation

Contraindications: Hypersensitivity, pregnancy (B), pheochromocytoma, lactation, CHF, child <18 yr

Precautions: Elderly, bronchial asthma, peptic ulcer, electrolyte imbalances, vascular disease

Pharmacokinetics:
PO: Onset 0.5-2 hr, peak 1½-2 hr, duration 4-14 hr, half-life 10-12 hr, excreted in urine (50% unchanged)

Interactions/ incompatibilities:
■ Increased hypotension: diuretics, other antihypertensives
■ Do not use with MAOIs
■ Increased orthostatic hypotension: alcohol, opioids

■ Decreased hypotensive effect: tricyclic antidepressants, phenothiazines, ephedrine, phenylpropanolamine

RESPIRATORY CARE CONSIDERATIONS:
Assess/evaluate:
■ Monitor patients with reversible airway obstruction or bronchospastic disease such as asthma or chronic bronchitis for presence of bronchospasm (wheezing, dyspnea, complaints of chest tightness) due to depletion of catecholamines.
■ Monitor effect on BP and pulse, especially if on positive pressure ventilatory support.
■ Assess effectiveness of beta-adrenergic bronchodilator therapy for possible antagonism and effect on BP to avoid increasing BP.
■ Consider use of nonadrenergic bronchodilator such as ipratropium bromide as alternative to beta adrenergic agents for asthmatics, COPD patients.

Patient education:
■ Do not use OTC products containing α-adrenergic stimulants (nasal decongestants, OTC cold preparations) unless directed by physician.
■ Caution patient that orthostatic hypotension commonly occurs.
■ Report symptoms of CHF: difficulty breathing, especially on exertion or when lying down, night cough, swelling of extremities.
■ Avoid hazardous activities (e.g., driving, using heavy equipment) if drowsiness occurs.

guanethidine monosulfate
(gwahn-eth'i-deen)
Guanethidine Sulfate, Ismelin
Func. class.:
Antihypertensive
Chem. class.: Antiadrenergic agent, peripheral

Action: Inhibits norepinephrine release, depleting norepinephrine stores in adrenergic nerve endings

Uses: Moderate to severe hypertension

Dosage and routes:
- *Adult:* PO 10 mg qd, increase by 10 mg qwk; may require 25-50 mg qd
- *Adult:* (Hospitalized) 25-50 mg; may increase by 25-50 mg/day or every other day
- *Child:* PO 200 µg/kg/day; increase q7-10d, not to exceed 3000 µg/kg/24 hr
Available forms: Tabs 10, 25 mg

Side effects/adverse reactions:
CV: Orthostatic hypotension, dizziness, weakness, lassitude, bradycardia, **CHF**, fatigue, angina, heart block, chest paresthesia
CNS: Depression
GI: Nausea, vomiting, *diarrhea*, constipation, dry mouth, weight gain, anorexia
INTEG: Dermatitis, loss of scalp hair
HEMA: **Thrombocytopenia, leukopenia**
EENT: Nasal congestion, ptosis, blurred vision
GU: Ejaculation failure, impotence, nocturia, edema, retention, increased BUN
RESP: Dyspnea

Contraindications: Hypersensitivity, pheochromocytoma, recent MI, CHF, cardiac failure, sinus bradycardia

Precautions: Pregnancy (B), lactation, peptic ulcer, asthma

Pharmacokinetics:
PO: Therapeutic level 1-3 wk; half-life 5 days, metabolized by liver, excreted in urine (metabolites), breast milk

Interactions/incompatibilities:
- Increased hypotension: diuretics, other antihypertensives
- Do not use with MAOIs
- Increased orthostatic hypotension: alcohol
- Decreased hypotensive effect: tricyclic antidepressants, phenothiazines, ephedrine, phenylpropanolamine, oral contraceptives, thiothixine, doxepin, haloperidol, amphetamines

Lab test interferences:
Increase: BUN
Decrease: Blood glucose, VMA excretion, urinary norepinephrine

RESPIRATORY CARE CONSIDERATIONS:
Assess/evaluate:
- Monitor patients with reversible airway obstruction or bronchospastic disease such as asthma or chronic bronchitis for presence of bronchospasm (wheezing, dyspnea, complaints of chest tightness) due to depletion of catecholamines.
- Monitor effect on BP and pulse, especially if on positive pressure ventilatory support.
- Assess effectiveness of beta-adrenergic bronchodilator

italic = common side effects   **bold** = life-threatening reactions

168 guanfacine HCl

therapy for possible antagonism and effect on BP to avoid increasing BP.
■ Consider use of nonadrenergic bronchodilator such as ipratropium bromide as alternative to beta-adrenergic agents for asthmatics, COPD patients.

Patient education:
■ Do not use OTC products containing α-adrenergic stimulants (nasal decongestants, OTC cold preparations) unless directed by physician.
■ Caution patient that orthostatic hypotension may occur.
■ Report symptoms of CHF: difficulty breathing, especially on exertion or when lying down, night cough, swelling of extremities
■ Avoid hazardous activities (e.g., driving, operating power equipment) if drowsiness occurs.

guanfacine HCl
(gwahn'fa-seen)
Tenex
Func. class.:
Antihypertensive
Chem. class.: α$_2$-adrenergic receptor agonist

Action: Stimulates central α-adrenergic receptors, resulting in decreased sympathetic outflow from brain

Uses: Hypertension in individual using a thiazide diuretic

Dosage and routes:
■ *Adult:* PO 1 mg/day hs; may increase dose in 2-3 wk to 2-3 mg/day
Available forms: Tabs 1 mg

Side effects/adverse reactions:
GI: Dry mouth, constipation, cramps, nausea, diarrhea
CNS: Somnolence, dizziness, headache, fatigue
GU: Impotence, urinary incontinence
EENT: Taste change, tinnitus, vision change, rhinitis, nasal congestion
MS: Leg cramps
RESP: Dyspnea
INTEG: Dermatitis, pruritus, purpura
CV: Bradycardia, chest pain

Contraindications: Hypersensitivity

Precautions: Pregnancy (B), lactation, children <12 yr, severe coronary insufficiency, recent MI, renal or hepatic disease, CVA

Pharmacokinetics: Peak 1-4 hr, 70% bound to plasma proteins, half-life 17 hr, eliminated via kidneys unchanged and as metabolites

Interactions/incompatibilities:
■ Increased sedation: CNS depressants, other antihypertensives
■ Decreased hypotensive effect: tricyclic antidepressants

RESPIRATORY CARE CONSIDERATIONS:
Assess/evaluate:
■ Evaluate BP and pulse for efficacy of hypertension treatment and to avoid hypotension, especially if on positive pressure ventilatory support.
■ Central-acting alpha-adrenergic agonists can cause drowsiness; increased sedative effect with CNS depressants

*Available in Canada only

such as alcohol, sedatives, tranquilizers, or many analgesics (opioid). Avoid hazardous activities.

■ Evaluate BP with COPD or asthmatic subjects who require beta agonists for reversible airway obstruction.

■ Assess for symptoms of CHF: edema, dyspnea, wet rales, BP.

■ Consider use of nonadrenergic bronchodilator such as ipratropium bromide as alternative to beta-adrenergic agents for asthmatics, COPD patients.

Patient education:
■ Do not use OTC products containing α-adrenergic stimulants (nasal decongestants, OTC cold preparations) unless directed by physician.

■ Caution patient that orthostatic hypotension may occur.

■ Report symptoms of CHF: difficulty breathing, especially on exertion or when lying down, night cough, swelling of extremities.

■ Avoid hazardous activities if drowsiness occurs.

heparin calcium/ heparin sodium

(hep'a-rin)
Calcilean,* Calciparine, Hepalean,* Heparin Sodium and 0.45% Sodium Chloride, Heparin Sodium and 0.9% Sodium Chloride, Heparin Lock Flush, Heparin Sodium, Hep-Lock, Liquaemin Sodium
Func. class.: Anticoagulant
Chem. class.: Sulfated mucopolysaccharides (bovine or porcine)

Action: Prevents conversion of fibrinogen to fibrin and prothrombin to thrombin by enhancing inhibitory effects of antithrombin III

Uses: Deep-vein thrombosis, pulmonary emboli, myocardial infarction, open heart surgery, disseminated intravascular clotting syndrome, atrial fibrillation with embolization, as an anticoagulant in transfusion and dialysis procedures, prevention of DVT/PE

Dosage and routes:
Deep vein thrombosis/MI
■ *Adult:* IV PUSH 5000-7000 U q4h then titrated to PTT or ACT level; IV BOL 5000-7500 U, then IV INF; IV INF after bolus dose, then 1000 U/hr titrated to PTT or ACT level
■ *Child:* IV INF 50 U/kg, maintenance 100 U/kg q4h or 20,000 U/m^2 qd
Pulmonary embolism
■ *Adult:* IV PUSH 7500-10,000 q4h then titrated to PTT or ACT level; IV BOL 7500-10,000, then IV INF; IV INF after bolus dose, then 1000 U/hr titrated to PTT or ACT level
■ *Child:* IV INF 50 U/kg, maintenance 100 U/kg q4h or 20,000 U/m^2 qd
Open heart surgery
■ *Adult:* IV INF 150-300 U/kg prophylaxis for DVT/PE
■ *Adult SC:* 5,000 units q8-12h
Available forms: Heparin sodium inj 1000, 2500, 5000, 7500, 10,000, 15,000, 20,000, 40,000 U/ml; heparin calcium inj 5000, 12,500, 20,000 U/dose

Side effects/adverse reactions:
CNS: Fever, chills
GI: Diarrhea, nausea, vomiting, anorexia, stomatitis, abdominal cramps, **hepatitis**

---

italic = common side effects   **bold** = life-threatening reactions

GU: Hematuria
HEMA: Hemorrhage, thrombocytopenia
INTEG: Rash, dermatitis, urticaria, alopecia, pruritus

Contraindications: Hypersensitivity, hemophilia, leukemia with bleeding, peptic ulcer disease, thrombocytopenic purpura, hepatic disease (severe), renal disease (severe), blood dyscrasias, severe hypertension, subacute bacterial endocarditis, acute nephritis

Precautions: Alcoholism, elderly, pregnancy (C)

Pharmacokinetics: Well absorbed (SC)
IV: Peak 5 min, duration 2-6 hr
SC: Onset 20-60 min, duration 8-12 hr
Half-life 1½ hr, excreted in urine, 95% bound to plasma proteins, does not cross placenta or alter breast milk, removed from the system via the lymph and spleen

**Interactions/
incompatibilities:**
▪ Decreased action of: corticosteroids
▪ Increased action of: diazepam
▪ Decreased action of heparin: digitalis, tetracyclines, antihistamines
▪ Increased action of heparin: oral anticoagulants, salicylates, dextran, steroids, nonsteroidal antiinflammatories
▪ Incompatible in sol with amikacin, ampicillin, atropine, cephalothin, chlordiazepoxide, chlorpromazine, chlortetracycline, codeine, dacarbazine, daunorubicin, diazepam, dobutamine, erythromycin, ergonovine, gentami-

cin hyaluronidase, hydrocortisone, hydroxyzine, insulin, kanamycin, levorphanol, meperidine, metaraminol, methadone, methicillin, morphine, penicillin G, polymyxin B, procainamide, prochlorperazine, promazine, promethazine, streptomycin, tetracycline, tobramycin, vancomycin, vinblastine

Lab test interferences:
Increase: T$_3$ uptake
Decrease: Uric acid

**RESPIRATORY CARE
CONSIDERATIONS:**
Assess/evaluate:
▪ Avoid or minimize arterial punctures for blood gas analysis.
▪ Use sites accessible to manual compression for arterial punctures.
▪ Use pressure dressings for arterial puncture after prolonged manual compression.
▪ Monitor for bleeding from any puncture sites.
▪ Assess possibility of bleeding with unexplained fall in hematocrit or BP.

Patient education:
▪ Instruct patient to notify health care personnel of any swelling, hematoma, or bleeding at a puncture site.

hepatitis B vaccine
Engerix-B, Recombivax HB
Func. class.: Vaccine
Chem. class.: Gamma globulin (pooled)

Action: Provides active immunity to hepatitis B

Uses: Prevention of hepatitis B virus

Dosage and routes:

- *Adult and child >10 yr:* IM 1 ml, then 1 ml after 1 mo, then 1 ml 6 mo after initial dose
- *Child 3 mo-10 yr:* IM 0.5 ml, then 0.5 ml after 1 mo, then 0.5 ml 6 mo after initial dose
- *Patients with decreased immunity:* IM 2 ml, then 2 ml after 1 mo, then 2 ml 6 mo after initial dose

Available forms: Inj IM 10 mg/0.5 ml, 20 µg/ml

Side effects/adverse reactions:

INTEG: Soreness at injection site, urticaria, erythema, swelling
SYST: Induration
CNS: Headache, dizziness, fever
GI: Nausea, vomiting

Contraindications: Hypersensitivity

Precautions: Pregnancy, elderly, lactation, children, active infection, compromised cardiac or pulmonary status

Interactions/incompatibilities:

- Immunosuppressants may decrease protection from HB vaccine
- HB vaccine may decrease response to yellow fever vaccine given concurrently
- HB vaccine may increase effect of anticoagulants

RESPIRATORY CARE CONSIDERATIONS:
Assess/evaluate:

- Personnel involved in respiratory care or critical care in general are well advised to obtain the hepatitis B vaccine, due to transmission of the virus by blood and serum-derived fluids and by direct contact with bodily fluids.

- Test for prior antibodies to hepatitis B may be performed before administering injection series.

hydralazine HCl

(hye'dral'a-zeen)
Alazine, Apresoline, Hydralazine HCl
Func. class.: Antihypertensive, direct-acting peripheral vasodilator
Chem. class.: Phthalazine

Action: Vasodilates arteriolar smooth muscle by direct relaxation; reduction in blood pressure with reflex increases in cardiac function

Uses: Essential hypertension; *parenteral:* severe essential hypertension, CHF

Dosage and routes:

- *Adult:* PO 10 mg qid 2-4 days, then 25 mg for rest of 1st wk, then 50 mg qid individualized to desired response, not to exceed 300 mg qd; IV/IM BOL 20-40 mg q4-6h, administer PO as soon as possible; IM 20-40 mg q4-6h
- *Child:* PO 0.75-3 mg/kg/day in 4 divided doses; max 7.5 mg/kg/24 hr, IV BOL 0.1-0.2 mg/kg q4-6h; IM 0.1-0.2 mg/kg q4-6h

Available forms: Inj IV, IM 20 mg/ml; tabs 10, 25, 50, 100 mg

Side effects/adverse reactions:

MISC: Nasal congestion, muscle cramps, *lupuslike symptoms*
CV: Palpitations, reflex tachycardia, angina, **shock,** *edema, rebound hypertension*
CNS: Headache, tremors, dizziness, anxiety, peripheral neuritis, depression

GI: Nausea, vomiting, anorexia, diarrhea, constipation
INTEG: Rash, pruritus
HEMA: Leukopenia, agranulocytosis, anemia
GU: Impotence, urinary retention, Na, H_2O retention

Contraindications: Hypersensitivity to hydralazines, coronary artery disease, mitral valvular rheumatic heart disease, rheumatic heart disease

Precautions: Pregnancy (C), CVA, advanced renal disease

Pharmacokinetics:
PO: Onset 20-30 min, peak 1 hr, duration 2-4 hr
IM: Onset 5-10 min, peak 1 hr, duration 2-4 hr
IV: Onset 5-20 min, peak 10-80 min, duration 2-6 hr, half-life 2-8 hr, metabolized by liver, less than 10% present in urine

Interactions/ incompatibilities:
- Increased tachycardia, angina: sympathomimetics (epinephrine, norepinephrine)
- Increased effects of: β-blockers
- Use MAOIs with caution in patients receiving hydralazine
- Incompatible with aminophylline, ampicillin, calcium disodium edetate, chlorothiazide, ethacrynic acid, hydrocortisone, mephentermine, methohexital, nitroglycerin, phenobarbital, verapamil, 10% fructose, $D_{10}LR$

RESPIRATORY CARE CONSIDERATIONS:
Assess/evaluate:
- Evaluate BP and pulse for efficacy of hypertension treatment and to avoid hypotension.
- Evaluate BP with COPD or asthmatic subjects who require beta agonists for reversible airway obstruction.
- Assess for symptoms of CHF: edema, dyspnea, wet rales, BP.
- Assess BP if on mechanical ventilatory support to minimize mean airway pressures which can increase hypotensive effect through impeded venous return and decreased cardiac output.

Patient education:
- Do not use OTC products containing α-adrenergic stimulants (nasal decongestants, OTC cold preparations) unless directed by physician.
- Report symptoms of CHF: difficult breathing, especially on exertion or when lying down, night cough, swelling of extremities.
- It is necessary to quit smoking to prevent excessive vasoconstriction
- Avoid hazardous activities until stabilized on medication; dizziness may occur.
- Make position changes slowly or fainting will occur.

hydrochlorothiazide
(hye-droe-klor-oh-thye'a-zide)
Diaqua, Diuchlor H,* Esidrix, Hydro-Chlor, Hydrochlorothiazide, HydroDiuril, Hydromal, Hydro-T, Hydrozide,* Neo-Codema,* Novohydrazide,* Oretic, Thiuretic, Urozide*
Func. class.: Thiazide diuretic
Chem. class.: Sulfonamide derivative

Action: Acts on distal tubule by increasing excretion of water, sodium, chloride, potassium

Uses: Edema, hypertension, diuresis, CHF

Dosage and routes:
- *Adult:* PO 25 - 100 mg/day
- *Child >6 mo:* PO 2.2 mg/kg/day in divided doses
- *Child <6 mo:* PO up to 3.3 mg/kg/day in divided doses
Available forms: Tabs 25, 50, 100 mg; sol 50 mg/5 ml, 100 mg/ml, 10 mg/ml

Side effects/adverse reactions:
GU: Frequency, polyuria, *uremia, glucosuria*
CNS: Drowsiness, paresthesia, depression, headache, *dizziness, fatigue, weakness*
GI: Nausea, vomiting, anorexia, constipation, diarrhea, cramps, pancreatitis, GI irritation, *hepatitis*
EENT: Blurred vision
INTEG: Rash, urticaria, purpura, photosensitivity, fever
META: Hyperglycemia, hyperuricemia, increased creatinine, BUN
HEMA: Aplastic anemia, hemolytic anemia, leukopenia, agranulocytosis, thrombocytopenia, neutropenia
CV: Irregular pulse, orthostatic hypotension, palpitations, volume depletion
ELECT: Hypokalemia, hypercalcemia, hyponatremia, hypochloremia, hypomagnesemia

Contraindications: Hypersensitivity to thiazides or sulfonamides, anuria, renal decompensation, hypomagnesemia

Precautions: Hypokalemia, renal disease, pregnancy (D), hepatic disease, gout, COPD, lupus erythematosus, diabetes mellitus

Pharmacokinetics:
PO: Onset 2 hr, peak 4 hr, duration 6 - 12 hr, excreted unchanged by kidneys, crosses placenta, enters breast milk

Interactions/ incompatibilities:
- Increased toxicity of: lithium, nondepolarizing skeletal muscle relaxants, digitalis
- Decreased effects of: antidiabetics
- Decreased absorption of thiazides: cholestyramine, colestipol
- Decreased hypotensive response: indomethacin, NSAIDs
- Hyperglycemia, hyperuricemia, hypotension: diazoxide

Lab test interferences:
Increase: BSP retention, amylase, parathyroid test
Decrease: PBI, PSP

RESPIRATORY CARE CONSIDERATIONS:
Assess/evaluate:
- Monitor serum electrolytes, especially potassium, to assess hypokalemia, which will cause metabolic alkalosis.
- Hypokalemia can also cause muscular weakness, possibly complicating weaning from mechanical ventilation.
- Monitor ECG for cardiac arrhythmias.
- Evaluate for dehydration, especially in COPD subjects or those with excess respiratory tract secretions.
- Monitor color, consistency of sputum.

---

italic = common side effects   **bold** = life-threatening reactions

- Evaluate breath sounds and respiratory pattern for pulmonary congestion.
- Evaluate chest radiograph if used in CHF, to assess clearing of infiltrates and pulmonary edema.

hydrocortisone/ hydrocortisone acetate/ hydrocortisone sodium phosphate/ hydrocortisone sodium succinate
(hye-dro-kor′ti-sone)
Cortef, Hydrocortone/ Cortef Acetate, Hydrocortone Acetate/Hydrocortone Phosphate/A-Hydrocort, Solu-Cortef, Cortenema
Func. class.: Corticosteroid
Chem. class.: Short-acting glucocorticoid

Action: Decreases inflammation by suppression of migration of polymorphonuclear leukocytes, fibroblasts, reversal of increased capillary permeability and lysosomal stabilization

Uses: Severe inflammation, adrenal insufficiency, ulcerative colitis, collagen disorders

Dosage and routes:
Adrenal insufficiency/ inflammation
- *Adult:* PO 5-30 mg bid-qid; IM/IV 100-250 mg (succinate), then 50-100 mg IM as needed; IM/IV 15-240 mg q12h (phosphate)
Shock
- *Adult:* 500 mg-2 g q2-6h (succinate)
- *Child:* IM/IV 0.16-1 mg/kg bid-tid (succinate)

Colitis
- *Adult:* ENEMA 100 mg nightly for 21 days
Available forms: Retention enema 100 mg/60 ml; tabs 5, 10, 20 mg; inj 25, 50 mg/ml; inj 50 mg/ml; phosphate inj 100, 250, 500, 1000 mg/vial; succinate inj 25, 50 mg/ml

Side effects/adverse reactions:
CNS: Depression, flushing, sweating, headache, mood changes
*CV: Hypertension, **circulatory collapse, thrombophlebitis, embolism**,* tachycardia, edema
EENT: Fungal infections, increased intraocular pressure, blurred vision
GI: Diarrhea, nausea, abdominal distention, ***GI hemorrhage***, increased appetite, *pancreatitis*
*HEMA: **Thrombocytopenia***
INTEG: Acne, poor wound healing, ecchymosis, petechiae
MS: Fractures, osteoporosis, weakness

Contraindications: Psychosis, hypersensitivity, idiopathic thrombocytopenia, acute glomerulonephritis, amebiasis, fungal infections, nonasthmatic bronchial disease, child <2 yr, AIDS, TB

Precautions: Pregnancy (C), diabetes mellitus, glaucoma, osteoporosis, seizure disorders, ulcerative colitis, CHF, myasthenia gravis, renal disease, esophagitis, peptic ulcer

Pharmacokinetics:
PO: Onset 1-2 hr, peak 1 hr, duration 1-1½ days
IM/IV: Onset 20 min, peak 4-8 hr, duration 1-1½ days
REC: Onset 3-5 days
Metabolized by liver, excreted in urine (17-OHCS, 17-KS), crosses placenta

Interactions/ incompatibilities:

- Decreased action of hydrocortisone: cholestyramine, colestipol, barbiturates, rifampin, ephedrine, phenytoin, theophylline
- Decreased effects of: anticoagulants, anticonvulsants, antidiabetics, ambenonium, neostigmine, isoniazid, toxoids, vaccines, anticholinesterases, salicylates, somatrem
- Increased side effects: alcohol, salicylates, indomethacin, amphotericin B, digitalis, cyclosporine, diuretics
- Increased action of hydrocortisone: salicylates, estrogens, indomethacin, oral contraceptives, ketoconazole, macrolide antibiotics

Phosphate

- Incompatible with amobarbital, calcium gluconate, cephalothin, chloramphenicol, erythromycin, diazepam, heparin, kanamycin, metaraminol, methicillin, pentobarbital, phentobarbital, phenytoin, phytonadione, prochlorperazine, promazine, tetracycline, vancomycin, Vit B complex with C, warfarin

Succinate

- Incompatible with aminophylline, amobarbital, ampicillin, bleomycin, chlorpromazine, colistimethate, dimenhydrinate, diphenhydramine, doxorubicin, ephedrine, heparin, hyaluronidase, hydralazine, hydroxyzine, kanamycin, lidocaine, meperidine, metaraminol, methicillin, nafcillin, netilmicin, phentobarbital, phenobarbital, prochlorperazine, promazine, promethazine, secobarbital, tetracycline, tolazoline, vancomycin, diazepam, phenytoin

Lab test interferences:

Increase: Cholesterol, Na, blood glucose, uric acid, Ca, urine glucose

Decrease: Ca, K, T_4 , T_3 , thyroid ^{131}I uptake test, urine 17-OHCS, 17-KS, PBI

False negative: Skin allergy tests

RESPIRATORY CARE CONSIDERATIONS:

Assess/evaluate:

- Monitor for side effects of increased corticosteroid level: Cushingoid symptoms (moon face, peripheral wasting, central edema).
- Monitor patients with latent tuberculosis or reactive skin tests for reactivation of the disease.
- Evaluate muscle weakness and steroid myopathy, especially in chronic lung disease patients.
- Evaluate cardiovascular system for hypertension, CHF.
- Monitor electrolytes; potassium and calcium loss can occur with hypokalemic alkalosis.
- Infection, including pneumonia, can occur.
- Increased corticosteroid levels can mask symptoms of infection.
- If asthma is present, monitor for breakthrough symptoms (bronchospasm, wheezing) if drug is discontinued.
- Evaluate possible adrenal insufficiency when transferring from systemic to inhaled aerosol corticosteroids in asthma.
- Monitor for symptoms of adrenal insufficiency: nausea, anorexia, fatigue, dizziness, dyspnea, weakness, joint pain.

---

italic = common side effects   **bold** = life-threatening reactions

hydroxyzine HCl/ hydroxyzine pamoate

(hye-drox′i-zeen)
Anxanil, Atarax, Atarax 100, Atozine, Durel, E-Vista, Hydroxacen, Hydroxyzine HCl, Hydroxyzine Pamoate, Hyzine-50, Quiess, Vamate, Vistacon, Vistaject-25, Vistaject-50, Vistaquel 50, Vistaril, Vistazine 50
Func. class.: Antianxiety
Chem. class.: Piperazine antihistamine

Action: Depresses activity in subcortical areas of the CNS. There is also skeletal muscle relaxation, bronchodilator activity, and antihistaminic, analgesic and antiemetic effects.

Uses: Anxiety preoperatively, postoperative prevention of nausea, vomiting, potentiation of narcotic analgesics, sedation, pruritus

Dosage and routes:
- *Adult:* PO 25-100 mg tid-qid
- *Child >6 yr:* 50-100 mg/day in divided doses
- *Child <6 yr:* 50 mg/day in divided doses
Preoperatively/postoperatively
- *Adult:* IM 25-100 mg q4-6h
- *Child:* IM 1.1 mg/kg q4-6h
Available forms: Tabs 10, 25, 50, 100 mg; caps 25, 50, 100 mg; syrup 10 mg/5 ml; oral susp 25 mg/5 ml IM inj 25, 50 mg/ml

Side effects/adverse reactions:
CNS: Dizziness, drowsiness, confusion, headache, tremors, fatigue, depression, *convulsions*
GI: Dry mouth

Contraindications: Hypersensitivity, pregnancy (C)

Precautions: Elderly, debilitated, hepatic disease, renal disease

Pharmacokinetics:
PO: Onset 15-30 min, duration 4-6 hr, half-life 3 hr

Interactions/ incompatibilities:
- Increased CNS depressant effect: barbiturates, narcotics, analgesics, alcohol

Lab test interferences: *False increase:* 17-OHCS

RESPIRATORY CARE CONSIDERATIONS:
Assess/evaluate:
- Note possibility of dry mouth; consider alternative to ipratropium bromide aerosol such as beta-adrenergic, if patient is on this bronchodilator, to avoid exacerbating dry mouth.
- Monitor for increased CNS depression if used with: alcohol, tricyclic antidepressants, narcotics, barbiturates, sedatives, hypnotics.
- Avoid hazardous activities while drug action persists.

Patient education:
- Caution individuals that other CNS depressants, including alcohol, narcotic analgesics, cough preparations, and antihistamines, may increase sedative effect, including respiratory depression.
- Dry mouth may occur.
- Avoid hazardous activities if drowsiness, dizziness occur.

*Available in Canada only

indapamide
(in-dap′a-mide)
Lozol, Lozide*
Func. class.: Diuretic—
thiazide-like
Chem. class.: Indoline

Action: Acts on proximal section of distal renal tubule by inhibiting reabsorption of sodium; may act by direct vasodilation caused by blocking of calcium channel

Uses: Edema, hypertension, diuresis

Dosage and routes:
■ *Adult:* PO 2.5 mg qd in AM; may be increased to 5 mg qd if needed
Available forms: Tabs 2.5 mg

Side effects/adverse reactions:
GU: Polyuria, dysuria, frequency
ELECT: Hypochloremic alkalosis, hypomagnesemia, hyperuricemia, hypercalcemia, hyponatremia, hypokalemia, hyperglycemia
CNS: Headache, dizziness, fatigue, weakness, paresthesias, depression
GI: Nausea, diarrhea, dry mouth, vomiting, anorexia, cramps, constipation, pancreatitis, abdominal pain, jaundice, hepatitis
EENT: Loss of hearing, tinnitus, blurred vision, nasal congestion, increased intraocular pressure
INTEG: Rash, pruritus, photosensitivity, alopecia, urticaria
MS: Cramps
*HEMA: **Thrombocytopenia, agranulocytosis, leukopenia, neutropenia,** anemia*
CV: Orthostatic hypotension, volume depletion, palpitations, dysrhythmias

Contraindications: Hypersensitivity, anuria, lactation

Precautions: Hypokalemia, dehydration, ascites, hepatic disease, severe renal disease, pregnancy (B)

Pharmacokinetics:
PO: Onset 1-2 hr, peak 2 hr, duration up to 36 hr, half-life 14-18 hr, excreted in urine, feces

Interactions/ incompatibilities:
■ Hyperglycemia, hyperuricemia, hypotension: diazoxide
■ Muscle relaxants, steroids, lithium, digitalis
■ Decreased K: steroids
■ Decreased effects: antidiabetics
■ Decreased absorption: cholestyramine, colestipol
■ Decreased hypotensive effect: indomethacin, NSAIDs

Lab test interferences:
Increase: Ca, parathyroid test

RESPIRATORY CARE CONSIDERATIONS:
Assess/evaluate:
■ Monitor serum electrolytes, especially potassium, to assess hypokalemia, which will cause metabolic alkalosis.
■ Hypokalemia can also cause muscular weakness, possibly complicating weaning from mechanical ventilation.
■ Monitor ECG for cardiac arrhythmias.
■ Evaluate for dehydration, especially in COPD subjects or those with excess respiratory tract secretions.
■ Monitor color, consistency of sputum.
■ Evaluate breath sounds and respiratory pattern for pulmonary congestion.

italic = common side effects   **bold** = life-threatening reactions

■ Evaluate chest radiograph, if used in CHF, to assess clearing of infiltrates and pulmonary edema.

indecainide HCl
(in-de-kane'ide)
Decabid
Func. class.: Antidysrhythmic (Class Ic)

Action: Unknown; able to slow conduction, reduce membrane responsiveness; inhibits automaticity, increases ratio of effective refractory period to action potential duration

Uses: Life-threatening dysrhythmias, sustained ventricular tachycardia

Dosage and routes:
■ *Adult:* PO 100-200 mg/day in divided dose q12h; 50 mg q12h initially, then increase dose by 25 mg increments q4d, max 400 mg/day
Available forms: Ext rel tabs 50, 75, 100 mg

Side effects/adverse reactions:
CV: Dysrhythmias, CHF
CNS: Headache, dizziness, lightheadedness
GI: Constipation, nausea
GU: Impotence
EENT: Blurred vision, diplopia

Contraindications: 2nd or 3rd degree AV block, right bundle branch block, cardiogenic shock, hypersensitivity

Precautions: Severe CHF, hypokalemia, hyperkalemia, sick-sinus syndrome, pregnancy (B), lactation, children, impaired hepatic or renal disease

Pharmacokinetics: Half-life 9-10 hr, metabolized by the liver, 63% of drug recovered in urine

Interactions/ incompatibilities:
■ Increased effect of indecainide: cimetidine
■ Increased serum concentrations of: digoxin

Lab test interferences:
Increase: CPK

RESPIRATORY CARE CONSIDERATIONS:
Assess/evaluate:
■ Monitor ECG; in case of increased QT and/or widening QRS, drug should be discontinued.
■ Monitor for dehydration or hypovolemia, I&O ratio, electrolytes (Na, K, Cl).
■ Monitor pulse and BP for hypotension, hypertension.
■ Monitor respiratory rate and pattern (labored, dyspnea).
■ Provide resuscitation support in the event of cardiac arrest.
■ Evaluate therapeutic response: decreased dysrhythmias.

Patient education:
■ Avoid hazardous activities if dizziness or blurred vision occurs.

indomethacin/ indomethacin sodium trihydrate
(in-doe-meth'a-sin)
Indomethacin, Indocin, Indocin SR, Indocin IV
Func. class.: Nonsteroidal antiinflammatory (NSAID)
Chem. class.: Propionic acid derivative

Action: Inhibits prostaglandin synthesis by decreasing enzyme needed for biosynthesis; analgesic, antiinflammatory, antipyretic

Uses: Rheumatoid arthritis, ankylosing rheumatoid spondylitis, acute gouty arthritis, closure of patent ductus arteriosus in premature infants

Dosage and routes:
Arthritis
■ *Adult:* PO/REC 25 mg bid-tid; may increase by 25 mg/day qwk, not to exceed 200 mg/day; SUS REL 75 mg qd, may increase to 75 mg bid
Acute arthritis
■ *Adult:* PO/REC 50 mg tid; use only for acute attack, then reduce dose
Patent ductus arteriosus
■ *Infant <2 days:* IV 0.2 mg/kg, then 0.1 mg/kg q12-24h
■ *Infant 2-7 days:* IV 0.2 mg/kg, then 0.2 mg × 2 doses after 12, 24h
■ *Infant >7 days:* IV 0.2 mg/kg, then 0.25 mg/kg × 2 doses after 12, 24 hr
Available forms: Caps 25, 50 mg; caps ext rel 75 mg; susp 25 mg/5 ml; rec supp 50 mg

Side effects/adverse reactions:
GI: Nausea, anorexia, vomiting, diarrhea, jaundice, *cholestatic hepatitis*, constipation, flatulence, cramps, dry mouth, peptic ulcer
CNS: Dizziness, drowsiness, fatigue, tremors, confusion, insomnia, anxiety, depression
CV: Tachycardia, peripheral edema, palpitations, dysrhythmias, hypertension

INTEG: Purpura, rash, pruritus, sweating
GU: **Nephrotoxicity, dysuria, hematuria, oliguria, azotemia**
HEMA: **Blood dyscrasias**
EENT: Tinnitus, hearing loss, blurred vision

Contraindications: Hypersensitivity, asthma, severe renal disease, severe hepatic disease, ulcer disease

Precautions: Lactation, children, bleeding disorders, GI disorders, cardiac disorders, hypersensitivity to other antiinflammatory agents, pregnancy (B) 1st and 2nd trimesters, depression

Pharmacokinetics:
PO: Onset 1-2 hr, peak 3 hr, duration 4-6 hr; metabolized in liver, kidneys; excreted in urine, bile, feces; crosses placenta; excreted in breast milk; 99% plasma protein binding

Interactions/incompatibilities:
■ Increased action of: coumarin, phenytoin, sulfonamides
■ Toxicity: lithium, methotrexate
■ Decreased action of: triamterene
■ Do not give with antacids

RESPIRATORY CARE CONSIDERATIONS
Assess/evaluate:
■ Verify presence of hemodynamically significant PDA using clinical findings: respiratory distress, continuous murmur, cardiomegaly, chest radiograph infiltrates.
■ Monitor arterial saturation (SaO$_2$ or SpO$_2$) or oxygen tension at pre- and post-ductal sites, which can include

italic = common side effects   **bold** = life-threatening reactions

the right upper thorax and the left lower quadrant of abdomen; equivalent saturations or oxygen tensions indicate effective reversal of patent ductus arteriosus.

- Echocardiograms, or doppler studies, provide more definitive assessment of status of ductus arteriosus.
- Evaluate improvement or change in arterial PaO_2.

---

iodinated glycerol

Iophen, Organidin, Par Glycerol, R-Gen
Func. class.: Expectorant
Chem. class.: Iodopropylidene glycerol isom

Action: Increases respiratory tract fluid by decreasing surface tension, adhesiveness, which increases removal of mucus; iodine directly stimulates mucus gland secretion through stomach vagal receptors.

Uses: Bronchial asthma, emphysema, bronchitis

Dosage and routes:
- *Adult:* PO 60 mg qid; SOL 20 gtts qid; ELIX 5 ml qid
- *Child:* PO up to half adult dose, depending on weight
Available forms: Tabs 30 mg; sol 50 mg/ml, 60 mg/5 ml

Side effects/adverse reactions:
EENT: Burning mouth, throat, eye irritation, swelling of eyelids
GI: Gastric irritation
ENDO: Iodism, goiter, myxedema
RESP: Pulmonary edema
INTEG: **Angioedema**, rash

CNS: Frontal headache, *CNS depression*, fever, parkinsonism

Contraindications: Hypersensitivity to iodides, pulmonary TB, pregnancy (X), hyperthyroidism, hyperkalemia, newborns, lactation, acute bronchitis

Precautions: Hypothyroidism, cystic fibrosis, lactation

Pharmacokinetics: Excreted in urine

Interactions/incompatibilities:
- Increased hypothyroid effects: lithium, antithyroid drugs
- Dysrhythmias, hyperkalemia: K-sparing diuretics, K-containing medication

Lab test interferences: May alter thyroid function tests

RESPIRATORY CARE CONSIDERATIONS
Assess/evaluate:
- Check with patient for presence of allergy to iodine.
- Monitor cough: type, frequency, character, including sputum production, with color, consistency, and amount.
- If respiratory infection is present, evaluate respiratory status: rate and pattern; ausculatate breath sounds, and assess chest radiograph when available and needed.
- Evaluate WBC, temperature if infection present, along with sputum culture to identify organism(s).
- Evaluate ability of patient to clear secretions prior to therapy: are tidal volume, expiratory force adequate?
- Assess need for concomitant bronchial hygiene techniques

such as postural drainage, chest percussion.

Patient education:
■ Drink large amount of non-diuresing fluids (e.g., water, juice, Gatorade) to facilitate mucociliary clearance.

ipecac syrup
(ip′e-kak)
Func. class.: Emetic
Chem. class.: Cephaelis ipecacuanha derivative

Action: Acts on chemoreceptor trigger zone to induce vomiting; irritates gastric mucosa

Uses: In poisoning to induce vomiting

Dosage and routes:
■ *Adult:* PO 15 ml, then 200-300 ml water
■ *Child >1 yr:* PO 15 ml, then 200-300 ml water
■ *Child <1 yr:* PO 5-10 ml, then 100-200 ml water; may repeat dose if needed
Available forms: Liq

Side effects/adverse reactions:
CNS: Depression, convulsions, coma
GI: Nausea, vomiting, bloody diarrhea
*CV: Circulatory failure, atrial fibrillation, **fatal myocarditis,** dysrhythmias*

Contraindications: Hypersensitivity, unconscious/semiconscious, depressed gag reflex, poisoning with petroleum products or caustic substances, convulsions

Precautions: Lactation, pregnancy (C)

Pharmacokinetics:
PO: Onset 15-30 min

Interactions/incompatibilities:
■ Do not administer with activated charcoal; effect will be decreased

RESPIRATORY CARE CONSIDERATIONS:
Assess/evaluate:
■ Assess sensorium, level of consciousness before administering. Inadequate airway reflexes or protection can lead to aspiration during emesis and pneumonia.
■ Place patient on side and monitor airway to prevent aspiration.
■ Monitor respiratory status before, during, after administration of emetic; check rate, rhythm, character. Respiratory depression can occur rapidly with elderly or debilitated patients.

ipratropium bromide
(eye-pra-troep′ee-um)
Atrovent
Func. class.:
Anticholinergic
Chem. class.: Synthetic quaternary ammonium compound

See Section III: Aerosol Agents for Oral Inhalation

iron dextran
Hydextran, Imferon, K-Feron
Func. class.: Hematinic
Chem. class.: Ferric hydroxide complex with dextran

Action: Iron is carried by transferrin to the bone marrow, where it is incorporated into hemoglobin

Uses: Iron deficiency anemia

Dosage and routes:
- *Adult and child:* IM 0.5 ml as a test dose by Z-track, then no more than the following per day
- *Adult <50 kg:* IM 100 mg
- *Adult >50 kg:* IM 250 mg
- *Infant <5 kg:* IM 25 mg
- *Child <9 kg:* IM 50 mg
- *Adult:* IV 0.5 ml test dose, then 100 mg qd after 2-3 days; IV 250/1000 ml of NaCl; give 25 mg test dose, wait 5 min, then infuse over 6-12 hr or follow equation:
0.3 × wt (lb) × 100-Hgb (g/dl) × 100 < If 30 lb (66 kg) should be given 80% of above formula dose
Available forms: Inj IM/IV 50 mg/ml, inj IM only 50 mg/ml

Side effects/adverse reactions:
CNS: Headache, paresthesia, dizziness, shivering, weakness, *seizures*
GI: Nausea, vomiting, metallic taste, abdominal pain
INTEG: Rash, pruritus, urticaria, fever, sweating, chills, brown skin discoloration, pain at injection site, necrosis, sterile abscesses, phlebitis
CV: Chest pain, *shock,* hypotension, tachycardia
RESP: Dyspnea
HEMA: Leukocytosis
OTHER: Anaphylaxis

Contraindications: Hypersensitivity, all anemias excluding iron deficiency anemia, hepatic disease

Precautions: Acute renal disease, children, asthma, lactation, rheumatoid arthritis (IV), infants < 4 mo, pregnancy (C)

Pharmacokinetics:
IM: Excreted in feces, urine, bile, breast milk; crosses placenta; most absorbed through lymphatics; can be gradually absorbed over weeks/months from fixed locations

Interactions/ incompatibilities:
- Not to mix with other drugs in syringe or sol
- Decreased reticulocyte response: chloramphenicol
- Increased toxicity: oral iron—do not use

Lab test interferences:
False increase: Serum bilirubin
False decrease: Serum Ca
False positive: 99kmTc diphosphate bone scan, iron test (large doses >2 ml)

RESPIRATORY CARE CONSIDERATIONS:
Assess/evaluate:
- Assess hemoglobin level to evaluate anemia and improvement in levels.
- Assess patient for fatigue and dyspnea on exertion due to inadequate tissue oxygenation.
- Evaluate total tissue oxygen transport: Total O_2 = Cardiac output X arterial O_2 content (use BP and pulse as index to cardiac output).
- Differentiate dyspnea caused by anemia with exertion from other possible causes (acute or chronic lung disease, including asthma, pneumothorax, pulmonary emboli, COPD progression).

- Determine cause of iron loss or anemia, including salicylates, sulfonamides.

isoetharine HCl/ isoetharine mesylate

(eye-soe-eth′a-reen)
Arm-a-Med Isoetharine HCl, Beta-2, Bronkometer, Bronkosol, Isoetharine HCl
Func. class.: β₂-adrenergic agonist
Chem. class.: Catecholamine

See Section III: Aerosol Agents for Oral Inhalation

isoniazid (INH)

(eye-soe-nye′a-zid)
Isoniazid, Isotamine,* Laniazid, Laniazid C.T., Nydrazid, PMS-Isoniazid*
Func. class.: Antitubercular
Chem. class.: Isonicotinic acid hydrazide

Action: Bactericidal interference with lipid, nucleic acid biosynthesis

Uses: Treatment, prevention of tuberculosis

Dosage and routes:
Treatment
- *Adult:* PO/IM 5 mg/kg qd as single dose for 9 mo to 2 yr, not to exceed 300 mg/day
- *Child and infants:* PO/IM 10-20 mg/kg qd as single dose for 18-24 mo, not to exceed 300 mg/day
Prevention
- *Adult:* PO 300 mg qd as single dose × 12 mo
- *Child and infants:* PO/IM 10 mg/kg qd as single dose for 12 mo, not to exceed 300 mg/day

Available forms: Tabs 50, 100, 300 mg; inj 100 mg/ml; powder, syrup 50 mg/5 ml

Side effects/adverse reactions:
Hypersensitivity: Fever, skin eruptions, lymphadenopathy, vasculitis
CNS: Peripheral neuropathy, memory impairment, *toxic encephalopathy, convulsions,* psychosis
EENT: Blurred vision, optic neuritis
HEMA: Agranulocytosis, hemolytic, aplastic anemia, thrombocytopenia, eosinophilia, methemoglobinemia
MISC: Dyspnea, B₆-deficiency, pellagra, hyperglycemia, metabolic acidosis, gynecomastia, rheumatic syndrome, SLE-like syndrome
GI: Nausea, vomiting, epigastric distress, *jaundice, fatal hepatitis*

Contraindications: Hypersensitivity, optic neuritis

Precautions: Pregnancy (C), renal disease, diabetic retinopathy, cataracts, ocular defects, hepatic disease, child <13 yr

Pharmacokinetics:
PO: Peak 1-2 hr, duration 6-8 hr
IM: Peak 45-60 min
Metabolized in liver, excreted in urine (metabolites), crosses placenta, excreted in breast milk

Interactions/ incompatibilities:
- Increased toxicity: alcohol, cycloserine, ethionamide, rifampin, carbamazepine

---

italic = common side effects   **bold** = life-threatening reactions

■ Decreased absorption: aluminum antacids

RESPIRATORY CARE CONSIDERATIONS:
Assess/evaluate:
■ Monitor bacteriologic response to therapy using drug-susceptibility testing.
■ Assess subject for adverse reactions to drug therapy for mycobacteria, such as visual acuity and color vision evaluation, liver enzymes, and peripheral neuropathy (numbness, tingling of extremities).
■ Respiratory care practitioners and other health care personnel should self-screen for infection with TB routinely and following exposure.
■ Proper environmental and personnel protection programs should be implemented when treating subjects with TB.
■ Consider the possibility of HIV infection in individuals with confirmed or suspected TB.

Patient education:
■ Compliance with dosage schedule, duration is necessary.
■ Scheduled appointments must be kept or relapse may occur.

isoproterenol HCl/
isoproterenol sulfate
(eye-soe-proe-ter′e-nole)
Dispos-a-Med Isoproterenol HCl, Isuprel, Isoproterenol HCl, Isuprel Glossets, Isuprel Mistometer, Medihaler-Iso, Norisodrine Aerotrol
Func. class.: Nonspecific beta-adrenergic agonist
Chem. class.: Catecholamine

See Section III: Aerosol Agents for Oral Inhalation

isosorbide dinitrate
(eye-soe-sor′bide)
Coronex,* Dilatrate-SR, Iso-Bid, Isordil Tembids, Isordil Titradose, Isosorbide Dinitrate, Isotrate Timecelles, Sorbitrate, Sorbitrate SA, Isordil, Isosorbide Dinitrate
Func. class.: Antianginal
Chem. class.: Nitrate

Action: Decreases preload, afterload, which is responsible for decreasing left ventricular end-diastolic pressure, systemic vascular resistance and reducing cardiac O_2 demand

Uses: Chronic stable angina pectoris, prophylaxis of angina pain

Dosage and routes:
■ *Adult:* PO 5-40 mg qid; SL 2.5-10 mg, may repeat q2-3h; CHEW TAB 5-10 mg prn or q2-3h as prophylaxis, sus rel 40-80 mg q8-12h
Available forms: Caps ext rel 40 mg; caps 40; tabs 5, 10, 20, 30, 40 mg; chew tabs 5, 10 mg; tabs ext rel 40 mg; SL tabs 2.5, 5, 10 mg

Side effects/adverse reactions:
MISC: Twitching, hemolytic anemia, *methemoglobinemia*
CV: Postural hypotension, tachycardia, *collapse,* syncope
GI: Nausea, vomiting
INTEG: Pallor, sweating, rash
CNS: Vascular headache, flushing, dizziness, weakness, faintness

Contraindications: Hypersensitivity to this drug or nitrates, severe anemia, increased intracranial pressure, cerebral hemorrhage, acute MI

Precautions: Postural hypotension, pregnancy (C), lactation, children

Pharmacokinetics:
Sus Action: Duration 6-8 hr
PO: Onset 15-30 min, duration 4-6 hr
SL: Onset 2-5 min, duration 1-4 hr
CHEW TAB: Onset 3 min, duration ½-3 hr, metabolized by liver, excreted in urine as metabolites (80%-100%)

Interactions/ incompatibilities:
■ Increased effects: β-blockers, diuretics, antihypertensives, alcohol products

Lab test interferences:
False decrease; nitrates may interfere with the Zlatkis-Zak color reaction test of serum cholesterol

RESPIRATORY CARE CONSIDERATIONS:
Assess/evaluate:
■ Therapeutic response: relief of chest pain (angina).
■ Monitor BP, pulse, and ECG if available.
■ Provide cardiopulmonary resuscitation if ventricular fibrillation or cardiac arrest occurs due to acute MI.
■ Note: alcohol or calcium channel blockers may increase risk of hypotension.
■ Evaluate for formation of methemoglobin and oxygen transport to tissues, in case of overdose or genetically abnormal hemoglobins.
■ Note possible respiratory adverse effects—bronchitis, pneumonia, URI—and monitor respiratory status (rate,

pattern, auscultation, patient report of breathing).

Patient education:
■ Prolonged chest pain may indicate MI: seek emergency treatment.
■ Make position changes slowly to prevent orthostatic hypotension.
■ Use analgesic (aspirin, acetaminophen) if headache occurs.

isosorbide mononitrate
(eye-soe-sor'bide)
Ismo
Func. class.: Antianginal
Chem. class.: Nitrate

Action: Decreases preload, afterload, resulting in decreased left ventricular end-diastolic pressure, systemic vascular resistance

Uses: Prevention of angina pectoris due to coronary artery disease

Dosage and routes:
■ *Adult:* PO 20 mg bid, 7 hr apart
Available forms: Tabs 20 mg

Side effects/adverse reactions:
MISC: Twitching, hemolytic anemia, methemoglobinemia
CV: Postural hypotension, tachycardia, *collapse*, syncope
GI: Nausea, vomiting
INTEG: Pallor, sweating, rash
CNS: Vascular headache, flushing, dizziness, weakness, faintness

Contraindications: Hypersensitivity to nitrates, severe anemia, increased intracranial pressure, cerebral hemorrhage, acute MI, closed-angle glaucoma

Precautions: Postural hypotension, pregnancy (C), lactation, children, glaucoma

Pharmacokinetics: Metabolized by the liver, excreted in urine as metabolites (80%-100%), half-life 4 hr

Interactions/ incompatibilities:
- Increased effects: β-blockers, diuretics, antihypertensives, alcohol, calcium channel blockers

Lab test interferences: False decrease; nitrates may interfere with the Zlatkis-Zak color reaction test of serum cholesterol.

RESPIRATORY CARE CONSIDERATIONS:
Assess/evaluate:
- Therapeutic response: relief of chest pain (angina).
- Monitor BP, pulse, and ECG if available.
- Provide cardiopulmonary resuscitation if ventricular fibrillation or cardiac arrest occurs due to acute MI.
- Note: alcohol or calcium channel blockers may increase risk of hypotension.
- Evaluate for formation of methemoglobin and oxygen transport to tissues, in case of overdose or genetically abnormal hemoglobins. Pulse oximetry will be inaccurate in presence of significant methemoglobin levels; check mixed venous oxygen level if available.
- Note possible respiratory adverse effects—bronchitis, pneumonia, URI—and monitor respiratory status (rate, pattern, auscultation, patient report of breathing).

Patient education:
- Prolonged chest pain may indicate MI: seek emergency treatment.
- Make position changes slowly to prevent orthostatic hypotension.
- Use analgesic (aspirin, acetaminophen) if headache occurs.

isoxsuprine HCl
(eye-sox'syoo-preen)
Isoxsuprine HCl, Vasodilan, Voxsuprine
Func. class.: Peripheral vasodilator
Chem. class.: Nylidrin-related agent

Action: α-adrenoreceptor antagonist with β-adrenoreceptor stimulating properties; may also act directly on vascular smooth muscle (propranolol does not block vasodilation); causes cardiac stimulation, uterine relaxation

Uses: Symptoms of cerebrovascular insufficiency, peripheral vascular disease including arteriosclerosis obliterans, thromboangiitis obliterans, Raynaud's disease

Dosage and routes:
- *Adult:* PO 10-20 mg tid or qid
Available forms: Tabs 10, 20 mg

Side effects/adverse reactions:
CV: Hypotension, tachycardia, palpitations, chest pain
CNS: Dizziness, weakness, tremors, anxiety
GI: Nausea, vomiting, abdominal pain, distention
INTEG: Severe rash, flushing

Contraindications: Hypersensitivity, postpartum, arterial bleeding

Precautions: Pregnancy (C), tachycardia

Pharmacokinetics:
PO: Peak 1 hr, duration 3 hr, half-life 1¼ hr, excreted in urine, crosses placenta

RESPIRATORY CARE CONSIDERATIONS:
Assess/evaluate:
- Evaluate BP and pulse for efficacy of hypertension treatment and to avoid hypotension.
- Evaluate BP with COPD or asthmatic subjects who require beta agonists for reversible airway obstruction.
- Assess for symptoms of CHF: edema, dyspnea, wet rales, BP.
- Assess BP if on mechanical ventilatory support, to minimize mean airway pressures which can increase hypotensive effect through impeded venous return and decreased cardiac output; minimize inspiratory times and optimal flow patterns and avoid large tidal volumes.

Patient education:
- Do not use OTC products containing α-adrenergic stimulants (nasal decongestants, OTC cold preparations) unless directed by physician.
- Report symptoms of CHF: difficult breathing, especially on exertion or when lying down, night cough, swelling of extremities.
- It is necessary to quit smoking to prevent excessive vasoconstriction.
- Avoid hazardous activities until stabilized on medication; dizziness may occur.
- Make position changes slowly or fainting will occur.

isradipine
(is-rad'-i-peen)
DynaCirc
Func. class.: Calcium channel blocker
Chem. class.: Dihydropyridine

Action: Inhibits calcium ion influx across cell membrane during cardiac depolarization; produces relaxation of coronary vascular smooth muscle, peripheral vascular smooth muscle; dilates coronary vascular arteries; increases myocardial oxygen delivery in patients with vasospastic angina

Uses: Essential hypertension, angina
Dosage and routes:
Hypertension:
- *Adult:* PO 1.25 mg bid; increase at 3-4 wk intervals up to 10 mg bid
Angina
- *Adult:* PO 2.5-7.5 mg tid
Available forms: Tabs 1.25 mg

Side effects/adverse reactions:
*HEMA: **Thrombocytopenia, leukopenia, anemia***
CV: Peripheral edema, tachycardia, hypotension, chest pain
GI: Nausea, vomiting, diarrhea, gastric upset, constipation, hepatitis
*GU: Nocturia, polyuria, **acute renal failure***
INTEG: Rash, pruritus, urticaria, photosensitivity, hair loss
CNS: Headache, fatigue, dizziness, fainting, sleep disturbances
MISC: Flushing

Contraindications: Sick sinus syndrome, 2nd or 3rd degree heart block, hypotension less than 90 mm Hg systolic, hypersensitivity

Precautions: CHF, hypotension, hepatic disease, pregnancy (C), lactation, children, renal disease, elderly

Pharmacokinetics: Metabolized in liver, metabolites excreted in urine and feces, secreted, in breast milk, peak plasma levels at 2-3 hr

Interactions/ incompatibilities:
▪ Increased effects of: digitalis, neuromuscular blocking agents, cyclosporine
▪ Increased effects of isradipine: cimetidine, carbamazepine

Lab test interferences: Elevated liver function tests have occurred

RESPIRATORY CARE CONSIDERATIONS:
Assess/evaluate:
▪ Therapeutic response: corrected arrhythmia, decreased anginal pain, decreased BP
▪ Monitor cardiovascular status: BP, pulse, respiration, ECG.
▪ Presence of adverse effects, especially dizziness or other signs of hypotension, bradycardia
▪ If on positive pressure ventilatory support, monitor cardiac output and/or BP, and adjust level of positive pressure to extent possible, if necessary to maintain adequate cardiac output.
▪ Monitor blood pressure if beta agonists are required to treat airway obstruction.

▪ Consider use of anticholinergic agent such as ipratropium bromide as an alternative to beta agonists, if bronchodilator therapy is needed; aerosol inhalation (MDI, SVN, DPI) of adrenergic bronchodilators will generally give lower systemic levels and fewer cardiovascular effects.

Patient education:
▪ Note: hand tremor can occur, such as seen with beta agonist bronchodilators.
▪ Change position slowly to avoid orthostatic hypotension.

labetalol
(la-bet'a-lole)
Normodyne, Trandate
Func. class.:
Antihypertensive
Chem. class.: alpha$_1$- and nonselective β-blocker

Action: Produces falls in BP without reflex tachycardia or significant reduction in heart rate through mixture of α-blocking and, β-blocking effects; elevated plasma renins are reduced

Uses: Mild to moderate hypertension

Dosage and routes:
Hypertension
▪ *Adult:* PO 100 mg bid; may be given with a diuretic; may increase to 200 mg bid after 2 days; may continue to increase q1-3 days; max 400 mg bid
Hypertensive crisis
▪ *Adult:* IV INF 200 mg/160 ml D$_5$W, run at 2 ml/min; stop infusion after desired response obtained, repeat q6-8h as needed; IV BOL

20 mg over 2 min, may repeat
40-80 mg q10min, not to
exceed 300 mg
Available forms: Tabs 100, 200,
300 mg, inj 5 mg/ml in 20
ml amps

Side effects/adverse reactions:

*CV: Orthostatic hypotension,
bradycardia,* **CHF,** *chest pain,*
ventricular dysrhythmias, AV
block
CNS: Dizziness, mental
changes, drowsiness, fatigue,
headache, catatonia, depression, anxiety, nightmares,
paresthesias, lethargy
GI: Nausea, vomiting, diarrhea
INTEG: Rash, alopecia, urticaria, pruritus, fever
HEMA: **Agranulocytosis, thrombocytopenia, purpura** (rare)
EENT: Tinnitus, visual changes,
sore throat, double vision, dry
burning eyes
GU: Impotence, dysuria, ejaculatory failure
RESP: **Bronchospasm,** dyspnea,
wheezing

Contraindications: Hypersensitivity to β-blockers, cardiogenic shock, heart block
(2nd or 3rd degree), sinus
bradycardia, CHF, bronchial
asthma

Precautions: Major surgery,
pregnancy (C), lactation, diabetes mellitus, renal disease,
thyroid disease, COPD, well-
compensated heart failure, CAD,
nonallergic bronchospasm

Pharmacokinetics:
PO: Onset 1-2 hr, peak 2-4
hr, duration 8-12 hr
IV: Peak 5 min
Half-life 6-8 hr, metabolized
by liver (metabolites inactive), excreted in urine and
bile, crosses placenta, excreted
in breast milk

Interactions/incompatibilities:
■ Increased bronchodilation:
β-adrenergic agonists
■ Increased hypotension:
diuretics, other antihypertensives, halothane, cimetidine,
nitroglycerin
■ Decreased effects: sym-
pathomimetics, lidocaine,
indomethacin, theophylline,
cimetidine
■ Increased hypoglycemia:
insulin
■ Incompatible with cefopera-
zone, nafcillin, $NaCO_3$ in sol
or syringe; mixing with other
drugs is not recommended

Lab test interferences:
False increase: Urinary catecholamines

RESPIRATORY CARE CONSIDERATIONS:
Assess/evaluate:
■ Avoid use with reversible
airway obstruction or bronchospastic disease such as
asthma or chronic bronchitis
due to potential for bronchospasm (wheezing, dyspnea,
complaints of chest tightness)
secondary to beta-blockade;
consider use of other classes
of antihypertensive agents for
these patients.
■ Monitor all subjects for
symptoms of increased airway
resistance (wheezing, tightness
in chest, difficulty breathing).
■ Monitor effect on BP and
pulse, especially if on positive
pressure ventilatory support.
■ Assess effectiveness of beta-
adrenergic bronchodilator
therapy for possible antagonism and effect on BP to
avoid increasing BP, if used.

italic = common side effects   **bold** = life-threatening reactions

- Consider use of nonadrenergic bronchodilator such as ipratropium bromide as alternative to beta-adrenergic agents for patients to avoid positive inotropic effect.

Patient education:
- Do not use OTC products containing α-adrenergic stimulants (nasal decongestants, OTC cold preparations) unless directed by physician.
- Caution patient that orthostatic hypotension may occur.
- Report symptoms of CHF: difficulty breathing, especially on exertion or when lying down, night cough, swelling of extremities.

---

levodopa
(lee-voe-doe′pa)
Dopar, Larodopa
Func. class.: Antiparkinson agent
Chem. class.: Catecholamine

Action: Decarboxylation to dopamine, which increases dopamine levels in brain

Uses: Parkinsonism, carbon monoxide poisoning, chronic manganese intoxication, cerebral arteriosclerosis

Dosage and routes:
- *Adult:* PO 0.5 - 1 g qd divided bid-qid with meals; may increase by up to 0.75 g q3 - 7d not to exceed 8 g/d unless closely supervised
Available forms: Caps 100, 250, 500 mg; tabs 100, 250, 500 mg

Side effects/adverse reactions:
HEMA: Hemolytic anemia, leukopenia, agranulocytosis
CNS: Involuntary choreiform movements, hand tremors, fatigue, headache, anxiety, twitching, numbness, weakness, confusion, agitation, insomnia, nightmares, psychosis, hallucination, hypomania, severe depression, dizziness
GI: Nausea, vomiting, anorexia, abdominal distress, dry mouth, flatulence, dysphagia, bitter taste, diarrhea, constipation
INTEG: Rash, sweating, alopecia
CV: Orthostatic hypotension, tachycardia, hypertension, palpitation
EENT: Blurred vision, diplopia, dilated pupils
MISC: Urinary retention, incontinence, weight change, dark urine

Contraindications: Hypersensitivity, narrow-angle glaucoma, undiagnosed skin lesions

Precautions: Renal disease, cardiac disease, hepatic disease, respiratory disease, MI with dysrhythmias, convulsions, peptic ulcer, pregnancy (C), asthma, endocrine disease, affective disorders, psychosis, lactation, children <12 yr

Pharmacokinetics:
PO: Peak 1 - 3 hr, excreted in urine (metabolites)

Interactions/incompatibilities:
- Hypertensive crisis: MAOIs, furazolidone
- Decreased effects of levodopa: anticholinergics, hydantoins, methionine, papaverine, pyridoxine, tricyclics, benzodiazepines
- Increased effects of levodopa: antacids, metoclopramide

Lab test interferences:
False positive: Urine ketones, urine glucose, Coombs' test
False negative: Urine glucose (glucose oxidase)

False increase: Uric acid, urine protein
Decrease: VMA

RESPIRATORY CARE CONSIDERATIONS:
Assess/evaluate:
- Blood pressure, respiration.
- Assess effect of concomitant beta agonist aerosol/oral therapy on blood pressure.
- Monitor effectiveness of drug therapy if on anticholinergic bronchodilator; although anticholinergics can decrease effect of levodopa, inhaled ipratropium should have limited effect on levodopa since action is contained topically in the lung with poor absorption and distribution.

Patient education:
- Beta-agonist bronchodilator therapy may worsen hand tremor.

lidocaine HCl
(lye-doe-kane)
Lidopen Auto-Injector, Xylocaine HCl IM for Cardiac Arrhythmias, Lidocaine HCl IV for Cardiac Arrhythmias, Xylocaine HCl IV for Cardiac Arrhythmias
Func. class.: Antidysrhythmic (Class IB)
Chem. class.: Aminoacylamide

Action: Increases electrical stimulation threshold of ventricle, His-Purkinje system, which stabilizes cardiac membrane, decreases automaticity

Uses: Ventricular tachycardia, ventricular dysrhythmias during cardiac surgery, myocardial infarction, digitalis toxicity, cardiac catheterization

Dosage and routes:
- *Adult:* IV BOL 50-100 mg over 2-3 min, repeat q3-5 min, not to exceed 300 mg in 1 hr: begin IV INF; IV INF 20-50 µg/kg/min; IM 200-300 mg in deltoid muscle
- *Elderly, CHF reduced liver function:* IV BOL give ½ adult dose
- *Child:* IV BOL 1 mg/kg, then IV INF 30 µg/kg/min
Available forms: IV INF 0.2%, 0.4%, 0.8%; IV Ad 4%, 10%, 20%; IV Dir 1%, 2%; IM 300 mg/ml, 10%

Side effects/adverse reactions:
CNS: Headache, dizziness, involuntary movement, confusion, tremor, drowsiness, euphoria, **convulsions**
EENT: Tinnitus, blurred vision
GI: Nausea, vomiting, anorexia
CV: Hypotension, bradycardia, **heart block, cardiovascular collapse, arrest**
RESP: Dyspnea, *respiratory depression*
INTEG: Rash, urticaria, edema, swelling
MISC: Febrile response, phlebitis at injection site

Contraindications: Hypersensitivity to amides, severe heart block, supraventricular dysrhythmias, Adams-Stokes syndrome, Wolff-Parkinson-White syndrome

Precautions: Pregnancy (B), lactation, children, renal disease, liver disease, CHF, respiratory depression, malignant hyperthermia

Pharmacokinetics:
IV: Onset 2 min, duration 20 min
IM: Onset 5-15 min, duration 1½ hr; half-life 8 min, 1-2 hr

italic = common side effects   **bold** = life-threatening reactions

(terminal); metabolized in liver; excreted in urine, crosses placenta

Interactions/incompatibilities:
- Increased neuromuscular blockade of: neuromuscular blockers, tubocurarine
- Increased effects of lidocaine: cimetidine, phenytoin, propranolol, metoprolol
- Decreased effects of lidocaine: barbiturates
- Incompatible with ampicillin, cefazolin, methohexital, phenytoin in syringe or sol; also incompatible with blood

Lab test interferences:
Increase: CPK

RESPIRATORY CARE CONSIDERATIONS:
Assess/evaluate:
- Monitor ECG; in case of increased QT and/or widening QRS, drug should be discontinued.
- Monitor for dehydration or hypovolemia, I&O ratio, electrolytes (Na, K, Cl).
- Assess pulse and BP for hypotension, hypertension.
- Respiratory rate and pattern (labored, dyspnea).
- Provide resuscitation support in the event of cardiac arrest, life-threatening arrhythmias.
- Evaluate therapeutic response: decreased dysrhythmias.
- Note: prolonged neuromuscular blockade may occur with succinylcholine when lidocaine is used.

Patient education:
- Make position change slowly to prevent orthostatic hypotension and fainting.

- Avoid hazardous activities if dizziness or blurred vision occurs.

lisinopril
(lyse-in′oh-pril)
Prinivil, Zestril
Func. class.: Angiotensin converting enzyme (ACE) inhibitor
Chem. class.: Enalaprilat lysine analog

Action: Selectively suppresses renin-angiotensin-aldosterone system; inhibits ACE, preventing conversion of angiotensin I to angiotensin II

Uses: Mild to moderate hypertension, adjunctive therapy of CHF

Dosage and routes:
- *Adult:* PO 10-40 mg qd; may increase to 80 mg qd if required
CHF
- *Adult* PO 5 mg initially with diuretics/digitalis
Available forms: Tabs 5, 10, 20 mg

Side effects/adverse reactions:
GI: Nausea, vomiting, anorexia, constipation, flatulence, GI irritation
GU: Proteinuria, renal insufficiency, sexual dysfunction, impotence
INTEG: Rash, pruritus
CNS: Vertigo, depression, stroke, insomnia, paresthesias, headache, fatigue, asthenia
EENT: Blurred vision, nasal congestion
RESP: Cough, dyspnea

Contraindications: Hypersensitivity

Precautions: Pregnancy (C), lactation, renal disease, hyperkalemia

Pharmacokinetics: Peak 6-8 hr, excreted unchanged in urine

Interactions/ incompatibilities:
- Increased hypotensive effect: diuretics, other hypertensives, probenecid
- Decreased effects of lisinopril: aspirin, indomethacin
- Increased K levels: K salt substitutes, K-sparing diuretics, K supplements
- Increased effects of: antihypertensives, reserpine, diuretics
- Increased hypersensitivity reactions: allopurinol

Lab test interferences:
Interfere: Glucose/insulin tolerance tests

RESPIRATORY CARE CONSIDERATIONS
Assess/evaluate:
- Therapeutic response: decrease in BP.
- Persistent cough and fever are common side effects of the ACE inhibitors, which should be differentiated from other possible causes, such as respiratory infection.
- Monitor for possible hypotension.
- Evaluate BP with COPD or asthmatic subjects who require beta agonists for reversible airway obstruction.
- Assess for symptoms of CHF: edema, dyspnea, wet rales, BP.

loratidine
(loer-at-i-deen)
Claritin
Func. class.: Antihistamine
Chem. class.: Selective histamine (H_1) receptor antagonist

Action: Blocks the action of histamine at H_1-receptor sites on blood vessels, GI, respiratory tract to decrease allergic inflammatory response and in general the pharmacologic effects of histamine. There is minimal anticholinergic (drying) and sedative effect compared to earlier antihistamines.

Uses: Seasonal rhinitis

Dosage and routes:
- *Adult:* PO 10 mg qd
Available forms: Tabs 10 mg

Side effects/adverse reactions:
CNS: Sedation (more common with increased doses)

Contraindications: Hypersensitivity, acute asthma attacks, lower respiratory tract disease

Precautions: Pregnancy (B), increased intraocular pressure, bronchial asthma

Pharmacokinetics: Peak 1½ hr, elimination half-life 14½ hr, metabolized in liver to active metabolites, excreted in urine

Interactions/ incompatibilities:
- Additive CNS depressant effects: alcohol, other CNS depressants

Lab test interference:
False negative: dermal reactivity indicators

RESPIRATORY CARE CONSIDERATIONS
Assess/evaluate:
- Note drying of the upper airway.
- Caution is suggested if used in asthma, although thickening

of lower respiratory tract secretions has not been established.
- Monitor nasal passages during long-term treatment for changes in mucus.
- Therapeutic response: decrease in runny nose.

Patient education:
- Sedative effect is less with loratadine than other antihistamines; however, avoid hazardous activities or use caution if drowsiness occurs.
- Additional CNS depression may occur with concomitant use of CNS depressants (tranquilizers, sedatives, or alcohol).

mannitol
(man'i-tole)
Mannitol, Osmitrol, Resectial
Func. class.: Osmotic diuretic
Chem. class.: Hexahydric alcohol

Action: Acts by increasing osmolarity of glomerular filtrate, which raises osmotic pressure of fluid in renal tubules; there is a decrease in reabsorption of water electrolytes, increase in urinary output, sodium, chloride excretion

Uses: Edema, promote systemic diuresis in cerebral edema, decrease intraocular pressure, improve renal function in acute renal failure, chemical poisoning

Dosage and routes:
Oliguria, prevention
- *Adult:* IV 50-100 g of a 5%-25% sol
Oliguria, treatment
- *Adult:* IV 300-400 mg/kg of a 20%-25% sol up to 100 g of a 15%-20% sol

Intraocular pressure/ intracranial pressure
- *Adult:* IV 1.5-2 g/kg of a 15%-25% sol over ½-1 hr
Renal failure
- *Adult:* IV 50-200 g/24 hr, adjusted to maintain output of 30-50 mg/hr
Diuresis in drug intoxication
- *Adult and child >12 yr:* 5%-10% sol continuously up to 200 g IV, while maintaining 100-500 ml output/hr
Available forms: Inj IV 5%, 10%, 15%, 20%, 25%

Side effects/adverse reactions:
GU: Marked diuresis, urinary retention, thirst
CNS: Dizziness, headache, *convulsions*, rebound increased ICP, confusion
GI: Nausea, *vomiting,* dry mouth, diarrhea
CV: Edema, thrombophlebitis, hypotension, hypertension, tachycardia, angina-like chest pains, fever, chills
RESP: Pulmonary congestion
ELECT: Fluid, electrolyte imbalances, acidosis, electrolyte loss, dehydration
EENT: Loss of hearing, blurred vision, nasal congestion, decreased intraocular pressure

Contraindications: Active intracranial bleeding, hypersensitivity, anuria, severe pulmonary congestion, edema, severe dehydration

Precautions: Dehydration, pregnancy (C), severe renal disease, CHF, lactation

Pharmacokinetics:
IV: Onset 30-60 min for diuresis, ½-1 hr for intraocular pressure, 25 min for cere-

brospinal fluid; duration 4-6 hr for intraocular pressure, 3-8 hr for cerebrospinal fluid; excreted in urine

Interactions/ incompatibilities:
- Decreased effect: lithium
- Increased effects of: EDTA
- Incompatible with whole blood, KCl, NaCl

Lab test interferences:
Interference: Inorganic phosphorus, ethylene glycol

RESPIRATORY CARE CONSIDERATIONS:
Assess/evaluate:
- Monitor serum electrolytes to detect hyponatremia. Such agents are generally free of pharmacologic effects due to their mode of action—osmosis.
- Evaluate for dehydration, especially in COPD subjects or those with excess respiratory tract secretions.
- Monitor color, consistency of sputum.
- Evaluate breath sounds and respiratory pattern for pulmonary congestion.

measles, mumps, and rubella virus vaccine, live
M-M-R-II
Func. class.: Vaccine
Chem. class.: Pooled gamma globulin

Action: Produces antibodies to measles, mumps, rubella

Uses: Prevention of measles, mumps, rubella

Dosage and routes:
- *Children >15 mos and adults:* SC 0.5 ml
Available forms: Inj SC measles 1000 TCID$_{50}$, mumps 20,000 TCID$_{50}$, rubella 1000 TCID$_{50}$ (0.5 ml)

Side effects/adverse reactions:
CNS: Fever, *subacute sclerosing panencephalitis and blindness associated with optic neuritis,* paresthesias
INTEG: Urticaria, erythema, burning, stinging at injection site
SYST: Lymphadenitis, **anaphylaxis,** malaise, sore throat, headache
MS: Osteomyelitis, arthralgia, arthritis

Contraindications: Hypersensitivity, blood dyscrasias, anemia, active infection, immunosuppression, egg, chicken allergy, pregnancy, febrile illness, neomycin allergy, neoplasms

Precautions: Elderly, lactation, children with TB

Interactions/ incompatibilities:
- Decreased response to: TB skin test
- Other live virus vaccines

RESPIRATORY CARE CONSIDERATIONS
Assess/evaluate:
- Monitor respiratory status if hypersensitivity reaction occurs; provide airway support, ventilation, oxygenation as indicated.
- Administer the tuberculin skin test before or simultaneously with vaccine; measles vaccine can temporarily decrease tuberculin skin sensitivity.
- Note: administering the vaccine does not exacerbate tuberculosis in children under treatment for TB.

M

mecamylamine HCl

(mek-a-mill'a-meen)

Inversine

Func. class.: Antihypertensive

Chem. class.: Ganglionic blocker

Action: Occupies receptor site, prevents acetylcholine from attaching to postsynaptic nerve ending in sympathetic and parasympathetic ganglia

Uses: Moderate to severe hypertension, malignant hypertension

Dosage and routes:
■ *Adult:* PO 2.5 mg bid, may increase in increments of 2.5 mg × 2 days until desired response; maintenance 25 mg/day in 3 divided doses

Available forms: Tabs 2.5 mg

Side effects/adverse reactions:

CV: Postural hypotension, irregular heart rate, *CHF*

CNS: Drowsiness, sedation, headache, tremors, weakness, syncope, paresthesia, dizziness, *convulsions*

EENT: Blurred vision, nasal congestion, dry mouth, dilated pupils

GU: Impotence, urinary retention, decreased libido

GI: Anorexia, glossitis, nausea, vomiting, constipation, *paralytic ileus*

Contraindications: Hypersensitivity, myocardial infarction, coronary insufficiency, renal disease, glaucoma, organic pyloric stenosis, uremia, uncooperative patients, mild/labile hypertension

Precautions: CVA, prostatic hypertrophy, bladder neck obstruction, urethral stricture, renal dysfunction (elevated BUN), cerebral dysfunction, pregnancy (C)

Pharmacokinetics:

PO: Onset ½-2 hr, duration 6-12 hr, excreted in urine, feces, breast milk; crosses placenta

Interactions/incompatibilities:
■ Increased effects: thiazide diuretics, antihypertensives, CNS depressants (alcohol, anesthetics, MAOIs), bethanechol

RESPIRATORY CARE CONSIDERATIONS:

Assess/evaluate:
■ Evaluate BP and pulse for efficacy of hypertension treatment and to avoid hypotension.
■ Evaluate BP with COPD or asthmatic subjects who require beta agonists for reversible airway obstruction.
■ Assess for symptoms of CHF: edema, dyspnea, wet rales, BP.
■ Assess BP if on mechanical ventilatory support, to minimize mean airway pressures which can increase hypotensive effect through impeded venous return and decreased cardiac output.

Patient education:
■ Do not use OTC products containing α-adrenergic stimulants (nasal decongestants, OTC cold preparations) unless directed by physician.
■ Report symptoms of CHF: difficult breathing, especially on exertion or when lying down, night cough, swelling of extremities.

*Available in Canada only

- Drug may cause dizziness or fainting; effect is increased with alcohol, exercise, or hot weather.

meclizine HCl
(mek´li-zeen)
Antivert, Antivert/25, Antivert/25 Chewable, Antivert-50, Antrizine, Bonamine,* Bonine, Dizmiss, Meclizine HCl, Meni-D, Ru-Vert-M
Func. class.: Antiemetic, Antihistamine, anticholinergic
Chem. class.: H_1-receptor antagonist, piperazine derivative

Action: There is reduced sensitivity of the labyrinthine apparatus. The inhibition of motion sickness and associated nausea/vomiting may be due to the anticholinergic property of the H_1 antagonist. There is also an anticholinergic drying effect and sedation.

Uses: Dizziness, motion sickness

Dosage and routes:
- *Adult:* PO 25-100 mg qd in divided doses or 1 hr before traveling
Available forms: Tabs 12.5, 25, 50 mg; chew tabs 25 mg; tabs film coated 25 mg

Side effects/adverse reactions:
CNS: Drowsiness, fatigue, restlessness, headache, insomnia
GI: Nausea, anorexia
EENT: Dry mouth, blurred vision

Contraindications: Hypersensitivity to cyclizines, shock, lactation

Precautions: Children, narrow-angle glaucoma, glaucoma, urinary retention, lactation, prostatic hypertrophy, elderly, pregnancy (B)

Pharmacokinetics:
PO: Duration 8-24 hr, half-life 6 hr

Interactions/ incompatibilities:
- Increased effect of: alcohol, tranquilizers, narcotics

Lab test interferences:
False negative: Allergy skin testing

RESPIRATORY CARE CONSIDERATIONS:
Assess/evaluate:
- Note drying of the upper airway.
- Caution is suggested if used in asthma, although thickening of lower respiratory tract secretions has not been established.
- Drowsiness may be a risk factor in subjects with sleep apnea.

Patient education:
- Avoid hazardous activities or use caution while drug action persists.
- Additional CNS depression may occur with concomitant use of CNS depressants (tranquilizers, sedatives, or alcohol).

mephentermine sulfate
(me-fen´ter-meen)
Wyamine
Func. class.: Adrenergic, direct and indirect acting
Chem. class.: Substituted phenylethylamine

Action: Causes increased contractility and heart rate by acting on β-receptors in heart;

also, acts on α-receptors, causing vasoconstriction in blood vessels; cardiac output is elevated, and systolic and diastolic pressures are increased

Uses: Shock and hypotension following variety of procedures

Dosage and routes:
Hypotension
- *Adult:* IV 15-45 mg depending on procedure

Hypotension/shock
- *Adult:* IV 0.5 mg/kg
- *Child:* IV 0.4 mg/kg

Available forms: Inj IV 15, 30 mg/ml

Side effects/adverse reactions:
CV: Palpitations, tachycardia, hypertension
CNS: Tremors, drowsiness, confusion, incoherence

Contraindications: Hypersensitivity to sympathomimetics

Precautions: Pregnancy (B), cardiac disorders, hyperthyroidism, diabetes mellitus, prostatic hypertrophy

Pharmacokinetics
IV: Onset immediate, duration ½-1 hr; metabolized in liver, excreted in urine

Interactions/ incompatibilities:
- Do not use with MAOIs or tricyclic antidepressants; hypertensive crisis may occur
- Decreased effect of mephentermine: methyldopa, urinary acidifiers, rauwolfia alkaloids
- Increased effect of mephentermine: urinary alkalizers
- Dysrhythmias: halothane, cyclopropaine, digitalis
- Incompatible with epinephrine, hydralazine

RESPIRATORY CARE CONSIDERATIONS:
Assess/evaluate:
- Therapeutic response: increased BP with stabilization.
- Monitor BP and pulse rate if administering adrenergic bronchodilators, for possible excess increase in BP.
- Evaluate tissue oxygen transport based on cardiac output and arterial O_2 content; correct any hypovolemia as quickly as possible to maintain BP and adequate tissue perfusion.
- If mechanical ventilatory support is instituted/present, minimize airway pressures to extent possible to avoid inhibiting venous return with high pressures, and causing decrease in cardiac output and BP.

metaproterenol sulfate
(met-a-proe-ter'e-nole)
Alupent, Arm-A-Med Metaproterenol Sulfate, Dey-Dose Metaproterenol Sulfate, Dey-Lute Metaproterenol Sulfate, Metaprel, Prometa
Func. class.: Selective β_2-agonist
Chem. class.: Resorcinol analogue of catecholamine

See also Section III: Aerosol Agents for Oral Inhalation, for detail on aerosol formulations

Action: Relaxes bronchial smooth muscle by direct action on β_2-adrenergic receptors

Uses: Bronchial asthma, bronchospasm

Dosage and routes:
- *Adult and child >12 yr:* MDI 2-3 puffs; may repeat q3-4h,

not to exceed 12 puffs/day;
SVN 0.3 ml of 5% solution,
with 2-3 cc normal saline to
dilute to volume, tid, qid.
Asthma/bronchospasm
▪ *Adult:* PO 20 mg q6-8h
▪ *Child >9 yr or >27 kg:* PO 20
mg q6-8h or 0.4-0.9 mg/
kg tid
▪ *Child 6-9 yr or <27 kg:* PO 10
mg q6-8h or 0.4-0.9 mg/
kg tid
Available forms: Tabs 10, 20
mg; MDI 0.65 mg/actuation;
syrup 10 mg/5 ml; SVN 0.6%,
5% solution

Side effects/adverse reactions:
CNS: Tremors, anxiety, insomnia, headache, dizziness, stimulation
CV: Palpitations, tachycardia, hypertension, dysrhythmias, *cardiac arrest*
GI: Nausea
RESP: Dyspnea

Contraindications: Hypersensitivity to sympathomimetics, narrow-angle glaucoma

Precautions: Pregnancy (C), cardiac disorders, hyperthyroidism, diabetes mellitus, prostatic hypertrophy

Pharmacokinetics: Well absorbed (PO)
PO: Onset 15-30 min, peak 1 hr, duration 4 hr, excreted in urine as metabolites
Inh: Onset 5 min, peak 1 hr, duration 4 hr

Interactions/ incompatibilities:
▪ Increased effects of both drugs: other sympathomimetics
▪ Decreased action of β-blockers, oral hypoglycemics

Lab test interferences:
Decrease: K

RESPIRATORY CARE CONSIDERATIONS:
Assess/evaluate:
▪ Assess effectiveness of drug therapy based on the indication(s) for the aerosol agent: presence of reversible airflow due to primary bronchospasm or other obstruction secondary to an inflammatory response and/or secretions, either acute or chronic.
▪ Monitor flow rates using office or bedside peak flow meters or laboratory reports of pulmonary function, especially before and after bronchodilator studies, to assess reversibility of airflow obstruction.
▪ Instruct and then verify correct use of aerosol delivery device (SVN, MDI, reservoir, DPI).
See Section I: Methods and Devices for Aerosol Delivery of Drugs
▪ Assess breathing rate and pattern.
▪ Assess breath sounds by auscultation before and after treatment.
▪ Assess pulse before and after treatment.
▪ Assess patient's subjective reaction to treatment for any change in breathing effort or pattern.
▪ Assess arterial blood gases or pulse oximeter saturation, as needed, for acute states with asthma or COPD to monitor changes in ventilation and gas exchange (oxygenation).
▪ Note effect of beta agonists on blood glucose (increase) and K^+ (decrease) laboratory values, if these are available.
▪ Monitor BP and pulse rate if subject is on other adrenergic

agents or tricyclic antidepressants.

- Long-term: monitor pulmonary function studies of lung volumes, capacities, and flows.

Patient education:
- Instruct asthmatic patients in use and interpretation of disposable peak flow meters to assess severity of asthmatic episodes.
- Instruct patients in use, assembly, and especially cleaning of aerosol inhalation devices.
- Caution patient that adrenergic catecholamines are relatively short-acting (1-2 hours); symptoms may return.
- Advise patient that adrenergic agonists do not protect against the late-phase reaction in asthma; symptoms may return or increase following use of adrenergic bronchodilator alone.
- Note: death has been associated with excessive use of inhaled adrenergic agents in severe acute asthma crises; individuals using such drugs should be instructed to contact a physician or an emergency room if there is no response to the usual dose of the inhaled agent.

methazolamide
(meth-a-zoe′la-mide)
Neptazane
Func. class.: Carbonic anhydrase inhibitor diuretic
Chem. class.: Sulfonamide derivative

Action: Decreases production of aqueous humor in eye, which lowers intraocular pressure

Uses: Open-angle glaucoma or preoperatively in narrow-angle glaucoma; can be used with miotic, osmotic agents

Dosage and routes:
- *Adult:* PO 50-100 mg bid or tid
Available forms: Tabs 25, 50 mg

Side effects/adverse reactions:
GU: Frequency, hypokalemia, polyuria, uremia, *glucosuria, hematuria,* dysuria, renal calculi
CNS: Drowsiness, paresthesia, anxiety, depression, headache, dizziness, confusion, stimulation, fatigue, *convulsions,* sedation, nervousness
GI: Nausea, vomiting, anorexia, constipation, diarrhea, melena, weight loss, hepatic insufficiency, metallic taste in mouth
EENT: Myopia, tinnitus
INTEG: Rash, pruritus, urticaria, fever, photosensitivity, Stevens-Johnson syndrome
ENDO: Hyperglycemia
HEMA: Aplastic anemia, hemolytic anemia, leukopenia, agranulocytosis, thrombocytopenia, purpura, pancytopenia

Contraindications: Hypersensitivity to sulfonamides, severe renal disease, severe hepatic disease, electrolyte imbalances (hyponatremia, hypokalemia), hyperchloremic acidosis, Addison's disease, severe COPD

Precautions: Hypercalciuria, pregnancy (C), diabetes mellitus

Pharmacokinetics:
PO: Onset 2-4 hr, peak 6-8 hr, duration 10-18 hr, excreted in urine, crosses placenta

**Interactions/
incompatibilities:**
- Decreased effectiveness of: lithium, barbiturates
- Increased action of: amphetamines, procainamide, quinidine, flecainide, ephedrine, pseudoephedrine
- Hypokalemia: with other diuretics, corticosteroids, amphotericin B
- Toxicity: salicylates

Lab test interferences:
False positive: Urinary protein

RESPIRATORY CARE CONSIDERATIONS:
Assess/evaluate:
- Monitor acid-base status: CA inhibitors can lead to metabolic acidosis due to HCO_3 loss and inhibited H^+ secretion.
- Monitor rate, depth, rhythm of respiration for increased levels to detect acidosis.
- Evaluate for dehydration, especially in COPD subjects or those with excess respiratory tract secretions.
- Monitor color, consistency of sputum in chronic bronchitic subjects.

methyldopa/ methyldopate
(meth-ill-doe′pa)
Aldomet, Amodopa, Dopamet,* Medimet,* Methyldopa/Methyldopate HCl, Novomedopa*
Func. class.:
Antihypertensive
Chem. class.: Centrally acting adrenergic inhibitor

Action: Stimulates central inhibitory α-adrenergic receptors or acts as false transmitter, resulting in reduction of arterial pressure

Uses: Hypertension

Dosage and routes:
- *Adult:* PO 250 mg bid or tid, then adjusted q2d as needed, 0.5-3 g qd in 2-4 divided doses (maintenance), not to exceed 3 g/day; IV 2,0 mg-500 mg in 100 ml D5W q6h, run over 30-60 min, not to exceed 1 g q6h
- *Child:* PO 10 mg/kg/day in 2-4 divided doses, not to exceed 65 mg/kg or 3 g/day, whichever is less; IV 20-40 mg/kg/day in 4 divided doses, not to exceed 65 mg/kg
Available forms: Tabs 125, 250, 500 mg; oral susp 250 mg/5ml; inj IV 50 mg/ml

Side effects/adverse reactions:
GI: Nausea, vomiting, diarrhea, constipation, hepatic dysfunction
CV: Bradycardia, myocarditis, orthostatic hypotension, angina, edema, weight gain
CNS: Drowsiness, weakness, dizziness, sedation, headache, depression, psychosis
EENT: Nasal congestion, eczema
HEMA: Leukopenia, thrombocytopenia, hemolytic anemia, positive Coombs' test
INTEG: Lupuslike syndrome
GU: Impotence, failure to ejaculate

Contraindications: Active hepatic disease, hypersensitivity, blood dyscrasias

Precautions: Pregnancy (C), liver disease, eclampsia, severe cardiac disease

Pharmacokinetics:
PO: Peak 2-4 hr, duration 12-24 hr

M

italic = common side effects   **bold** = life-threatening reactions

IV: Peak 2 hr, duration 10-16 hr, metabolized by liver, excreted in urine

Interactions/ incompatibilities:
- Increased pressor effect: sympathomimetic amines (norepinephrine, phenylpro-panolamine)
- Increased hypotension: levodopa
- Increased sedation: halo-peridol
- Increased action of: anesthetics

RESPIRATORY CARE CONSIDERATIONS:
Assess/evaluate:
- Evaluate BP and pulse for efficacy of hypertension treatment and to avoid hypotension, especially if on positive pressure ventilatory support.
- Central-acting alpha-adrenergic agonists can cause drowsiness, increased sedative effect with CNS depressants such as alcohol, sedatives, tranquilizers, or many analgesics (opioid). Avoid hazardous activities.
- Evaluate BP with COPD or asthmatic subjects who require beta agonists for reversible airway obstruction.
- Assess for symptoms of CHF: edema, dyspnea, wet rales, BP.
- Consider use of nonadrenergic bronchodilator such as ipratropium bromide as alternative to beta-adrenergic agents for asthmatics, COPD patients.

Patient education:
- Do not use OTC products containing α-adrenergic stimulants (nasal deconges-tants, OTC cold preparations) unless directed by physician.
- Caution patient that orthostatic hypotension may occur.
- Report symptoms of CHF: difficulty breathing, especially on exertion or when lying down, night cough, swelling of extremities.
- Avoid hazardous activities if drowsiness occurs.

methylene blue
(meth′i-leen)
Methylene Blue, Urolene Blue
Func. class.: Urinary tract antiseptic
Chem. class.: Antiseptic dye

Action: Oxidation-reduction action with opposite actions on hemoglobin depending on concentration; with increased concentration, converts ferrous ion of reduced hemoglobin to ferric form and methemoglobin is thus produced; prolonged administration accelerates destruction of erythrocytes

Uses: Oxalate urinary tract calculi; urinary tract infections caused by *E. coli, Klebsiella, Enterobacter, P. mirabilis, P. vulgaris, P. morganii, Serratia, Citrobacter, cyanide poisoning, methemoglobinemia*

Dosage and routes:
- *Adult:* PO 65-130 mg pc with full glass of water
Cyanide poisoning/ methemoglobinemia
- *Adult and child:* IV 1-2 mg/kg of 1% sol; inject slowly over 5 min or more
Available forms: Tabs 65 mg, inj 10 mg/ml

Side effects/adverse reactions:

CV: Cyanosis, CV abnormalities
INTEG: Pruritus, rash, urticaria, photosensitivity, profuse sweating
CNS: Dizziness, headache, drowsiness, mental confusion, fever with large doses
GI: Nausea, vomiting, abdominal pain, diarrhea
GU: Bladder irritation

Contraindications: Hypersensitivity to this drug, renal insufficiency

Precautions: Anemia, renal disease, hepatic disease, G-6-PD deficiency, pregnancy (C)

Pharmacokinetics:
PO/IV: Excreted in urine, bile, feces

RESPIRATORY CARE CONSIDERATIONS:
Assess/evaluate:

■ Monitor hemoglobin for possible anemia, which can be caused by hemolysis action with prolonged administration.
■ Assess patient for cyanosis.
■ Assess cardiovascular status: BP, pulse.
■ Note inaccuracy of pulse oximetry readings for arterial O_2 saturation in presence of methemoglobin, and use cooximeter measures.
■ Monitor respiratory rate and pattern, sensorium, and heart rate in presence of cyanide poisoning to assess efficacy of treatment.
■ Optimal measure of effect in cyanide poisoning is mixed venous O_2, if available.

methylprednisolone/ methylprednisolone acetate/ methylprednisolone sodium succinate
(meth-il-pred-niss'-oh-lone)
Medrol/Depo-Medrol, Duralone, Medralone, Rep-Pred/A-Methapred, Solu-Medrol
Func. class.: Corticosteroid
Chem. class.: Glucocorticoid, immediate acting

Action: Decreases inflammation by suppression of migration of polymorphonuclear leukocytes, fibroblasts, reversal of increased capillary permeability, and lysosomal stabilization

Uses: Severe inflammation, shock, adrenal insufficiency, collagen disorders

Dosage and routes:
Adrenal insufficiency/ inflammation
■ *Adult:* PO 2-60 mg in 4 divided doses; IM 40-80 mg (acetate); IM/IV 10-250 mg (succinate); intraarticular: 4-30 mg (acetate)
■ *Child:* IV 117 µg-1.66 mg/kg in 3-4 divided doses (succinate)
Shock
■ *Adult:* IV 100-250 mg q2-6h (succinate)
Available forms: Tabs 2, 4, 6, 8, 16, 24, 32 mg; inj 20, 40, 80 mg/ml acetate; inj 40, 125, 500, 1000 mg/vial succinate

Side effects/adverse reactions:
CNS: Depression, flushing, sweating, headache, mood changes
CV: Hypertension, *circulatory collapse, thrombophlebitis, embolism,* tachycardia

italic = common side effects   **bold** = life-threatening reactions

EENT: Fungal infections, increased intraocular pressure, blurred vision
GI: Diarrhea, nausea, abdominal distention, GI hemorrhage, increased appetite, pancreatitis
HEMA: Thrombocytopenia
INTEG: Acne, poor wound healing, ecchymosis, petechiae
MS: Fractures, osteoporosis, weakness

Contraindications: Psychosis, hypersensitivity, idiopathic thrombocytopenia, acute glomerulonephritis, amebiasis, fungal infections, nonasthmatic bronchial disease, child <2 yr, AIDS, TB

Precautions: Pregnancy (C), diabetes mellitus, glaucoma, osteoporosis, seizure disorders, ulcerative colitis, CHF, myasthenia gravis, renal disease, esophagitis, peptic ulcer

Pharmacokinetics: Well absorbed PO, IM
PO: Peak 1-2 hr, duration 1½ day
IM: Peak 4-8 days, duration 1-4 wk
INTRAARTICULAR: Peak 1 wk
Half-life > 3-½ hr; crosses placenta, enters breast milk in small amounts; metabolized in liver, excreted by the kidneys (unchanged)

Interactions/ incompatibilities:
▪ Decreased action of methylprednisolone: cholestyramine, colestipol, barbiturates, rifampin, ephedrine, phenytoin, theophylline
▪ Decreased effects of: anticoagulants, anticonvulsants, antidiabetics, ambenonium, neostigmine, isoniazid, toxoid, vaccines, anticholinesterases, salicylates, somatrem
▪ Increased side effects: alcohol, salicylates, indomethacin, amphotericin B, digitalis, cyclosporine, diuretics
▪ Increased action of methylprednisolone: salicylates, estrogens, indomethacin, oral contraceptives, ketoconazole, macrolide antibiotics
▪ Incompatible with aminophylline, calcium gluconate, cephalothin, chlorpromazine, cytarabine, digitoxin, diphenhydramine, glycopyrrolate, insulin, meperidine, metaraminol, nafcillin, penicillin G, promethazine, tetracycline, thiopental, tolazine

Lab test interferences:
Increase: Cholesterol, Na, blood glucose, uric acid, Ca, urine glucose
Decrease: Ca, K, T_4, T_3, thyroid ^{131}I uptake test, urine 17-OHCS, 17-KS, PBI
False negative: Skin allergy tests

RESPIRATORY CARE CONSIDERATIONS:
Assess/evaluate:
▪ Monitor for side effects of increased corticosteroid level: Cushingoid symptoms (moon face, peripheral wasting, central edema).
▪ Monitor patients with latent tuberculosis or reactive skin tests for reactivation of the disease.
▪ Evaluate muscle weakness and steroid myopathy, especially in chronic lung disease patients.
▪ Evaluate cardiovascular system for hypertension, CHF.
▪ Monitor electrolytes: potassium and calcium loss can oc-

cur, with hypokalemic alkalosis.
- Infection, including pneumonia, can occur.
- Increased corticosteroid levels can mask symptoms of infection.
- If asthma is present, monitor for breakthrough symptoms (bronchospasm, wheezing) if drug is discontinued.
- Evaluate possible adrenal insufficiency when transferring from systemic to inhaled aerosol corticosteroids in asthma.
- Monitor for symptoms of adrenal insufficiency: nausea, anorexia, fatigue, dizziness, dyspnea, weakness, joint pain.

metipranolol HCl
(met-ee-pran′oh-lole)
Optipranolol
Func. class.: Nonselective β-adrenergic blocker
Chem. class.: L-isomer

Action: Reduces production of aqueous humor by unknown mechanism

Uses: Ocular hypertension, chronic open-angle glaucoma

Dosage and routes:
- *Adult:* Instill 1 gtt bid
Available forms: Sol 0.3%

Side effects/adverse reactions:
CNS: Weakness, fatigue, depression, anxiety, headache, confusion
GI: Nausea, anorexia, dyspepsia
EENT: Eye irritation, conjunctivitis, keratitis
INTEG: Rash, urticaria
CV: Bradycardia, hypertension, *MI, atrial fibrillation, angina, palpitations*

RESP: Bronchospasm, dyspnea, bronchitis, coughing, rhinitis

Contraindications: Hypersensitivity, asthma, 2nd or 3rd degree heart block, right ventricular failure, congenital glaucoma (infants)

Pharmacokinetics:
INSTILL: Onset 15-30 min, peak 1-2 hr, duration 24 hr

Interactions/incompatibilities:
- Increased effect: propranolol, metoprolol

RESPIRATORY CARE CONSIDERATIONS:
Assess/evaluate:
- Topical ophthalmic agents are absorbed systemically and can cause the same adverse reactions seen with systemic administration of beta-blocking agents.
- Monitor patients with reversible airway obstruction or bronchospastic disease such as asthma or chronic bronchitis for presence of bronchospasm (wheezing, dyspnea, complaints of chest tightness).

metocurine iodide
(met-oh-kyoo′reen)
Metubine Iodide
Func. class.: Neuromuscular blocker (nondepolarizing)
Chem. class.: Methyl analog of tubocurarine, an isoquinoline

Action: Inhibits transmission of nerve impulses at the neuromuscular junction by binding with cholinergic receptor sites, antagonizing action of acetylcholine, and causing muscle weakness or paralysis, depending on dose.

italic = common side effects   **bold** = life-threatening reactions

Uses: Facilitation of endotracheal intubation; skeletal muscle relaxation during mechanical ventilation, surgery, or general anesthesia; reduction of fractures/dislocations

Dosage and routes:
- *Adult:* IV 2-4 mg if given cyclopropane as an anesthetic; 1.5-3 mg if given ether as an anesthetic; 4-7 mg if given nitrous oxide
Available forms: Inj IV 2 mg/ml

Side effects/adverse reactions:
CV: Bradycardia, tachycardia, increased, decreased BP
RESP: Prolonged apnea, bronchospasm, cyanosis, respiratory depression
EENT: Increased secretions
INTEG: Rash, flushing, pruritus, urticaria

Contraindications: Hypersensitivity to iodides

Precautions: Pregnancy (C), cardiac disease, hepatic disease, renal disease, lactation, children <2 yr, electrolyte imbalances, dehydration, neuromuscular disease (myasthenia gravis), respiratory disease, or patients in which histamine release is a definite hazard (e.g., asthma)

Pharmacokinetics:
IV: Peak 3-5 min, duration 35-90 min, half-life 3½ hr, excreted in urine, bile (½ unchanged), crosses placenta

Interactions/ incompatibilities:
- Increased neuromuscular blockade: aminoglycosides, clindamycin, lincomycin, quinidine, local anesthetics, polymyxin antibiotics, lithium, narcotic analgesics, thiazides, enflurane, isoflurane, magnesium sulfate
- Dysrhythmias: theophylline
- Do not mix with barbiturates in sol or syringe; unstable in alkaline sol

RESPIRATORY CARE CONSIDERATIONS:
Assess/evaluate:
- Provide airway and ventilatory support before administering drug.
- Note possible interaction with the following antibiotics, which can increase neuromuscular blockade: the aminoglycosides, the polymyxins, clindamycin, and lincomycin.
- Use with mechanical ventilation; assess patient for adequate and preferably optimal ventilator settings *before* paralyzing. If patient is "fighting" the ventilator, provide adequately high flow rates and tidal volumes, short inspiratory times, and reasonable I:E ratios, check the sensitivity in assist-control mode, provide sufficiently high rates to avoid patient fatigue; consider paralysis if these measures fail.
- Drug can cause histamine release; assess airway resistance, especially in asthmatic patients.
- Assess ventilator patients for pain, hypoxemia, or ventilator malfunction, if restless and anxious, before instituting muscle paralysis.
- Assess need of patient and provide for pain control and sedation during neuromuscular blockade. *Neuromuscular blocking agents do not provide analgesia or sedation.*

- Close eyelids and provide eye lubricant during prolonged paralysis.
- Since usual signs of pain or anxiety (restlessness, tachynea, distress, thrashing) are blocked, monitor vital signs closely and overall patient appearance and state to detect problems (e.g., IV infiltration).
- Check ventilator alarm settings for sufficient limits and sensitivity; a disconnect alarm is critical.
- Assess reversal of drug before attempting to wean from mechanical ventilatory support.

Administer:
- Administer by IV, not by IM, for more consistent absorption and distribution, and to avoid the pain associated with IM injection of the drug.
- Reversal: neostigmine or edrophonium, preceded by atropine to inhibit muscarinic response especially in upper airway.

metolazone
(me-tole′a-zone)
Diulo, Mykrox, Zaroxolyn
Func. class.: Diuretic
Chem. class.: Thiazide-like quinazoline derivative

Action: Acts on distal tubule by increasing excretion of water, sodium, chloride, potassium, magnesium

Uses: Edema, hypertension, CHF

Dosage and routes:
Edema
- *Adult:* PO 5-20 mg/day
Hypertension
- *Adult:* PO 2.5-5 mg/day

Available forms: Tabs 0.5, 2.5, 5, 10 mg

Side effects/adverse reactions:
GU: Frequency, polyuria, *uremia, glucosuria*
CNS: Drowsiness, paresthesia, anxiety, depression, headache, *dizziness, fatigue, weakness*
GI: Nausea, vomiting, anorexia, constipation, diarrhea, cramps, pancreatitis, GI irritation, *hepatitis*
EENT: Blurred vision
INTEG: Rash, urticaria, purpura, photosensitivity, fever
META: Hyperglycemia, hyperuricemia, increased creatinine, BUN
*HEMA: **Aplastic anemia, hemolytic anemia, leukopenia, agranulocytosis, thrombocytopenia,** neutropenia*
CV: Irregular pulse, orthostatic hypotension, palpitations, volume depletion
ELECT: Hypokalemia, hypomagnesemia, hypercalcemia, hyponatremia, hypochloremia

Contraindications: Hypersensitivity to thiazides or sulfonamides, anuria, pregnancy (D), lactation

Precautions: Hypokalemia, renal disease, hepatic disease, gout, COPD, lupus erythematosus, diabetes mellitus

Pharmacokinetics:
PO: Onset 1 hr, peak 2 hr, duration 12-24 hr, half-life 8 hr, excreted unchanged by kidneys, crosses placenta, enters breast milk

Interactions/ incompatibilities:
- Synergism: furosemide
- Increased toxicity of: lithium, nondepolarizing skeletal muscle relaxants

italic = common side effects   **bold** = life-threatening reactions

- Decreased effects of: antidiabetics, methenamine
- Decreased absorption of: thiazides, cholestyramine, colestipol
- Decreased hypotensive response: indomethacin
- Hyperglycemia, hyperuricemia, hypotension: diazoxide

Lab test interferences:
Increase: BSP retention, Ca, amylase, parathyroid test
Decrease: PBI, PSP

RESPIRATORY CARE CONSIDERATIONS:
Assess/evaluate:
- Monitor serum electrolytes, especially potassium, to assess hypokalemia, which will cause metabolic alkalosis.
- Hypokalemia can also cause muscular weakness, possibly complicating weaning from mechanical ventilation.
- Monitor ECG for cardiac arrhythmias.
- Evaluate for dehydration, especially in COPD subjects or those with excess respiratory tract secretions.
- Monitor color, consistency of sputum.
- Evaluate breath sounds and respiratory pattern for pulmonary congestion.

---

metoprolol tartrate
(met-oh´proe-lole)
Betaloc,* Lopresor,* Lopressor
Func. class.:
Antihypertensive
Chem. class.: β₁-blocker

Action: Lowers BP by β-blocking effects; elevated plasma renins are reduced; blocks β₂-adrenergic receptors in bronchial, vascular smooth muscle only at high doses

Uses: Mild to moderate hypertension, acute myocardial infarction to reduce cardiovascular mortality, angina pectoris

Dosage and routes:
Hypertension
- *Adult:* PO 50 mg bid, or 100 mg qd; may give up to 200-450 mg in divided doses
Myocardial infarction
- *Adult:* (early treatment) IV bol 5 mg q2min × 3, then 50 mg PO 15 min after last dose and q6h × 48 hr, (late treatment) PO maintenance 100 mg bid for 3 mo
Available forms: Tabs 50, 100 mg; inj IV 1 mg/ml

Side effects/adverse reactions:
CV: Hypotension, *bradycardia, CHF, palpitations,* dysrhythmias, *cardiac arrest, AV block*
CNS: Insomnia, dizziness, mental changes, hallucinations, *depression,* anxiety, headaches, nightmares, confusion, fatigue
GI: Nausea, vomiting, colitis, cramps, *diarrhea,* constipation, flatulence, dry mouth, *hiccups*
INTEG: Rash, purpura, alopecia, dry skin, urticaria, pruritus
HEMA: Agranulocytosis, eosinophilia, thrombocytopenia, purpura
EENT: Sore throat, dry burning eyes
GU: Impotence
RESP: Bronchospasm, dyspnea, wheezing

Contraindications: Hypersensitivity to β-blockers, cardiogenic shock, heart block (2nd, 3rd degree), sinus bradycardia, CHF, bronchial asthma

---

*Available in Canada only

Precautions: Major surgery, pregnancy (C), lactation, diabetes mellitus, renal disease, thyroid disease, COPD, heart failure, CAD, nonallergic bronchospasm, hepatic disease

Pharmacokinetics:
PO: Peak 2-4 hr, duration 13-19 hr, half-life 3-4 hr, metabolized in liver (metabolites), excreted in urine, crosses placenta, enters breast milk

Interactions/ incompatibilities:
■ Increased hypotension, bradycardia: reserpine, hydralazine, methyldopa, prazosin
■ Decreased antihypertensive effects: indomethacin, sympathomimetics
■ Increased hypoglycemic effects: insulin
■ Decreased bronchodilation: theophyllines, β-agonists
■ Incompatible with any drug in syringe or sol

Lab test interferences:
Increase: Liver function tests, renal function tests

RESPIRATORY CARE CONSIDERATIONS:
Assess/evaluate:
■ Avoid use with reversible airway obstruction or bronchospastic disease such as asthma or chronic bronchitis due to potential for bronchospasm (wheezing, dyspnea, complaints of chest tightness) secondary to beta-blockade; consider use of other classes of antihypertensive agents for these patients.
■ Monitor all subjects for symptoms of increased airway resistance (wheezing, tightness in chest, difficulty breathing).

■ Monitor effect on BP and pulse, especially if on positive pressure ventilatory support.
■ Assess effectiveness of beta-adrenergic bronchodilator therapy for possible antagonism and effect on BP to avoid increasing BP, if used.
■ Consider use of nonadrenergic bronchodilator such as ipratropium bromide as alternative to beta-adrenergic agents for patients to avoid positive inotropic effect.

Patient education:
■ Do not use OTC products containing α-adrenergic stimulants (nasal decongestants, OTC cold preparations) unless directed by physician
■ Caution patient that orthostatic hypotension may occur.
■ Report symptoms of CHF: difficulty breathing, especially on exertion or when lying down, night cough, swelling of extremities

metyrosine
(me-tye′roe-seen)
Demser
Func. class.: Antihypertensive
Chem. class.: Adrenergic blocker

Action: Inhibits enzyme tyrosine hydroxylase which catalyzes the first step in the production of catecholamines such as norepinephrine, resulting in decreased endogenous levels of catecholamines.

Uses: Pheochromocytoma

Dosage and routes:
■ *Adult and child >12 yr:* PO 250 mg qid, may increase by 250-500 mg qd to a max of 4 g/day in divided doses

italic = common side effects   **bold** = life-threatening reactions

Available forms: Caps 250 mg

Side effects/adverse reactions:
CNS: Sedation, drowsiness, dizziness, headache, depression, EPS, hallucinations, psychosis, agitation
INTEG: Rash, urticaria
EENT: Dry mouth, nasal stuffiness
GU: Dysuria, *oliguria, hematuria,* enuresis, impotence
GI: Nausea, vomiting, anorexia, diarrhea, abdominal pain
MISC: Breast swelling

Contraindications: Hypersensitivity, essential hypertension, children <12 yr

Precautions: Pregnancy (C), lactation, hepatic disease, renal disease

Pharmacokinetics:
PO: Onset 2 days, duration 3-4 days, half-life 3.4-3.7 hr, excreted in urine

Interactions/ incompatibilities:
■ Increased sedation: alcohol, barbiturates, antipsychotics, other CNS depressants
■ Decreased effects of: levodopa
■ Extrapyramidal effects: phenothiazines, haloperidol

Lab test interferences:
False increase: Urinary catecholamines

RESPIRATORY CARE CONSIDERATIONS:
Assess/evaluate:
■ Evaluate BP and pulse for efficacy of hypertension treatment and to avoid hypotension.
■ Avoid use with COPD or asthmatic subjects who require beta-agonists for reversible airway obstruction.

■ Assess for symptoms of CHF: edema, dyspnea, wet rales, BP.
■ Assess BP if on mechanical ventilatory support to minimize mean airway pressures which can increase hypotensive effect through impeded venous return and decreased cardiac output.

Patient education:
■ Maintain adequate fluid intake, especially with chronic pulmonary disease such as bronchitis.
■ Avoid alcohol and other CNS depressants.
■ Use caution with hazardous activities such as driving if drowsiness occurs.

mexiletine HCl
(mex-il'e-teen)
Mexitil
Func. class.: Antidysrhythmic (Class IB)
Chem. class.: Lidocaine analog

Action: Increases electrical stimulation threshold of ventricle, His-Purkinje system, which stabilizes cardiac membrane

Uses: Ventricular tachycardia, ventricular dysrhythmias during cardiac surgery, myocardial infarction

Dosage and routes:
■ *Adult:* PO 200-400 mg q8h
Available forms: Caps 150, 200, 250 mg

Side effects/adverse reactions:
CNS: Headache, dizziness, confusion, *convulsions,* tremors, psychosis, nervousness, paresthesias, weakness, fa-

tigue, coordination difficulties, change in sleep habits

EENT: Blurred vision, hearing loss, tinnitus

GI: Nausea, vomiting, anorexia, diarrhea, abdominal pain, *hepatitis*, dry mouth, peptic ulcer, altered taste, GI bleeding

CV: Hypotension, bradycardia, angina, PVCs, *heart block, cardiovascular collapse, arrest,* sinus node slowing, *left ventricular failure,* syncope, *cardiogenic shock*

RESP: Dyspnea, *fibrosis, embolism,* pneumonia

INTEG: Rash, alopecia, dry skin

HEMA: **Thrombocytopenia, leukopenia, agranulocytosis, hypoplastic anemia,** systemic lupus erythematosus syndrome

GU: Urinary hesitancy, decreased libido

MISC: Edema, arthralgia, fever

Contraindications: Hypersensitivity to amides, cardiogenic shock, blood dyscrasias, severe heart block

Precautions: Pregnancy (C), lactation, children, renal disease, liver disease, CHF, respiratory depression, myasthenia gravis

Pharmacokinetics:
PO: Peak 2-3 hr, half-life 12 hr, metabolized by liver, excreted unchanged by kidneys (10%), excreted in breast milk

Interactions/ incompatibilities:
■ Decreased effects: cimetidine
■ Decreased levels of mexiletine: phenytoin, phenobarbital, rifampin

Lab test interferences:
Increase: CPK

RESPIRATORY CARE CONSIDERATIONS:
Assess/evaluate:
■ Monitor ECG; in case of increased QT and/or widening QRS, drug should be discontinued.
■ Monitor for dehydration or hypovolemia, I&O ratio, electrolytes (Na, K, Cl).
■ Monitor BP for hypotension or hypertension, pulse rate.
■ Monitor respiratory rate and pattern (labored, dyspnea).
■ Provide resuscitation support in the event of cardiac arrest.
■ Evaluate therapeutic response: decreased dysrhythmias.

Patient education:
■ Make position change slowly to prevent orthostatic hypotension and fainting.
■ Avoid hazardous activities if dizziness or blurred vision occurs.

midazolam HCl
(mid'-az-zoe-lam)
Versed
Func. class.: General anesthetic
Chem. class.: Benzodiazepine, short-acting
Controlled Substance Schedule IV

Action: Benzodiazepines bind to specific benzodiazepine receptors in the CNS and appear to facilitate transmission of the inhibitory neurotransmitter GABA and others, to produce sleep and alter memory, motor, sensory, and cognitive functions.

Uses: Preoperative sedation, general anesthesia induction, sedation for diagnostic endo-scopic procedures, intubation

Dosage and routes:
Preoperative sedation
- *Adult:* IM 0.07 - 0.08 mg/kg ½ - 1 hr before general anesthesia
Induction of general anesthesia
- *Adult:* IV (unpremedicated patients) 0.3 - 0.35 mg/kg over 30 sec, wait 2 min, follow with 25% of initial dose if needed; (premedicated patients) 0.15 - 0.35 mg/kg over 20 - 30 sec, allow 2 min for effect
Available forms: Inj l, 5 mg/ml

Side effects/adverse reactions:
CNS: Retrograde amnesia, euphoria, confusion, headache, anxiety, insomnia, slurred speech, paresthesia, tremors, weakness, chills
RESP: Coughing, *apnea, bronchospasm, laryngospasm,* dyspnea
CV: Hypotension, PVCs, tachycardia, bigeminy, nodal rhythm
EENT: Blurred vision, nystagmus, diplopia, blocked ears, loss of balance
GI: Nausea, vomiting, increased salivation, hiccups
INTEG: Urticaria, pain, swelling at injection site, rash, pruritus

Contraindications: Pregnancy (D), hypersensitivity to benzodiazepines, shock, coma, alcohol intoxication, acute narrow-angle glaucoma

Precautions: COPD, CHF, chronic renal failure, chills, elderly, debilitated

Pharmacokinetics:
IM: Onset 15 min, peak ½ - 1 hr
IV: Onset 3 - 5 min, onset of anesthesia 1½ - 2½ min; protein binding 97%; half-life 1.2 - 12.3 hr; metabolized in liver; metabolites excreted in urine; crosses placenta, blood-brain barrier

Interactions/incompatibilities:
- Prolonged respiratory depression: alcohol, barbiturates, other CNS depressants
- Increased hypnotic effect: fentanyl, narcotic agonists, analgesics, droperidol
- Incompatible with dimenhydrinate, pentobarbital, perphenazine, prochlorperazine, rantidine

RESPIRATORY CARE CONSIDERATIONS:
Assess/evaluate:
- Monitor for possible respiratory depression, which is dose dependent.
- Note possible apnea with higher doses, including during recovery period. Monitor patient for respiratory rate and depth.
- Increased CNS depression will result when used with alcohol, tricyclic antidepressants, narcotics, barbiturates, sedatives, hypnotics.
- Avoid hazardous activities while drug action persists.
- Reversal: use the benzodiazepine receptor antagonist, flumazenil.

Patient education:
- Caution individuals that other CNS depressants, including alcohol, narcotic analgesics, cough preparations, and antihistamines, may increase effect, including respiratory depression.
- Avoid hazardous activities if drowsiness, dizziness occurs.

M

milrinone lactate
(mill-re'-none)
Primacor
Func. class.: Inotropic/
vasodilator agent with
phosphodiesterase activity
Chem. class.: Bipyridine
derivative

Action: Positive inotropic
agent with vasodilator properties; reduces preload and afterload by direct relaxation on
vascular smooth muscle

Uses: Short-term management of CHF that has not responded to other medication;
can be used with digitalis

Dosage and routes:
■ *Adult:* IV BOL 50 µg/kg
given over 10 min; start infusion of 0.375 - 0.75 µg/kg/min;
reduce dose in renal impairment
Available forms: Inj 1 mg/ml

**Side effects/adverse
reactions:**
HEMA: **Thrombocytopenia**
*MISC: Headache, hypokalemia,
tremor*
*CV: Dysrhythmias, hypotension,
chest pain*
*GI: Nausea, vomiting, anorexia,
abdominal pain,* **hepatotoxicity,**
jaundice

Contraindications: Hypersensitivity to this drug, severe
aortic disease, severe pulmonic valvular disease, acute
myocardial infarction

Precautions: Lactation, pregnancy (C), children, renal disease, hepatic disease, atrial
flutter/fibrillation, elderly

Pharmacokinetics:
IV: Onset 2 - 5 min, peak 10
min, duration variable, half-

life 4 - 6 hr, metabolized in
liver, excreted in urine as drug
and metabolites 60% - 90%

**Interactions/
incompatibilities:**
■ Excessive hypotension:
antihypertensives

RESPIRATORY CARE
CONSIDERATIONS:
Assess/evaluate:
■ Monitor blood pressure and
heart rate carefully; milrinone
can cause hypotension due to
vasodilator effect.
■ Prior vigorous diuretic
therapy may lead to hypotension due to decreases in cardiac filling pressure.
■ Monitor fluid and electrolytes; hypokalemia due to diuretic therapy can predispose
to arrhythmias.
■ Improved cardiac output
may necessitate decreases in
diuretics.
■ If on positive pressure ventilatory support, minimize
mean airway pressures to
extent possible, to maintain
good cardiac output.
■ Therapeutic response: increased cardiac output, decreased PCWP, adequate CVP,
improved systemic blood pressure, decreased dyspnea, edema.

minoxidil
(mi-nox-i-dill)
Loniten, Minodyl, Minoxidil,
Rogaine
Func. class.:
Antihypertensive
Chem. class.: Vasodilator—
peripheral

Action: Directly relaxes arteriolar smooth muscle, causing
vasodilation

Uses: Severe hypertension not responsive to other therapy (use with diuretic); topically to treat alopecia

Dosage and routes:
- *Adult:* PO 5 mg/day not to exceed 100 mg daily, usual range 10-40 mg/day in single doses
- *Child <12 yr:* (initial) 0.2 mg/kg/day; (effective range) 0.25-1 mg/kg/day; (max) 50 mg/day
Alopecia
- *Adult:* Apply topically, rub into scalp daily
Available forms: Tabs 2.5, 10 mg, top 20 mg/ml

Side effects/adverse reactions:
CV: Severe rebound hypertension, tachycardia, angina, increased T wave, *CHF, pulmonary edema, pericardial effusion,* edema, sodium, water retention
CNS: Drowsiness, dizziness, sedation, headache, depression, fatigue
GI: Nausea, vomiting
GU: Gynecomastia, breast tenderness
INTEG: Pruritus, *Stevens-Johnson syndrome,* rash, hirsutism
HEMA: Hct, Hgb, initial decrease in erythrocyte count

Contraindications: Acute MI, dissecting aortic aneurysm, hypersensitivity, pheochromocytoma

Precautions: Pregnancy (C), lactation, children, renal disease, CAD, CHF

Pharmacokinetics:
PO: Onset 30 min, peak 2-3 hr, duration 75 hr, half-life 4.2 hr, metabolized in liver, metabolites excreted in urine, feces

Interactions/ incompatibilities:
- Orthostatic hypotension: guanethidine

Lab test interferences:
Increase: Renal function studies
Decrease: Hgb/Hct/RBC

RESPIRATORY CARE CONSIDERATIONS:
Assess/evaluate:
- Evaluate BP and pulse for efficacy of hypertension treatment and to avoid hypotension.
- Evaluate BP with COPD or asthmatic subjects who require beta agonists for reversible airway obstruction.
- Assess for symptoms of CHF: edema, dyspnea, wet rales, BP.
- Assess BP if on mechanical ventilatory support to minimize mean airway pressures which can increase hypotensive effect through impeded venous return and decreased cardiac output; minimize inspiratory times and optimize flow patterns and avoid large tidal volumes.

Patient education:
- Do not use OTC products containing α-adrenergic stimulants (nasal decongestants, OTC cold preparations) unless directed by physician.
- Report symptoms of CHF: difficult breathing, especially on exertion or when lying down, night cough, swelling of extremities.
- It is necessary to quit smoking to prevent excessive vasoconstriction

*Available in Canada only

- Avoid hazardous activities until stabilized on medication; dizziness may occur
- Make position changes slowly or fainting will occur

mivacurium chloride
(miv-a-kure'ee-um)
Mivacron
Func. class.: Nondepolarizing neuromuscular blocker
Chem. class.: An isoquinoline

Action: Inhibits transmission of nerve impulses at the neuromuscular junction by binding with cholinergic receptor sites, antagonizing action of acetylcholine, and causing muscle weakness or paralysis, depending on dose.

Uses: Facilitation of endotracheal intubation, skeletal muscle relaxation during mechanical ventilation, surgery, or general anesthesia

Dosage and routes:
- *Adult:* IV 0.15 mg/kg; maintenance q15 min
- *Child:* 2-12 IV 0.2 mg/kg for a 10 min block
Available forms: 5, 10 ml single-use vial (2 mg/ml); premixed infusion in D_5W 50 ml flex container

Side effects/adverse reactions:
CV: Decreased BP, bradycardia, tachycardia
RESP: Prolonged apnea, bronchospasm, wheezing, respiratory depression
EENT: Diplopia
MS: Weakness, prolonged skeletal muscle relaxation, *paralysis*
INTEG: Rash, urticaria

Contraindications: Hypersensitivity

Precautions: Pregnancy (C), renal or hepatic disease, lactation, children < 3 mo, fluid and electrolyte imbalances, neuromuscular disease, respiratory disease, obesity, elderly

Pharmacokinetics: Rapidly hydrolyzed by plasma cholinesterases, peak 2-3 min, reversal within 15-30 min

Interactions/incompatibilities:
- Increased neuromuscular blockade: aminoglycosides, quinidine, local anesthetics, polymyxin
- Antibiotics, enflurane, isoflurane, tetracyclines, halothane, Mg, colistin, procainamide, bacitracin, lincomycin, clindamycin, lithium

RESPIRATORY CARE CONSIDERATIONS:
Assess/evaluate:
- Provide airway and ventilatory support before administering drug.
- Note possible interaction with the following antibiotics, which can increase neuromuscular blockade: the aminoglycosides, the polymyxins, clindamycin, and lincomycin.
- Use with mechanical ventilation; assess patient for adequate and preferably optimal ventilator settings *before* paralyzing. If patient is "fighting" the ventilator, provide adequately high flow rates and tidal volumes, short inspiratory times, and reasonable I:E ratios, check the sensitivity in assist-control mode, provide sufficiently high rates to avoid

italic = common side effects   **bold** = life-threatening reactions

patient fatigue; consider paralysis if these measures fail.

- Assess ventilator patients for pain, hypoxemia, or ventilator malfunction, if restless and anxious, before instituting muscle paralysis.
- Assess need of patient and provide for pain control and sedation during neuromuscular blockade; *neuromuscular blocking agents do not provide analgesia or sedation.*
- Close eyelids and provide eye lubricant during prolonged paralysis.
- Since usual signs of pain or anxiety (restlessness, tachynea, distress, thrashing) are blocked, monitor vital signs closely and overall patient appearance and state to detect problems (e.g., IV infiltration).
- Check ventilator alarm settings for sufficient limits and sensitivity; a disconnect alarm is critical.
- Assess reversal of drug before attempting to wean from mechanical ventilatory support.

Administer:
- Administer by IV, not by IM, for more consistent absorption and distribution and to avoid the pain associated with IM injection of the drug.
- Reversal: neostigmine or edrophonium, preceded by atropine to inhibit muscarinic response especially in upper airway.

moricizine
(mor iss' i-zeen)
Ethmozine
Func. class.: Antidysrhythmic, class I
Chem. class.: Phenothiazine

Action: Decreased rate of rise of action potential, prolonging refractory period and shortening the action potential duration; depression of inward influx if sodium mediates the effects; drug may slow atrial and AV nodal conduction

Uses: Symptomatic vertricular and life-threatening dysrhythmias

Dosage and routes:
- *Adult:* PO 10-15 mg/kg/day in 2-3 divided doses
Available forms: Film-coated tabs 200, 250, 300 mg

Side effects/adverse reactions:
GI: Nausea, abdominal pain, vomiting, diarrhea
CNS: Dizziness, headache, fatigue, perioral numbness, euphoria, nervousness, sleep disorders, depression, tinnitus, fatigue
RESP: Dyspnea, hyperventilation, *apnea*, asthma, pharyngitis, cough
GU: Sexual dysfunction, difficult urination, dysuria, incontinence
CV: Palpitations, chest pain, *CHF*, hypertension, syncope, dysrythmias, bradycardia, *MI*, thrombophlebitis
MISC: Sweating, musculoskeletal pain

Contraindications: 2nd or 3rd degree AV block, right bundle branch block, cardiogenic shock, hypersensitivity,

Precautions: CHF, hypokalemia, hyperkalemia, sick sinus syndrome, pregnancy (B), lactation, children, impaired hepatic and renal function, cardiac dysfunction

Pharmacokinetics: Half-life 1.5-3.5 hr, peak 0.5-2.2 hr, metabolized by liver, metabolites excreted in feces and urine, protein binding >90%

Interactions/ incompatibilities:
■ Increased plasma levels of moricizine: amantadine
■ Digoxin or propranolol may enhance some of cardiac effects of moricizine; moricizine may decrease effects of theophylline

Lab test interferences:
Increase: CPK

RESPIRATORY CARE CONSIDERATIONS

Assess/evaluate:
■ Monitor ECG; in case of increased QT and/or widening QRS; drug should be discontinued.
■ Assess for dehydration or hypovolemia, I&O ratio, electrolytes (Na, K, Cl).
■ BP for hypotension or hypertension, pulse rate.
■ Monitor respiratory rate and pattern for dyspnea, hyperventilation, apnea, asthmatic response, pharnygitis, cough, sinusitis.
■ Provide resuscitation support in the event of cardiac arrest, life threatening arrhythmias.
■ Evaluate therapeutic response: decreased dysrhythmias.

Patient education:
■ Make position change slowly to prevent orthostatic hypotension and fainting.
■ Avoid hazardous activities if dizziness or blurred vision occurs.

italic = common side effects

nadolol
(nay-doe'-lole)
Corgard
Func. class.: Antihypertensive, antianginal
Chem. class.: Nonselective β-adrenergic receptor blocker

Action: Long-acting, nonselective β-adrenergic receptor blocking agent; blockade of beta$_1$ cardiac receptors causes a decrease in cardiac output and myocardial work.

Uses: Chronic stable angina pectoris, mild to moderate hypertension, prophylaxis of migraine headaches

Dosage and routes:
■ *Adult:* PO 40 mg qd, increase by 40-80 mg q3-7d; maintenance 40-240 mg/day for angina, 40-320 mg/day for hypertension
Available forms: Oral tabs 20, 40, 80, 120, 160 mg

Side effects/adverse reactions:
RESP: Dyspnea, respiratory dysfunction, *bronchospasm,* cough, wheezing, nasal stuffiness, pharyngitis, *laryngospasm*
CV: Bradycardia, hypotension, *CHF,* palpitations, AV block, chest pain, peripheral ischemia, flushing, edema, vasodilation, conduction disturbances
HEMA: Agranulocytosis, thrombocytopenia
GI: Nausea, vomiting, diarrhea, colitis, constipation, cramps, dry mouth, flatulence, hepatomegaly, pancreatitis, taste distortion

bold = life-threatening reactions

218   naphazoline HCl

INTEG: Rash, pruritus, fever
CNS: Depression, hallucinations, dizziness, fatigue, lethargy, paresthesias, headache
EENT: Sore throat

Contraindications: Hypersensitivity to this drug, cardiac failure, cardiogenic shock, 2nd or 3rd degree heart block, bronchospastic disease, sinus bradycardia, CHF, COPD

Precautions: Diabetes mellitus, pregnancy (C), renal disease, lactation, hyperthyroidism, peripheral vascular disease, myasthenia gravis

Pharmacokinetics:
PO: Onset variable, peak 3-4 hr, duration 17-24 hr, half-life 16-20 hr, not metabolized, excreted in urine (unchanged), bile, breast milk

Interactions/ incompatibilities:
▪ Increased effects of: reserpine, digitalis, ergots, neuromuscular blocking agents, calcium channel blockers
▪ Increased hypotensive effects: other hypotensive agents, diuretics, phenothiazines
▪ Decreased effects of: norepinephrine, xanthines, isoproterenol, thyroid

Lab test interferences:
Increase: Serum K, serum uric acid, ALT/AST, alk phosphatase, LDH blood glucose, cholesterol

RESPIRATORY CARE CONSIDERATIONS:
Assess/evaluate:
▪ Avoid use with reversible airway obstruction or bronchospastic disease such as asthma or chronic bronchitis due to potential for broncho-

spasm (wheezing, dyspnea, complaints of chest tightness) secondary to beta-blockade; consider use of other classes of antihypertensive agents for these patients.
▪ Monitor all subjects for symptoms of increased airway resistance (wheezing, tightness in chest, difficulty breathing).
▪ Monitor effect on BP and pulse, especially if on positive pressure ventilatory support.
▪ Assess effectiveness of beta-adrenergic bronchodilator therapy for possible antagonism and effect on BP to avoid increasing BP, if used.
▪ Consider use of nonadrenergic bronchodilator such as ipratropium bromide as alternative to beta-adrenergic agents for patients to avoid positive inotropic effect.

Patient education:
▪ Do not use OTC products containing α-adrenergic stimulants (nasal decongestants, OTC cold preparations) unless directed by physician.
▪ Caution patient that orthostatic hypotension may occur.
▪ Report symptoms of CHF: difficulty breathing, especially on exertion or when lying down, night cough, swelling of extremities.

naphazoline HCl
(naf-az'oh-leen)
Privine
Func. class.: Nasal decongestant
Chem. class.: Sympathomimetic amine

Action: Produces vasoconstriction (rapid, long-acting)

*Available in Canada only

of arterioles through alpha-adrenergic stimulation, thereby decreasing fluid exudation, mucosal engorgement

Uses: Nasal congestion

Dosage and routes:
- *Adult:* Instill 2 gtts or sprays to nasal mucosa q3-4h
- *Child 6-12 yr:* Instill 1-2 gtts or sprays, repeat q3-4h prn, not to exceed 5 days
Available forms: Sol 0.025, 0.05%

Side effects/adverse reactions:
GI: Nausea, vomiting, anorexia
EENT: Irritation, burning, sneezing, stinging, dryness, rebound congestion
INTEG: Contact dermatitis
CNS: Anxiety, restlessness, tremors, weakness, insomnia, dizziness, fever, headache

Contraindications: Hypersensitivity to sympathomimetic amines

Precautions: Child <6 yr, elderly, diabetes, cardiovascular disease, hypertension, hyperthyroidism, increased ICP, prostatic hypertrophy, pregnancy (C), glaucoma

Interactions/ incompatibilities:
- Hypertension: MAOIs, β-adrenergic blockers
- Hypotension: methyldopa, mecamylamine, reserpine

RESPIRATORY CARE CONSIDERATIONS:
Assess/evaluate:
- Therapeutic response: decreased nasal congestion.
- Assess subject's BP for possible increases if using beta agonist bronchodilator simultaneously.

Patient education:
- Environmental humidification may help to decrease nasal congestion, dryness.
- Warn patient that rebound nasal congestion can occur.
- Use for short-term symptoms only; prolonged rhinitis should be evaluated by physician, ENT specialist, or allergist.

nedocromil inhaler
(ned-o-kroe′-mill)
Tilade
Func. class.: Antiasthmatic, inflammatory mediator inhibitor
Chem. class.: disodium salt of a pyranoquinolone

See Section III: Aerosol Agents for Oral Inhalation

neostigmine bromide/neostigmine methylsulfate
(nee-oh-stig′meen)
Neostigmine Bromide, Neostigmine Methylsulfate, Prostigmin
Func. class.: Cholinergic stimulant, cholinesterase inhibitor
Chem. class.: Quaternary compound

Action: An indirect-acting cholinergic, which inhibits cholinesterase, preventing the destruction of acetylcholine; this increases concentration at sites where acetylcholine is released and facilitates neuromuscular transmission

Uses: Myasthenia gravis, non-depolarizing neuromuscular blocker antagonist, bladder distention, postoperative ileus

Dosage and routes:
Myasthenia gravis
- *Adult:* PO 15-375 mg/day; IM/IV 0.5-2 mg q1-3h
- *Child:* PO 2 mg/kg/day q3-4h

Tubocurarine antagonist
- *Adult:* IV 0.5-2 mg slowly, may repeat if needed (give 0.6-1.2 mg atropine before this drug)

Abdominal distention/ postoperative ileus
- *Adult:* IM/SC 0.25-1 mg q4-6h depending on condition

Available forms: Tabs 15 mg; inj IM, SC, IV 1:1000, 1:2000, 1:4000

Side effects/adverse reactions:
INTEG: Rash, urticaria, flushing
CNS: Dizziness, headache, sweating, weakness, *convulsions,* incoordination, *paralysis,* drowsiness, LOC
GI: Nausea, *diarrhea, vomiting, cramps,* increased peristalsis, salivary and gastric secretions
CV: Tachycardia, dysrhythmias, bradycardia, hypotension, AV block, ECG changes, *cardiac arrest,* syncope
GU: Frequency, incontinence, urgency
RESP: Respiratory depression, bronchospasm, constriction, laryngospasm, respiratory arrest, dyspnea
EENT: Miosis, blurred vision, lacrimation, visual changes

Contraindications: Obstruction of intestine, renal system, pregnancy (C), bromide sensitivity, peritonitis

Precautions: Bradycardia, hypotension, seizure disorders, bronchial asthma, coronary occlusion, hyperthyroidism, dysrhythmias, peptic ulcer, megacolon, poor GI motility, lactation, children

Pharmacokinetics:
PO: Onset 45-75 min, duration 2½-4 hr
IM/SC: Onset 10-30 min, duration 2½-4 hr
IV: Onset 4-8 min; duration 2-4 hr, metabolized in liver, excreted in urine

Interactions/ incompatibilities:
- Decreased action of: gallamine, metocurine, pancuronium, tubocurarine, atropine
- Increased action of: decamethonium, succinylcholine
- Decreased action of neostigmine: aminoglycosides, anesthetics, procainamide, quinidine, mecamylamine, polymyxin, magnesium
- Considered incompatible with drugs in sol or syringe

RESPIRATORY CARE CONSIDERATIONS:
Assess/evaluate:
- Therapeutic response: reversal of neuromuscular blockade or improved muscle function, especially diaphragmatic contractile force as evidenced by tidal volume, vital capacity, grip strength.
- In reversing neuromuscular blockade, maintain airway and ventilatory support until complete recovery of adequate ventilation is seen in spontaneous respiratory rate and pattern.
- Monitor for exacerbation of asthma or airway resistance in COPD subjects, due to parasympathetic induced bronchoconstriction.
- Assess respiratory rate and pattern, breath sounds for wheezing.

■ Assess subjective response of patient for difficulty in breathing, tightness in chest.
■ Assess pulse for bradycardia and BP for decrease.
■ Note: use of a cholinergic agent can intensify and prolong a depolarizing blockade induced by succinylcholine, due to the inactivation of acetylcholine needed for neuromuscular transmission.

nicardipine HCl
(nye-card′i-peen)
Cardene, Cardene IV, Cardene SR
Func. class.: Calcium channel blocker
Chem. class.: Dihydropyridine

Action: Inhibits calcium ion influx across cell membrane during cardiac depolarization; produces relaxation of coronary vascular smooth muscle, peripheral vascular smooth muscle; dilates coronary vascular arteries; increases myocardial oxygen delivery in patients with vasospastic angina

Uses: Chronic stable angina pectoris, hypertension

Dosage and routes:
Angina
■ *Adult:* PO 20 mg tid initially, may increase after 3 days (range 20-40 mg tid)
Hypertension
■ *Adult:* PO 20 mg tid initially, then increase after 3 days (range 20-40 mg tid); IV dilute to 0.1 mg/ml, give 5 mg/hr initially, then increase by 2.5 mg/hr q15 min to a maximum of 15 mg/hr

Available forms: Caps 20, 30 mg; caps SR 30, 45, 60 mg; inj 2.5 mg/ml (10 ml)

Side effects/adverse reactions:
CV: Dysrhythmia, edema, CHF, bradycardia, hypotension, palpitations, *MI, pulmonary edema*
GI: Nausea, vomiting, diarrhea, gastric upset, constipation, *hepatitis,* abdominal cramps
GU: Nocturia, polyuria, *acute renal failure*
INTEG: Rash, pruritus, urticaria, photosensitivity, hair loss
CNS: Headache, fatigue, drowsiness, dizziness, anxiety, depression, weakness, insomnia, confusion, paresthesia, somnolence
OTHER: Blurred vision, flushing, nasal congestion, sweating, shortness of breath, gynecomastia, hyperglycemia, sexual difficulties

Contraindications: Sick sinus syndrome, 2nd or 3rd degree heart block, hypotension less than 90 mm Hg systolic, hypersensitivity

Precautions: CHF, hypotension, hepatic injury, pregnancy (C), lactation, children, renal disease, elderly

Pharmacokinetics:
PO: Onset 10 min, peak 1-2 hr, half-life 2-5 hr, metabolized by liver, excreted in urine (98% as metabolites)

Interactions/ incompatibilities:
■ Increased effects of: digitalis, neuromuscular blocking agents, theophylline
■ Increased effects of nicardipine: cimetidine

N

RESPIRATORY CARE CONSIDERATIONS:
Assess/evaluate:
- Therapeutic response: corrected arrhythmia, decreased anginal pain, decreased BP.
- Monitor cardiovascular status: BP, pulse, respiration, ECG.
- Evaluate presence of adverse effects, especially dizziness or other signs of hypotension, bradycardia.
- If on positive pressure ventilatory support, monitor cardiac output and/or BP, and adjust level of positive pressure to extent possible, if necessary to maintain adequate cardiac output.
- Monitor BP if beta agonists are required to treat airway obstruction.
- Consider use of anticholinergic agent such as ipratropium bromide as an alternative to beta agonists, if bronchodilator therapy is needed; aerosol inhalation (MDI, SVN, DPI) of adrenergic bronchodilators will generally give lower systemic levels and fewer cardiovascular effects.

Patient education:
- Note: hand tremor can occur, such as seen with beta agonist bronchodilators.
- Change position slowly to avoid orthostatic hypotension.

nicotine polacrilex (nicotine resin complex)
(nik′o-teen poe-lah-kri′-lecks)
Nicorette, Nicorette DS
Func. class.: Smoking deterrent
Chem. class.: Ganglionic cholinergic agonist

Action: Nicotine polacrilex is nicotine bound to a resin in a chewing gum base. Nicotine stimulates acetylcholine receptors at autonomic ganglia, and in the adrenal medulla, the neuromuscular junction, and the brain. Generally sympathetic effects predominate with ganglionic agonist activity and from release of circulating epinephrine: tachycardia, increased blood pressure, peripheral vasoconstriction. Fine motor tremor and hand unsteadiness occur. Nausea and vomiting occur until tolerance develops, probably due to toxic medullary stimulation. Other CNS effects include increased alertness and cognitive performance and a "reward" effect via stimulation of the limbic system; these may be the basis for the positive reinforcement with use of nicotine. Use of nicotine polacrilex can satisfy cravings for nicotine in addicted subjects with lower plasma levels than those with smoking.

Uses: Withdrawal from nicotine in addicted individuals as an alternative to cigarette smoking

Dosage and routes:
- *Adult:* Gum 1 piece chewed × ½ hr as needed to abstain from smoking, not to exceed 30/day
Available forms: 2 mg/piece of gum

Side effects/adverse reactions:
RESP: Breathing difficulty, cough, hoarseness, sneezing, wheezing
EENT: Jaw ache, irritation in buccal cavity

*Available in Canada only

CNS: Dizziness, vertigo, insomnia, headache, confusion, convulsions, depression, euphoria, numbness, tinnitus
GI: Nausea, vomiting, anorexia, indigestion, diarrhea, abdominal pain, constipation, eructation
CV: Dysrhythmias, tachycardia, palpitations, edema, flushing, hypertension

Contraindications: Hypersensitivity, immediate post MI recovery period, severe angina pectoris, pregnancy (X)

Precautions: Vasospastic disease, dysrhythmias, diabetes mellitus, children, hyperthyroidism, pheochromocytoma, coronary disease, esophagitis, peptic ulcer, lactation, children, hepatic/renal disease

Pharmacokinetics: Onset 15-30 min, metabolized in liver, excreted in urine, half-life 2-3 hr, 30-120 hr (terminal)

Interactions/ incompatibilities:
- Decreased absorption: glutethimide
- Increased absorption: SC insulin
- Decreased metabolism of: propoxyphene
- Smoking cessation increases diuretic effects of: furosemide
- Increased blood levels with cessation of smoking: caffeine, theophylline, petazocine, imipramine, oxazepam, propranolol, acetaminophen

RESPIRATORY CARE CONSIDERATIONS:
Assess/evaluate:
- Therapeutic response: decrease in urge to smoke, decreased need for gum after 3-6 mo.

- Monitor for adverse reaction: irritation of buccal cavity, dislike of taste, jaw ache.
- Monitor cardiovascular status (heart rate, rhythm, blood pressure) with use of nicotine, especially if on beta agonists for airway obstruction, to avoid hypertension, tachycardia, cardiac irritation.

Patient education:
- Chew gum slowly for 30 min to promote buccal absorption of the drug; do not chew more than 45 min.
- The gum is as toxic as cigarettes; it is to be used only to deter smoking.
- Cigarette smoking or other tobacco forms, such as snuff and chewing tobacco, will add further nicotine to the system and can increase its effects.
- Do not use during pregnancy; birth defects may occur.
- Review all aspects of drug; give package insert to patient and explain.
- Advise considering the use of the nicotine drug in the context of a smoking cessation program to maximize chance of withdrawal from smoking.
- Use of beta agonists may cause or worsen hand tremor.

nicotine transdermal system
Habitrol, Nicoderm, Nicotrol, Prostep
Func. class.: Smoking deterrent
Chem. class.: Ganglionic cholinergic agonist

Action: Nicotine stimulates acetylcholine receptors at autonomic ganglia and in the adrenal medulla, the neuromuscular junction, and the brain. Generally sympathetic effects predominate with ganglionic agonist activity and from release of circulating epinephrine: tachycardia, increased blood pressure, peripheral vasoconstriction. Fine motor tremor and hand unsteadiness occur. Nausea and vomiting occur until tolerance develops, probably due to toxic medullary stimulation. Other CNS effects include increased alertness and cognitive performance and a "reward" effect via stimulation of the limbic system; these may be the basis for the positive reinforcement with use of nicotine. Use of nicotine transdermal patch can satisfy cravings for nicotine in addicted subjects with lower plasma levels than those with smoking.

Uses: Deter cigarette smoking and smoking cessation

Dosage and routes:
- *Nicotrol:* 15 mg/day × 12 wk; 10 mg/day × 2 wk; 5 mg/day × 2 wk
- *Prostep:* 22 mg/day × 4-8 wk 11 mg/day × 2-4 wk
Available forms: Transdermal patch delivering 7, 14, 21 mg, 15 mg, 10 mg, 5 mg, 22 mg, and 11 mg/day patches depending on product

Side effects/adverse reactions:
RESP: Cough, pharyngitis, sinusitis
MISC: Back pain, pain, chest pain
INTEG: Erythema, pruritus, burning at application site, cutaneous hypersensitivity, sweating, rash

GI: Diarrhea, dyspepsia, constipation, nausea, abdominal pain, vomiting
MS: Arthralgia, myalgia
EENT: Dry mouth, abnormal taste
CNS: Abnormal dreams, insomnia, nervousness, headache, dizziness, paresthesia

Contraindications: Hypersensitivity, children, pregnancy (D), nonsmokers, during immediate postmyocardial infarction period, life-threatening dysrhythmias, severe or worsening angina pectoris

Precautions: Skin disease, angina pectoris, myocardial infarction, renal or hepatic insufficiency, peptic ulcer, accelerated hypertension, serious cardiac dysrhythmias, hyperthyroidism, pheochromocytoma, insulin-dependent diabetes, elderly

Pharmacokinetics: Half-life 3-4 hr, protein binding <5%, 30% is excreted unchanged in urine

Interactions/ incompatibilities:
- Decreased absorption: glutethimide
- Decreased dose at cessation of smoking: acetaminophen, caffeine, imipramine, oxazepam, pentazocine, propranolol, theophylline, insulin, adrenergic antagonists
- Increased dose at cessation of smoking: adrenergic agonists
- Decreased metabolism of: propoxyphene
- Increased diuretic effects of: furosemide
- Increased absorption: SC insulin

RESPIRATORY CARE CONSIDERATIONS:
Assess/evaluate:
- Therapeutic response: decrease in urge to smoke, absence of nicotine withdrawal symptoms.
- Monitor for adverse reactions: irritation, pruritus, burning at patch site.
- Monitor BP when initiating drug therapy for increases; evaluate if used with adrenergic bronchodilators or anticholinergic bronchodilators.

Patient education:
- Discuss all aspects of drug; give package insert to patient and explain.
- The patch is as toxic as cigarettes; it is to be used only to deter smoking.
- Do not use during pregnancy; birth defects may occur.
- Smoking during use of drug can increase level of nicotine in body, causing toxic reaction (tremor, increased heart rate, vasoconstriction).
- Use of beta agonists may cause or worsen hand tremor.
- Advise considering the use of the nicotine drug in the context of a smoking cessation program, to maximize chance of withdrawal from smoking.

nifedipine
(nye-fed'i-peen)
Adalat, Nifedipine, Procardia, Procardia XL
Func. class.: Calcium-channel blocker
Chem. class.: Dihydropyridine

Action: Inhibits calcium ion influx across cell membrane during cardiac depolarization; relaxes coronary vascular smooth muscle; dilates coronary arteries; increases myocardial oxygen delivery in patients with vasospastic angina; dilates peripheral arteries

Uses: Chronic stable angina pectoris, vasospastic angina, hypertension (sus rel only)

Dosage and routes:
- *Adult PO immediate release:* 10 mg tid, increase in 10 mg increments q4-6h, not to exceed 180 mg/24h or single dose of 30 mg
Adult PO sus rel: 30-60 mg/qd, may increase q7-14d, doses >120 mg not recommended
Available forms: Caps 10, 20 mg, tabs sus rel 30, 60, 90 mg

Side effects/adverse reactions:
CNS: Headache, fatigue, drowsiness, dizziness, anxiety, depression, weakness, insomnia, lightheadedness, paresthesia, tinnitus, blurred vision, nervousness
CV: Dysrhythmias, edema, CHF, hypotension, palpitations, *MI, **pulmonary edema,** tachycardia
GI: Nausea, vomiting, diarrhea, gastric upset, constipation, increased liver function studies, dry mouth
GU: Nocturia, polyuria
INTEG: Rash, pruritus, flushing, photosensitivity, hair loss
MISC: Flushing, sexual difficulties, cough, fever, chills

Contraindications: Hypersensitivity

Precautions: CHF, hypotension, sick sinus syndrome, 2nd or 3rd degree heart block, hypotension less than 90 mm Hg systolic, hepatic injury,

---

italic = common side effects   **bold** = life-threatening reactions

pregnancy (C), lactation, children, renal disease

Pharmacokinetics: Well absorbed PO
PO-SR: Duration 24 hrs
PO: Onset 20 min, peak ½-6 hr, duration 6-8 hrs, half-life 2-5 hr, metabolized by liver, excreted in urine (98% as metabolites)

Interactions/incompatibilities:
■ Increased effects of: theophylline, β-blockers, antihypertensives, digitalis
■ Increased nifedipine level: cimetidine
■ Decreased effects: quinidine

RESPIRATORY CARE CONSIDERATIONS:
Assess/evaluate:
■ Therapeutic response: decreased anginal pain, decreased BP
■ Monitor cardiovascular status: BP, pulse, respiration, ECG.
■ Monitor for adverse effects, especially dizziness or other signs of hypotension, bradycardia.
■ If on positive pressure ventilatory support, monitor cardiac output and/or BP and adjust level of positive pressure to extent possible, if necessary to maintain adequate cardiac output.
■ Monitor blood pressure if beta agonists are required to treat airway obstruction.
■ Consider use of anticholinergic agent such as ipratropium bromide as an alternative to beta agonists, if bronchodilator therapy is needed; aerosol inhalation (MDI, SVN, DPI) of adrenergic bronchodilators will generally give lower systemic

levels and fewer cardiovascular effects.

Patient education:
■ Note: hand tremor can occur, such as seen with beta agonist bronchodilators.
■ Change position slowly to avoid orthostatic hypotension.

nitroglycerin

(nye-troe-gli'ser-in)
Nitro-Bid IV, Nitroglycerin, Tridil, Nitrostat, Nitro-Bid Plateau Caps, Nitrocine Timecaps, Nitroglyn, Nitrong, Nitro-Bid, Nitrol, Deponit, Minitran, Nitrodisc, Nitro-Dur, Nitroglycerin Transdermal, Nitrocine, Transderm-Nitro, Nitrolingual, Nitrogard
Func. class.: Coronary vasodilator
Chem. class.: Nitrate

Action: Decreases preload, afterload, which is responsible for decreasing left ventricular end-diastolic pressure, systemic vascular resistance

Uses: Chronic stable angina pectoris, prophylaxis of angina pain, CHF associated with acute MI, controlled hypotension in surgical procedures

Dosage and routes:
■ *Adult:* SL dissolve tablet under tongue when pain begins; may repeat q5min until relief occurs; take no more than 3 tabs/15 min; use 1 tab prophylactically 5-10 min before activities; sus cap q6-12h on empty stomach; TOP 1-2 in q8h, increase to 4 in q4h as needed; IV 5 µg/min, then increase by 5 µg/min q3-5min; if no response after 20 µg/min, increase by 10-20

μg/min until desired response; trans apply a pad qd to a site free of hair
Available forms: Buccal tabs 1, 2, 3 mg; aero 0.4 mg/meter spray; caps 2.5, 6.5, 9 mg; tabs ext rel 2.6, 6.5, 9 mg; inj 0.5, 0.8, 5, 10 mg/ml; SL tabs 0.15, 0.3, 0.4, 0.6 mg; top oint 2%; trans derm syst 2.5, 5, 7.5, 10, 15 mg/24 hr

Side effects/adverse reactions:

CV: Postural hypotension, tachycardia, *collapse,* syncope
GI: Nausea, vomiting
INTEG: Pallor, sweating, rash
CNS: Headache, flushing, dizziness

Contraindications: Hypersensitivity to this drug or nitrites, severe anemia, increased intracranial pressure, cerebral hemorrhage

Precautions: Postural hypotension, pregnancy (C), lactation

Pharmacokinetics:

SUS REL: Onset 20-45 min, duration 3-8 hr
SL: Onset 1-3 min, duration 30 min
TRANS DER: Onset ½-1 hr, duration 12-24 hr
IV: Onset immediately, duration variable
TRANSMUC: Onset 3 min, duration 10-30 min
AEROSOL: Onset 2 min, duration 30-60 min
TOP OINT: Onset 30-60 min, duration 2-12 hr
Metabolized by liver, excreted in urine

Interactions/ incompatibilities:

■ Increased effects: β-blockers, diuretics, antihypertensives, anticoagulants, alcohol

■ Decreased heparin: IV nitroglycerin
■ Incompatible with any drug in sol or syringe

RESPIRATORY CARE CONSIDERATIONS:

Assess/evaluate:

■ Therapeutic response: relief of chest pain (angina).
■ Monitor BP, pulse, and ECG if available.
■ Provide cardiopulmonary resuscitation if ventricular fibrillation or cardiac arrest occurs due to acute MI.
■ Note: alcohol or calcium channel blockers may increase risk of hypotension.
■ Evaluate for formation of methemoglobin and oxygen transport to tissues in case of overdose or genetically abnormal hemoglobins.
■ Monitor respiratory status (rate, pattern, auscultation, patient report of dyspnea) for signs of CHF.

Patient education:

■ Prolonged chest pain may indicate MI; seek emergency treatment.
■ Make position changes slowly to prevent orthostatic hypotension.
■ Use analgesic (aspirin, acetaminophen) if headache occurs.

nitroprusside sodium
(nye-troe-pruss′ide)
Nitropress, Nipride, Sodium Nitroprusside
Func. class.: Antihypertensive
Chem. class.: Peripheral vasodilator

Action: Directly relaxes arteriolar, venous smooth muscle, resulting in reduction in cardiac preload, afterload

Uses: Hypertensive crisis, to decrease bleeding by creating hypotension during surgery, acute CHF

Dosage and routes:
- *Adult:* IV INF dissolve 50 mg in 2-3 ml of D_5W, then dilute in 250-1000 ml of D_5W; run at 0.5-8 µg/kg/min
Available forms: Inj IV 50 mg

Side effects/adverse reactions:
GI: Nausea, vomiting, abdominal pain
CNS: Dizziness, headache, agitation, twitching, decreased reflexes, *LOC,* restlessness
EENT: Tinnitus, blurred vision
GU: Impotence
INTEG: Pain, irritation at injection site, sweating
CV: Palpitation, severe hypotension, dyspnea
MISC: Cyanide, thiocyanate toxicity

Contraindications: Hypersensitivity, hypertension (compensatory)

Precautions: Pregnancy (C), lactation, children, fluid, electrolyte imbalances, hepatic disease, renal disease, hypothyroidism, elderly

Pharmacokinetics:
IV: Onset 1-2 min, duration 1-10 min, half-life 4 days in patients with abnormal renal function, metabolized in liver, excreted in urine

Interactions/ incompatibilities:
- Severe hypotension: ganglionic blockers, volatile liquid anesthetics, halothane, enflurane, circulatory depressants
- Incompatible with any drug in syringe or sol

RESPIRATORY CARE CONSIDERATIONS:
Assess/evaluate:
- Evaluate BP and pulse for efficacy of hypertension treatment and to avoid hypotension.
- Evaluate BP with COPD or asthmatic subjects who require beta agonists for reversible airway obstruction.
- Assess BP if on mechanical ventilatory support to minimize mean airway pressures which can increase hypotensive effect through impeded venous return and decreased cardiac output.
- Note: alcohol or calcium channel blockers may increase risk of hypotension.
- Evaluate thiocyanate levels and oxygen transport to tissues (acid-base balance, lactic acidosis, mixed venous O_2 if available).

norepinephrine injection
(nor-ep-i-nef'rin)
Levophed
Func. class.: Adrenergic
Chem. class.: Catecholamine

Action: Acts on α receptors, causing vasoconstriction in blood vessels; BP is elevated, coronary blood flow improves, cardiac output increases; also causes increased contractility and heart rate by acting on β receptors in heart

Uses: Acute hypotension

Dosage and routes:
- *Adult:* IV INF 8-12 µg/min titrated to BP
Available forms: Inj IV 1 mg/ml

Side effects/adverse reactions:
CNS: Headache, anxiety, dizziness, insomnia, restlessness, tremor
CV: Palpitations, tachycardia, hypertension, ectopic beats, angina
GI: Nausea, vomiting
INTEG: Necrosis, tissue sloughing with extravasation, **gangrene**
RESP: Dyspnea
GU: Decreased urine output

Contraindications: Hypersensitivity, ventricular fibrillation, tachydysrhythmias, pheochromocytoma, pregnancy (D)

Precautions: Lactation, arterial embolism, peripheral vascular disease, hypertension, hyperthyroidism, elderly, heart disease

Pharmacokinetics:
IV: Onset 1-2 min, metabolized in liver, excreted in urine (inactive metabolites), crosses placenta

Interactions/ incompatibilities:
■ Do not use within 2 wk of MAOIs, or hypertensive crisis may result
■ Dysrhythmias: general anesthetics
■ Decreased action of norepinephrine: αblockers
■ Increased BP: oxytocics
■ Increased pressor effect: tricyclic antidepressant, MAOIs
■ Incompatible with alkaline solutions: Na, HCO₃

RESPIRATORY CARE CONSIDERATIONS:
Assess/evaluate:
■ Therapeutic response: increased BP with stabilization.

■ Monitor BP and pulse rate for possible excess increase in BP if administering adrenergic bronchodilators.
■ Evaluate tissue oxygen transport based on cardiac output and arterial O₂ content; correct any hypovolemia as quickly as possible to maintain BP and adequate tissue perfusion.
■ If mechanical ventilatory support is instituted/present, minimize airway pressures to extent possible to avoid inhibiting venous return with high pressures and causing decrease in cardiac output and BP.

nylidrin HCl
(nye'li-drin)
Arlidin, Rolidrin
Func. class.: Peripheral vasodilator, β-adrenergic agonist
Chem. class.: β-adrenergic agonist—phenylisopropylamine

Action: Acts on β-adrenergic receptors to dilate arterioles in skeletal muscles; increases cardiac output; may have direct vasodilatory effect on vascular smooth muscle

Uses: Arteriosclerosis obliterans, thromboangiitis obliterans, diabetic vascular disease, night leg cramps, Raynaud's disease, ischemic ulcer, frostbite, acrocyanosis, acroparesthesia, thrombophlebitis, primary cochlear cell ischemia, cochlear stria ischemia, muscular or ampullar ischemia, other disturbances from labyrinth artery spasm or obstruction

Dosage and routes:
- *Adult:* PO 3-12 mg tid or qid
Available forms: Tabs 6, 12 mg

Side effects/adverse reactions:
CV: Postural hypotension, palpitations
CNS: Dizziness, anxiety, tremors, weakness, nervousness
GI: Nausea, vomiting
INTEG: Flushing

Contraindications: Hypersensitivity, paroxysmal tachycardia, progressive angina pectoris, thyrotoxicosis, MI

Precautions: CHF, pregnancy (C)

Pharmacokinetics:
PO: Onset 10 min, peak 30 min, duration 2 hr, slowly metabolized in liver, excreted in urine, therapeutic effect may take several weeks

Interactions/ incompatibilities:
- Increased hypotension: phenothiazines, other vasodilators, antihypertensives

RESPIRATORY CARE CONSIDERATIONS:
Assess/evaluate:
- Monitor BP, pulse during treatment until stable.
Take BP lying, standing; orthostatic hypotension is common.
- Therapeutic response: ability to walk without pain, increased pulse volume, increased temperature in extremities or orientation, long- and short-term memory.
- Assess effect of beta agonist bronchodilators, if needed for airway obstruction, on blood pressure and heart rate.

- Consider use of anticholinergic bronchodilator as alternative to beta agonists.

Patient education:
- It is necessary to quit smoking to prevent excessive vasoconstriction.
- Avoid hazardous activities until stabilized on medication; dizziness may occur.
- Palpitations should subside as therapy continues.

oxtriphylline
(ox-trye'fi-lin)
Choledyl, Choledyl SA, Novotriphyl,* Oxtriphylline
Func. class.: Bronchodilator
Chem. class.: Choline salt of theophylline

Action: Weak bronchodilator effect through unclear mechanism, possibly due to antagonistic effect on adenosine receptors; stimulation of central ventilatory drive and strengthened diaphragmatic contractility are observed to occur; 64% theophylline

Uses: Acute bronchial asthma, reversible bronchospasm in chronic bronchitis and COPD

Dosage and routes:
- *Adult and child >12 yr:* PO 200 mg qid
- *Child 2-12 yr:* PO 4 mg/kg q6h; may be increased to desired response, therapeutic level
Available forms: Elix 100 mg/5 ml; syr 50 mg/5 ml; tabs 100, 200, 400, 600 mg

Side effects/adverse reactions:
*CNS: Anxiety, restlessness, insomnia, dizziness, **convulsions,** headache, lightheadedness*

CV: Palpitations, sinus tachycardia, hypotension
GI: Nausea, vomiting, anorexia, diarrhea, bitter taste, dyspepsia
RESP: Increased rate
INTEG: Flushing, urticaria, alopecia

Contraindications: Hypersensitivity to xanthines, tachydysrhythmias

Precautions: Elderly, CHF, cor pulmonale, hepatic disease, active peptic ulcer disease, diabetes mellitus, hyperthyroidism, hypertension, children, pregnancy (C), glaucoma, prostatic hypertrophy

Pharmacokinetics:
SOL: Peak 1 hr, metabolized in liver, excreted in urine, breast milk; crosses placenta

Interactions/ incompatibilities:
- Increased action of oxtriphylline: cimetidine, erythromycin, troleandomycin, oral contraceptive, propranolol
- May increase effects of: anticoagulants, coffee (substances with caffeine)
- Cardiotoxicity: β-blockers
- Decreased effect of: lithium
- Decreased theophylline level: rifampin, phenytoin

RESPIRATORY CARE CONSIDERATIONS:
Assess/evaluate:
- Therapeutic response: decreased dyspnea, improved respiratory rate and pattern.
- Monitor theophylline blood levels (therapeutic level is 10-20 μg/ml); toxicity may occur with small increase above 20 μg/ml, especially in elderly patients; 10-12

mcg/ml may be optimal in COPD patients.
- Monitor fluid intake for onset of diuresis; dehydration may result in elderly or children.
- Monitor respiratory rate, rhythm, depth; auscultate lung fields bilaterally; notify physician of abnormalities.
- Assess for allergic reactions: rash, urticaria. If these occur, drug should be discontinued.
- Assess side effects reported, and evaluate blood level for toxic range.

Patient education:
- Take doses as prescribed, do not skip dose.
- Check OTC medications, current prescription medications for ephedrine, which will increase CNS stimulation. Do not drink alcohol or caffeine products (tea, coffee, chocolate, colas) which will increase diuresis or add to the xanthine level (caffeine).
- Avoid hazardous activities; dizziness may occur.
- If GI upset occurs, take drug with 8 oz water; avoid food, since absorption may be decreased.
- Notify physician of toxicity: insomnia, anxiety, nausea, vomiting, rapid pulse, convulsions.
- Cigarette smoking will increase metabolism of the drug, lowering blood levels.
- Increase fluid intake if sputum becomes thicker when taking drug.
- Use non-diuresing liquids, such as water, juice, Gatorade, milk rather than diuretic products such as caffeinated coffee, tea or colas.

---

italic = common side effects   **bold** = life-threatening reactions

oxymetazoline HCl (nasal)

(ox-i-met-az'oh-leen)

Afrin, Afrin Children's Nose Drops, Allerest 12-Hour Nasal, Chlorphed-LA, Coricidin Nasal Mist, Dristan Long Lasting, Duramist Plus, Duration, Genasal, NTZ Long-Acting Nasal, Nafrine,* Neo-Synephrine 12 Hour, Nostrilla, Oxymetazoline HCl, Sinarest 12-Hour, Sinex Long-Acting, Twice-A-Day Nasal, 4-Way Long Acting Nasal

Func. class.: Nasal decongestant

Chem. class.: Sympathomimetic amine

Action: Produces vasoconstriction (rapid, long-acting) of arterioles by alpha-adrenergic stimulation, thereby decreasing fluid exudation, mucosal engorgement

Uses: Nasal congestion

Dosage and routes:
- *Adult and child >6 yr:* instill 2-3 gtts or sprays to each nostril bid
- *Child 2-6 yr:* instill 2-3 gtts or sprays 0.025% sol bid, not to exceed 3 days

Available forms: Sol 0.025%, 0.05%

Side effects/adverse reactions:
GI: Nausea, vomiting, anorexia
EENT: Irritation, burning, sneezing, stinging, dryness, rebound congestion
INTEG: Contact dermatitis
CNS: Anxiety, restlessness, tremors, weakness, insomnia, dizziness, fever, headache

Contraindications: Hypersensitivity to sympathomimetic amines

Precautions: Child <6 yr, elderly, diabetes, cardiovascular disease, hypertension, hyperthyroidism, increased ICP, prostatic hypertrophy, pregnancy (C), glaucoma

Interactions/ incompatibilities:
- Hypertension: MAOIs, β-adrenergic blockers
- Hypotension: methyldopa, mecamylamine, reserpine

RESPIRATORY CARE CONSIDERATIONS:
Assess/evaluate:
- Therapeutic response: decreased nasal congestion.
- Assess subject's BP for possible increases if using beta agonist bronchodilator simultaneously.

Patient education:
- Environmental humidification may help to decrease nasal congestion, dryness.
- Warn patient that rebound nasal congestion can occur.
- Use for short-term symptoms only; prolonged rhinitis should be evaluated by physician, ENT specialist, or allergist.

pancreatin

(pan'kree-a-tin)

Elzyme 303 Enseals

Func. class.: Digestant

Chem. class.: Pancreatic enzyme concentrate—bovine/porcine

Action: Pancreatic enzyme needed for proper digestion and GI absorption of fats

Uses: Enzyme replacement therapy in subjects with exocrine pancreatic secretion insufficiency, cystic fibrosis (digestive aid)

Dosage and routes:
- *Adult:* PO 8000-24,000 USP U with meals

Available forms: Tab 650, 2000, 12,000 U

Side effects/adverse reactions:
GI: Anorexia, nausea, vomiting, diarrhea, glossitis, anal soreness
GU: Hyperuricuria, hyperuricemia
INTEG: Rash, hypersensitivity
EENT: Buccal soreness

Contraindications: Hypersensitivity to pork, chronic pancreatic disease

Precautions: Pregnancy (C), lactation

Interactions/ incompatibilities:
- Decreased absorption: cimetidine, antacids, oral iron

RESPIRATORY CARE CONSIDERATIONS:
Assess/evaluate:
- Although not a direct-acting respiratory agent, digestive enzymes are critical for proper nutrition in cystic fibrosis to maintain health and avoid malnutrition with attendant immune depression.
- Therapeutic response: weight gain, appearance, energy level of subjects with CF.
- Monitor concomitantly the respiratory status to avoid infections, improve secretion clearance.
- Assess fluid intake to help maintain normalcy of respiratory tract secretions.

italic = common side effects

pancrelipase
(pan-kre-li'pase)
Cotazym Capsules, Cotazym-S Capsules, CREON Capsules, Entolase-HP, Festal II Tablets, Ilozyme Tables, Ku-Zyme HP Capsules, Pancrease Capsules, Pancrease MT 4, Pancrease MT 10, Pancrease MT 16, Pancrease MT 25, Ultrase MT 12, Ultrase MT 20, Ultrase MT 24, Viokase Powder, Viokase Tablets, Zymase
Func. class.: Digestant
Chem. class.: Pancreatic enzyme—bovine/porcine

Action: Pancreatic enzyme needed for proper digestion and GI absorption of fats

Uses: Enzyme replacement therapy in subjects with exocrine pancreatic secretion insufficiency, cystic fibrosis (digestive aid)

Dosage and routes:
- *Adult and child:* PO 1-3 caps/tabs ac or with meals, or 1 caps/tab with snack or 1-2 pdr pkt ac

Available forms: Tab 8000, 11,000, 30,000 U; caps 8000, 30,000 U; enteric coated caps 4000, 5000, 20,000, 25,000 U; powd 16,800 U

Side effects/adverse reactions:
GI: Anorexia, nausea, vomiting, diarrhea
GU: Hyperuricuria, hyperuricemia

Contraindications: Allergy to pork, chronic pancreatic disease

Precautions: Pregnancy (C)

bold = life-threatening reactions

Interactions/incompatibilities:
- Decreased absorption: cimetidine, antacids, oral iron

RESPIRATORY CARE CONSIDERATIONS:
Assess/evaluate:
- Although not a direct-acting respiratory agent, digestive enzymes are critical for proper nutrition in cystic fibrosis to maintain health and avoid malnutrition with attendant immune depression.
- Therapeutic response: weight gain, appearance, energy level of subjects with CF.
- Monitor concomitantly the respiratory status to avoid infections, improve secretion clearance.
- Assess fluid intake to help maintain normalcy of respiratory tract secretions.

pancuronium bromide

(pan-kyoo-roe'nee-um)
Pancuronium Bromide,
Pavulon
Func. class.: Neuromuscular blocker (nondepolarizing)
Chem. class.: Modified steroid nucleus

Action: Inhibits transmission of nerve impulses at the neuromuscular junction by binding with cholinergic receptor sites, antagonizing action of acetylcholine, and causing muscle weakness or paralysis, depending on dose.

Uses: Facilitation of endotracheal intubation, skeletal muscle relaxation during mechanical ventilation, surgery, or general anesthesia

Dosage and routes:
- *Adult:* IV 0.04-0.1 mg/kg, then 0.01 mg/kg q ½-1hr
- *Child >10 yr:* IV 0.04-0.1 mg/kg, then 1/5 initial dose q ½-1hr
Available forms: Inj IV, IM, 1, 2 mg/ml

Side effects/adverse reactions:
CV: Bradycardia; tachycardia; increased, decreased BP; ventricular extra systoles
RESP: **Prolonged apnea, bronchospasm, cyanosis, respiratory depression**
EENT: Increased secretions
MS: Weakness to prolonged skeletal muscle relaxation
INTEG: Rash, flushing, pruritus, urticaria, sweating, salivation

Contraindications: Hypersensitivity to bromide ion

Precautions: Pregnancy (C), renal disease, cardiac disease, lactation, children <2 yr, electrolyte imbalances, dehydration, neuromuscular disease, respiratory disease

Pharmacokinetics:
IV: Onset 30-45 sec, peak 3-5 min, metabolized (small amounts), excreted in urine (unchanged), crosses placenta

Interactions/incompatibilities:
- Increased neuromuscular blockade: aminoglycosides, clindamycin, lincomycin, quinidine, local anesthetics, polymyxin antibiotics, lithium, narcotic analgesics, thiazides, enflurane, isoflurane
- Dysrhythmias: theophylline
- Incompatible with barbiturates in solution or syringe

Lab test interferences:
Decrease: Cholinesterase

P

RESPIRATORY CARE CONSIDERATIONS:
Assess/evaluate:
- Provide airway and ventilatory support before administering drug.
- Note possible interaction with the following antibiotics, which can increase neuromuscular blockade: the aminoglycosides, the polymyxins, clindamycin, and lincomycin.
- Use with mechanical ventilation, assess patient for adequate and preferably optimal ventilator settings *before* paralyzing. If patient is "fighting" the ventilator, provide adequately high flow rates and tidal volumes, short inspiratory times, and reasonable I:E ratios, check the sensitivity in assist-control mode, provide sufficiently high rates to avoid patient fatigue; consider paralysis if these measures fail.
- Assess ventilator patients for pain, hypoxemia, or ventilator malfunction, if restless and anxious, before instituting muscle paralysis.
- Assess need of patient and provide for pain control and sedation during neuromuscular blockade, *neuromuscular blocking agents do not provide analgesia or sedation.*
- Close eyelids and provide eye lubricant during prolonged paralysis.
- Since usual signs of pain or anxiety (restlessness, tachynea, distress, thrashing) are blocked, monitor vital signs closely and overall patient appearance and state to detect problems (e.g., IV infiltration).

- Check ventilator alarm settings for sufficient limits and sensitivity; a disconnect alarm is critical.
- Assess reversal of drug before attempting to wean from mechanical ventilatory support.

Administer:
- Administer by IV, not by IM, for more consistent absorption and distribution and to avoid the pain associated with IM injection of the drug.
- Reversal: neostigmine or edrophonium, preceded by atropine to inhibit muscarinic response especially in upper airway.

papaverine HCl
(pa-pav′er-een)
Cerespan, Genabid, Papaverine HCl, Pavabid HP Capsulets, Pavabid Plateau Caps, Pavarine Spancaps, Pavased, Pavatine, Pavatym, Paverolan Lanacaps
Func. class.: Peripheral vasodilator
Chem. class.: Opium alkaloid (no narcotic activity)

Action: Relaxes all smooth muscle; possibly due to inhibition of cyclic nucleotide phosphodiesterase, which increases intracellular cAMP, causing vasodilation

Uses: Arterial spasm resulting in cerebral and peripheral ischemia; myocardial ischemia associated with vascular spasm or dysrhythmias; angina pectoris; peripheral pulmonary embolism; visceral

italic = common side effects　　　**bold** = life-threatening reactions

236   papaverine HCl

spasm as in ureteral, biliary, GI colic PVD

Dosage and routes:
- *Adult:* PO 100-300 mg 3-5 times day; sus rel 150-300 mg q8-12h; IM/IV 30-120 mg q3h prn
Available forms: Cap time-release 150, 200, 300 mg; tabs 30, 60, 100, 150, 200, 300 mg; inj IM/IV 30 mg/ml

Side effects/adverse reactions:
CV: Tachycardia, increased BP
RESP: Increased depth of respirations
CNS: Headache, dizziness, drowsiness, sedation, vertigo, malaise
GI: Nausea, anorexia, abdominal pain, constipation, diarrhea, jaundice, altered liver enzymes, *hepatotoxicity*
INTEG: Flushing, sweating, rash

Contraindications: Hypersensitivity, complete AV heart block

Precautions: Cardiac dysrhythmias, glaucoma, pregnancy (C), lactation, drug dependency, children

Pharmacokinetics:
PO: Onset 30 sec, peak 1-2 hr, duration 3-4 hr
SUS REL: Onset erratic
90% bound to plasma proteins, metabolized in liver, excreted in urine (inactive metabolites)

Interactions/incompatibilities:
- Decreased effect of: levodopa
- Increased hypotension: antihypertensives, vasodilators, diazoxide, alcohol
- Incompatible with alkaline sol, aminophylline, iodides, bromides

RESPIRATORY CARE CONSIDERATIONS:
Assess/evaluate:
- Evaluate BP and pulse for efficacy of hypertension treatment and to avoid hypotension.
- Evaluate BP with COPD or asthmatic subjects who require beta agonists for reversible airway obstruction.
- Assess for symptoms of CHF: edema, dyspnea, wet rales, BP.
- Assess BP if on mechanical ventilatory support to minimize mean airway pressures which can increase hypotensive effect through impeded venous return and decreased cardiac output; minimize inspiratory times and optimize flow patterns and avoid large tidal volumes.
- Hepatic hypersensitivity reaction: nausea, vomiting, jaundice; drug should be discontinued if this occurs.

Patient education:
- Do not use OTC products containing α-adrenergic stimulants (nasal decongestants, OTC cold preparations) unless directed by physician.
- Report symptoms of CHF: difficult breathing, especially on exertion or when lying down, night cough, swelling of extremities.
- It is necessary to quit smoking to prevent excessive vasoconstriction.
- Avoid hazardous activities until stabilized on medication; dizziness may occur.
- Make position changes slowly or fainting will occur.

paramethasone acetate

(par-a-meth′a-sone)
Haldrone
Func. class.: Corticosteroid
Chem. class.: Glucocorticoid, long acting

Action: Decreases inflammation by suppression of migration of polymorphonuclear leukocytes, fibroblasts, reversal to increase capillary permeability and lysosomal stabilization

Uses: Severe inflammation, collagen disorders, respiratory, dermatologic disorders, adrenal insufficiency

Dosage and routes:
- *Adult:* PO 0.5-6 mg tid-qid
- *Child:* PO 58-800 μg/kg/day in divided doses tid-qid
Available forms: Tabs 2 mg

Side effects/adverse reactions:
INTEG: Acne, poor wound healing, ecchymosis, petechiae
CNS: Depression, flushing, sweating, headache, mood changes
*CV: Hypertension, **circulatory collapse, thrombophlebitis, embolism,*** tachycardia, edema
*HEMA: **Thrombocytopenia***
MS: Fractures, osteoporosis, weakness
GI: Diarrhea, nausea, abdominal distention, *GI hemorrhage,* increased appetite, *pancreatitis*
EENT: Fungal infections, increased intraocular pressure, blurred vision

Contraindications: Psychosis, hypersensitivity, idiopathic thrombocytopenia, acute glomerulonephritis, amebiasis, fungal infections, nonasthmatic bronchial disease, child <2 yr, AIDS, TB

Precautions: Pregnancy (C), diabetes mellitus, glaucoma, osteoporosis, seizure disorders, ulcerative colitis, CHF, myasthenia gravis, renal disease, esophagitis, peptic ulcer

Pharmacokinetics:
PO: Peak 1-2 hr, duration 2 days
IM: Peak 3-4 hr

Interactions/ incompatibilities:
- Decreased action of paramethasone: cholestyramine, colestipol, barbiturates, rifampin, ephedrine, phenytoin, theophylline
- Decreased effects of: anticoagulants, anticonvulsants, antidiabetics, ambenonium, neostigmine, isoniazid, toxoids, vaccines
- Increased side effects: alcohol, salicylates, indomethacin, amphotericin B, digitalis preparations
- Increased action of paramethasone: salicylates, estrogens, indomethacin

Lab test interferences:
Increase: Cholesterol, Na, blood glucose, uric acid, Ca, urine glucose
Decrease: Ca, K, T_4, T_3, thyroid ^{131}I uptake test, urine 17-OHCS, 17-KS, PBI
False negative: Skin allergy tests

RESPIRATORY CARE CONSIDERATIONS:
Assess/evaluate:
- Monitor for side effects of increased corticosteroid level: Cushingoid symptoms (moon face, peripheral wasting, central edema).

---

italic = common side effects   **bold** = life-threatening reactions

- Monitor patients with latent tuberculosis or reactive skin tests for reactivation of the disease.
- Evaluate muscle weakness and steroid myopathy, especially in chronic lung disease patients.
- Evaluate cardiovascular system for hypertension, CHF.
- Monitor electrolytes, potassium and calcium loss can occur, with hypokalemic alkalosis.
- Infection, including pneumonia, can occur.
- Increased corticosteroid levels can mask symptoms of infection.
- If asthma is present, monitor for breakthrough symptoms (bronchospasm, wheezing) if drug is discontinued.
- Evaluate possible adrenal insufficiency when transferring from systemic to inhaled aerosol corticosteroids in asthma.
- Symptoms of adrenal insufficiency: nausea, anorexia, fatigue, dizziness, dyspnea, weakness, joint pain.

pargyline HCl
(par'gi-leen)
Eutonyl
Func. class.:
Antihypertensive
Chem. class.: MAOI

Action: Inhibits monoamine oxidase, decreasing BP

Uses: Moderate to severe hypertension

Dosage and routes:
- *Adult:* PO 25 mg daily; increase by 10 mg q7d, not to exceed 200 mg; maintenance dosage: 25-50 mg daily

Available forms: Tabs 10, 25, 50 mg

Side effects/adverse reactions:
CV: Orthostatic hypotension, tachycardia, chest pain, bradycardia, fluid retention, *CHF*
CNS: Drowsiness, dizziness, sedation, headache, depression, insomnia, weakness, fatigue, confusion, blurred vision, EPS
GI: Nausea, vomiting, anorexia, constipation, weight gain
EENT: Dry mouth
GU: Impotence
MS: Arthralgia
MISC: Sweating, increased appetite, hypoglycemia

Contraindications: Hypersensitivity, malignant hypertension, paranoid schizophrenia, severe pulmonary failure, pheochromocytoma, hyperthyroidism, advanced renal failure, children <12 yr

Precautions: Pregnancy (C), lactation, impaired renal function, liver disease, CAD, parkinsonism, diabetes mellitus

Pharmacokinetics: Excreted in urine, therapeutic response may take 4 days-3 weeks

Interactions/incompatibilities:
- Hypertensive crisis: amphetamine, cyclopentamide, ephedrine, pseudoephedrine, metaraminol, methylphenidate, phenylpropanolamine, levodopa, methyldopa, reserpine, tryptamine, tyramine foods
- Hypotension and increased sedation: barbiturates, alcohol, narcotics, CNS depressants, antihypertensive agents
- May potentiate effects: doxapram, narcotics, phenothi-

azines, other psychotropic agents, tricyclic antidepressants

RESPIRATORY CARE CONSIDERATIONS:
Assess/evaluate:
■ Use beta agonists with caution in the presence of MAOIs and monitor BP for increases, including a hypertensive crisis.
■ Note: cold agents that contain adrenergics (e.g., ephedrine, phenylephrine, phenylpropanolamine) may also interact with MAOIs to increase BP.

Patient education:
■ Avoid high-tyramine foods: cheese (aged), sour cream, beer, wine, pickled products, liver, raisins, bananas, figs, avocados, meat tenderizers, chocolate, yogurt, or an increase in caffeine.
■ Report headache, palpitation, neck stiffness.
■ Avoid OTC cold medications that contain ephedrine or sympathomimetic amines, which can increase BP.

pentaerythritol tetranitrate
(pen-ta-er-ith′ri-tole)
Duotrate, Duotrate 45, P.E.T.N., Pentylan, Peritrate, Peritrate SA
Func. class.: Vasodilatory, coronary
Chem. class.: Nitrate

Action: Decreases preload, afterload, which is responsible for decreasing left ventricular end-diastolic pressure, systemic vascular resistance

Uses: Chronic stable angina pectoris, prophylaxis of angina pain

Dosage and routes:
■ *Adult:* PO 10-20 mg tid or qid, max 40 mg qid; sus rel 30-80 mg q12h
Available forms: Caps ext rel 30, 45, 80 mg; tabs 10, 20, 40, 80 mg; tabs ext rel 80 mg

Side effects/adverse reactions:
CV: Postural hypotension, palpitations, tachycardia, *collapse,* syncope
GI: Nausea, vomiting, abdominal pain
INTEG: Pallor, sweating, rash
CNS: Headache, flushing, dizziness, restlessness, weakness, faintness
MISC: Muscle twitching, **hemolytic anemia, methemoglobinemia**

Contraindications: Hypersensitivity to this drug or nitrates, severe anemia, increased intracranial pressure, cerebral hemorrhage, acute MI

Precautions: Postural hypotension, pregnancy (C), lactation, children

Pharmacokinetics:
PO: Onset 30 min, duration 4-5 hr
SUS REL: Onset 30 min, duration 12 hr
Metabolized by liver, excreted in urine, half-life 10 min

Interactions/ incompatibilities:
■ Increased effects: β-blockers, diuretics, antihypertensives, alcohol

RESPIRATORY CARE CONSIDERATIONS:
Assess/evaluate:
■ Therapeutic response: relief of chest pain (angina).

P

---

italic = common side effects   **bold** = life-threatening reactions

- Monitor BP, pulse, and ECG if available.
- Provide cardiopulmonary resuscitation if ventricular fibrillation or cardiac arrest occurs due to acute MI.
- Note: alcohol or calcium channel blockers may increase risk of hypotension.
- Evaluate for formation of methemoglobin and oxygen transport to tissues in case of overdose or genetically abnormal hemoglobins. Pulse oximetry will be inaccurate in presence of significant methemoglobin levels; check mixed venous oxygen level if available.
- Note possible respiratory adverse effects—bronchitis, pneumonia, URI—and monitor respiratory status (rate, pattern, auscultation, patient report of breathing).

Patient education:
- Prolonged chest pain may indicate MI: seek emergency treatment.
- Make position changes slowly to prevent orthostatic hypotension.
- Use analgesic (aspirin, acetaminophen) if headache occurs.

pentamidine isethionate
(pen-tam′i-deen)
Pentam 300, Pentacarinat,*
NebuPent
Func. class.: Antiprotozoal
Chem. class.: Aromatic diamide derivative

See also Section III: Aerosol Agents for Oral Inhalation

Action: Interferes with DNA/RNA synthesis in protozoa

Uses: *P. carinii* infections; inhaled formulation is prophylactic only, not acute treatment

Dosage and routes:
- *Adult and child:* IV/IM 4 mg/kg/day × 2 wk; SVN 300 mg/6ml sterile water via specific nebulizer given q4wk for prevention (see Aerosol Agents)
Available forms: Inj IV, IM, aerosol 300 mg/vial

Side effects/adverse reactions:
CV: Hypotension, ventricular tachycardia, ECG abnormalities
HEMA: Anemia, *leukopenia, thrombocytopenia*
INTEG: Sterile abscess, pain at injection site, pruritus, urticaria, rash
GU: Acute renal failure, increased serum creatinine, renal toxicity
GI: Nausea, vomiting, anorexia, increased AST, ALT, *acute pancreatitis*, metallic taste
CNS: Disorientation, hallucinations, dizziness, confusion
RESP: Cough, shortness of breath, *bronchospasm* (with aerosol)
MISC: Fatigue, chills, night sweats
META: Hyperkalemia, hypocalcemia, hypoglycemia

Precautions: Blood dyscrasias, hepatic disease, renal disease, diabetes mellitus, cardiac disease, hypocalcemia, pregnancy (C), hypertension, hypotension, lactation, children

Pharmacokinetics: Excreted unchanged in urine (66%)

Interactions/ incompatibilities
- Nephrotoxicity: aminoglycosides, amphotericin B, colis-

tin, cisplatin, methoxyflurane, polymyxin B, vancomycin
- Considered incompatible with any drug in sol or syringe

RESPIRATORY CARE CONSIDERATIONS:
Assess/evaluate:
- Monitor efficacy of pentamidine prophylaxis in preventing episodes of PCP or acute treatment in resolving pneumonia.
- Assess breathing rate and pattern.
- Assess breath sounds by auscultation before and after treatment.
- Assess pulse before and after treatment.
- Assess patient's subjective reaction to treatment for any change in breathing effort or pattern.
- Assess chest radiograph for clearance or worsening of infiltrates.
- Assess arterial blood gases as a guide to need for ventilatory support, if indicated.
- Use ABGs or pulse oximetry to titrate supplemental oxygen.
- Evaluate blood studies, blood glucose, CBC, platelets.
- Monitor subjects for onset of adverse reactions noted.
- Patient should be lying down when receiving drug by injectable route severe hypotension may develop; monitor BP during administration and several times after until BP is stable.
- Screen HIV subjects for tuberculosis and treat accordingly.
- Health care workers should self-monitor for TB regularly, and following exposure to untreated active case.
For details on aerosol treatment: see Section III.

pentoxifylline
(pen-tox-i'fi-leen)
Trental
Func. class.: Hemorrheologic agent
Chem. class.: Dimethylxanthine derivative

Action: Decreases blood viscosity, stimulates prostacyclin formation, increases blood flow by increasing flexibility of RBCs; decreases RBC hyperaggregation; reduces platelet aggregation, decreases fibrinogin concentration

Uses: Intermittent claudication related to chronic occlusive vascular disease

Dosage and routes:
- *Adult:* PO 400 mg tid with meals
Available forms: Tabs, controlled-release 400 mg

Side effects/adverse reactions:
MISC: Epistaxis, flulike symptoms, laryngitis, nasal congestion, leukopenia, malaise, weight changes
EENT: Blurred vision, earache, increased salivation, sore throat, conjunctivitis
CNS: Headache, anxiety, tremors, confusion, dizziness
GI: Dyspepsia, nausea, vomiting, anorexia, bloating, belching, constipation, cholecystitis, dry mouth, thirst, bad taste
INTEG: Rash, pruritus, urticaria, brittle fingernails
CV: Angina, dysrhythmias, palpitation, hypotension, chest pain, dyspnea, edema

Contraindications: Hypersensitivity to this drug or xanthines

italic = common side effects   **bold** = life-threatening reactions

Precautions: Pregnancy (C), angina pectoris, cardiac disease, lactation, children, impaired renal function

Pharmacokinetics:
PO: Peak 1 hr, half-life ½-1 hr, degradation in liver, excreted in urine

Interactions/incompatibilities:
- Increased PT: warfarin

RESPIRATORY CARE CONSIDERATIONS:
Assess/evaluate:
- Caution: although pentoxifylline differs from thrombolytic or anticoagulant agents, there have been reports of bleeding and prolonged prothrombin time (PT) with or without concomitant use of anticoagulants; minimize or avoid arterial punctures, and if such is performed, apply manual compression and pressure dressing, with inspection for bleeding.
- Evaluate respiratory side effects: laryngitis, flu-like symptoms, epistaxis, or nasal congestion—and rule out other causes such as viral infection.
- Monitor cardiovascular side effects, such as angina/chest pain, edema, hypotension, dyspnea, to distinguish from CHF.
- Monitor hematocrit and hemoglobin to insure adequate oxygen transport capability.

phenoxybenzamine HCl

(fen-ox-ee-ben′za-meen)
Dibenzyline
Func. class.:
Antihypertensive
Chem. class.: α-adrenergic blocker

Action: α-adrenergic blocker that binds to α-adrenergic receptors, blocking alpha-adrenergic induced vasoconstriction in peripheral blood vessels; lowers peripheral resistance, lowers blood pressure

Uses: Pheochromocytoma

Dosage and routes:
- *Adult:* PO 10 mg bid, increase by 10 mg qod until optimal dose is reached, usual range: 20-40 mg bid-tid
Available forms: Caps 10 mg

Side effects/adverse reactions:
GI: Dry mouth, nausea, vomiting, diarrhea
CV: Postural hypotension, tachycardia, palpitations
CNS: Dizziness, flushing, drowsiness, sedation, weakness, confusion, headache, malaise
GU: Inhibition of ejaculation
EENT: Nasal congestion, dry mouth, miosis
INTEG: Allergic contact dermatitis

Contraindications: Hypersensitivity, CHF, angina, cerebral vascular insufficiency, coronary arteriosclerosis

Precautions: Severe renal disease, severe pulmonary disease, pregnancy (C)

Pharmacokinetics:
PO: Onset 2 hr, peak 4-6 hr, duration 3-4 days, half-life 24 hr, metabolized in liver, excreted in urine, bile

Interactions/incompatibilities:
- Hypotensive response: epinephrine, antihypertensives

---

*Available in Canada only

RESPIRATORY CARE CONSIDERATIONS:
Assess/evaluate:
- Evaluate BP and pulse for efficacy of hypertension treatment and to avoid hypotension.
- Evaluate BP with COPD or asthmatic subjects who require beta agonists for reversible airway obstruction.
- Assess for symptoms of CHF: edema, dyspnea, wet rales, BP.
- Assess BP if on mechanical ventilatory support to minimize mean airway pressures which can increase hypotensive effect through impeded venous return and decreased cardiac output; minimize inspiratory times and optimize flow patterns and avoid large tidal volumes.
- Note: since alpha receptors are blocked, other adrenergic agents that stimulate both types of sympathetic receptors or beta receptors, such as epinephrine, may cause exaggerated response of tachycardia and hypotension.
- Treatment of overdose with epinephrine can cause worsening of hypotension, as outlined previously; use leg elevation, discontinue the drug, support circulation.

Patient education:
- Do not use OTC products containing α-adrenergic stimulants (nasal decongestants, OTC cold preparations) or other sympathomimetics unless directed by physician.
- Report symptoms of CHF: difficult breathing, especially on exertion or when lying down, night cough, swelling of extremities.

- It is necessary to quit smoking to prevent excessive vasoconstriction.
- Avoid hazardous activities until stabilized on medication; dizziness may occur.
- Make position changes slowly, or fainting will occur.

phentolamine mesylate
(fen-tole′a-meen)
Regitine, Rogitine*
Func. class.: Antihypertensive
Chem. class.: α-adrenergic blocker

Action: α-adrenergic blocker, binds to α-adrenergic receptors, blocking alpha-adrenergic induced vasoconstriction in peripheral blood vessels, lowering peripheral resistances, lowering blood pressure

Uses: Hypertension, pheochromocytoma, prevention, treatment of dermal necrosis following extravasation of norepinephrine or dopamine

Dosage and routes:
Treatment of hypertensive episodes in pheochromocytoma
- *Adult:* 5 mg IV/IM, repeat if necessary
- *Child:* 1 mg IV/IM, repeat if necessary
- *Adult:* 2.5 mg IV, if negative repeat with 5 mg IV
- *Child:* 0.5 mg IV, if negative repeat with 1 mg IV
Prevention, treatment of necrosis
- *Adult:* 5 - 10 mg/10 ml NS injected into area of norepinephrine extravasation within 12 hr
Available forms: Inj IM, IV 5 mg/ml; tabs 25, 50 mg (only injectable form available in US)

---

italic = common side effects   **bold** = life-threatening reactions

Side effects/adverse reactions:
GI: Dry mouth, nausea, vomiting, diarrhea, abdominal pain
CV: Hypotension, tachycardia, angina, dysrhythmias, myocardial infarction
CNS: Dizziness, flushing, weakness
EENT: Nasal congestion

Contraindications: Hypersensitivity, myocardial infarction, coronary insufficiency, angina

Precautions: Pregnancy (C), lactation

Pharmacokinetics:
IV: Peak 2 min, duration 10-15 min
IM: Peak 15-20 min, duration 3-4 hr, metabolized in liver, excreted in urine

Interactions/ incompatibilities:
- Increased effects of: epinephrine, antihypertensives
- Incompatible with iron salts

RESPIRATORY CARE CONSIDERATIONS:
Assess/evaluate:
- Monitor effect on BP and pulse, especially if on positive pressure ventilatory support.
- Assess effectiveness of beta-adrenergic bronchodilator therapy for possible antagonistic effect on BP to avoid increasing BP, or decreasing BP due to beta receptor stimulation of vascular smooth muscle in the presence of blocked alpha receptors.
- Consider use of nonadrenergic bronchodilator such as ipratropium bromide as alternative to beta-adrenergic agents for asthmatics, COPD patients.

- Note: since alpha-receptors are blocked, other adrenergic agents that stimulate both types of sympathetic receptors or beta receptors, such as epinephrine, may cause exaggerated response of tachycardia and hypotension.
- Treatment of overdose with epinephrine can cause worsening of hypotension, as outlined previously; use leg elevation, discontinue the drug, support circulation.

Patient education:
- Do not use OTC products containing α-adrenergic stimulants (nasal decongestants, OTC cold preparations) or other sympathomimetics unless directed by physician. Report symptoms of CHF: difficulty breathing, especially on exertion or when lying down, night cough, swelling of extremities

phenylephrine HCl
(fen-ill-ef′rin)
Neo-Synephrine
Func. class.: Adrenergic, direct acting
Chem. class.: Substituted phenylethylamine

Action: Powerful and selective α_1-receptor agonist causing contraction of blood vessels

Uses: Hypotension, paroxysmal supraventricular tachycardia, shock, maintain BP during spinal anesthesia

Dosage and routes:
Hypotension
- *Adult:* SC/IM 2-5 mg, may repeat q10-15 min if needed IV 0.1-0.5 mg, may repeat q10-15 min if needed

- *PVCs*
- *Adult:* IV BOL 0.5 mg given rapidly, not to exceed prior dose by >0.1 mg; total dose >1 mg
Shock
- *Adult:* IV INF 10 mg/500 ml D₅W given 100-180 gtts/min, then 40-60 gtts/min titrated to BP
Available forms: Inj IV, SC, IM, 1% (10 mg/ml)

Side effects/adverse reactions:
CNS: Headache, anxiety, tremor, insomnia, dizziness
CV: Palpitations, tachycardia, hypertension, ectopic beats, angina, reflex bradycardia
GI: Nausea, vomiting
INTEG: Necrosis, tissue sloughing with extravasation, **gangrene**

Contraindications: Hypersensitivity, ventricular fibrillation, tachydysrhythmias, pheochromocytoma, narrow-angle glaucoma

Precautions: Pregnancy (C), lactation, arterial embolism, peripheral vascular disease, elderly, hyperthyroidism, bradycardia, myocardial disease, severe arteriosclerosis

Pharmacokinetics:
IV: Duration 20-30 min
IM/SC: Duration 45-60 min

Interactions/ incompatibilities:
- Do not use within 2 wk of MAOIs, or hypertensive crisis may result
- Dysrhythmias: general anesthetics, bretylium
- Decreased action of phenylephrine: α-blockers
- Increase in BP: oxytocics
- Increased pressor effect: tricyclic antidepressant, MAOIs, guanethidine

- Incompatible with alkaline solutions: NaHCO₃, iron salts, phenytoin

RESPIRATORY CARE CONSIDERATIONS:
Assess/evaluate:
- Therapeutic response: increased BP with stabilization.
- Monitor BP and pulse rate if administering adrenergic bronchodilators for possible excess increase in BP.
- Evaluate tissue oxygen transport based on cardiac output and arterial O₂ content; correct any hypovolemia as quickly as possible to maintain BP and adequate tissue perfusion.
- If mechanical ventilatory support is instituted/present, minimize airway pressures to extent possible to avoid inhibiting venous return with high pressures and causing decrease in cardiac output and BP.

phenylephrine HCl (nasal)
(fen-ill-ef'rin)
Alconefrin, Alconefrin-25, Alconefrin-50, Duration, Neo-Synephrine, Nostril, Rhinall-10, Sinex, St. Joseph Measured Dose
Func. class.: Nasal decongestant
Chem. class.: Sympathomimetic amine

Action: Produces vasoconstriction (rapid, long-acting) of arterioles by alpha-adrenergic stimulation, thereby decreasing fluid exudation, mucosal engorgement

Uses: Nasal congestion

italic = common side effects   **bold** = life-threatening reactions

Dosage and routes:
- *Adult:* INSTILL 2-3 gtts or sprays to nasal mucosa bid (0.25%-1%); TOP apply to nasal mucosa q3-4h prn
- *Child 6-12 yr:* INSTILL 1-2 gtts or sprays (0.25%) q3-4h prn
- *Child <6 yr:* INSTILL 2-3 gtts or sprays (0.125%) q3-4h prn

Available forms: Sol 0.125%, 0.16%, 0.2%, 0.25%, 0.5%, 1%; jelly 0.5%

Side effects/adverse reactions:
GI: Nausea, vomiting, anorexia
EENT: Irritation, burning, sneezing, stinging, dryness, rebound congestion
INTEG: Contact dermatitis
CNS: Anxiety, restlessness, tremors, weakness, insomnia, dizziness, fever, headache

Contraindications: Hypersensitivity to sympathomimetic amines

Precautions: Child <6 yr, elderly, diabetes, cardiovascular disease, hypertension, hyperthyroidism, increased ICP, prostatic hypertrophy, pregnancy (C), glaucoma

Interactions/ incompatibilities:
- Hypertension: MAOIs, β-adrenergic blockers
- Hypotension: methyldopa, mecamylamine, reserpine

RESPIRATORY CARE CONSIDERATIONS:
Assess/evaluate:
- Therapeutic response: decreased nasal congestion.
- Assess subject's BP for possible increases if using beta agonist bronchodilator simultaneously.

Patient education:
- Environmental humidification may help to decrease nasal congestion, dryness.
- Warn patient that rebound nasal congestion can occur.
- Use for short-term symptoms only; prolonged rhinitis should be evaluated by physician, ENT specialist, or allergist.

physostigmine salicylate
(fi-zoe-stig′meen)
Antilirium
Func. class.: Antidote, reversible anticholinesterase (indirect-acting cholinergic)
Chem. class.: Tertiary amine

Action: Increases acetylcholine at cholinergic nerve terminals by inhibition of cholinesterase enzymes; reverses central, peripheral anticholinergic effects

Uses: To reverse CNS effects of diazepam, anticholinergic, tricyclic antidepressant, Alzheimer's disease, hereditary ataxia

Dosage and routes:
Overdose of anticholinergics
- *Adult:* IM/IV 2 mg; give no more than 1 mg/min; may repeat
- *Pediatric:* IM/IV inj 0.02 mg/kg, not more than 0.5 mg/min; may repeat at 5-10 min intervals until max dose of 2 mg
Postanesthesia
- *Adult:* IM/IV 0.5-1 mg; give no more than 1 mg/min (IV); can repeat at 10 to 30 min intervals
Available forms: Inj IM, IV 1 mg/ml

*Available in Canada only

Side effects/adverse reactions:
INTEG: Rash, urticaria
CNS: Dizziness, headache, sweating, weakness, *convulsions,* incoordination, *paralysis,* hallucination, delirium, drowsiness
GI: Nausea, diarrhea, vomiting, cramps, increased salivary and gastric secretions
CV: Bradycardia, hypotension, syncope
GU: Frequency, incontinence, urgency
RESP: Respiratory depression, bronchospasm, constriction, dyspnea
EENT: Miosis, blurred vision, lacrimation

Contraindications: Hypotension, obstruction of intestine or renal system, asthma, gangrene, CV disease, choline esters, depolarizing neuromuscular blocking agents, diabetes

Precautions: Seizure disorders, bronchial asthma, coronary occlusion, hyperthyroidism, dysrhythmias, peptic ulcer, megacolon, poor GI motility, pregnancy (C), Parkinson's disease, bradycardia, lactation

Pharmacokinetics:
IM/IV: Peak 5 min, duration 45-60 min, crosses blood-brain barrier, excreted in urine

Interactions/ incompatibilities:
■ Decreased action of: gallamine, metocurine, pancuronium, tubocurarine, atropine
■ Increased action of: decamethonium, succinylcholine
■ Decreased action of physostigmine: aminoglycosides, anesthetics, procainamide, quinidine
■ Considered incompatible with any drug in sol or syringe

RESPIRATORY CARE CONSIDERATIONS:
Assess/evaluate:
■ Monitor for exacerbation of asthma or airway resistance in COPD subject due to parasympathetic induced bronchoconstriction.
■ Assess respiratory rate and pattern, breath sounds for wheezing.
■ Assess subjective response of patient for difficulty in breathing, tightness in chest.
■ Assess pulse for bradycardia and BP for decrease.
■ Note: use of a cholinergic agent can intensify and prolong a depolarizing blockade induced by succinylcholine, due to the inactivation of acetylcholine needed for neuromuscular transmission.

pinacidil
(pye-na'si-dil)
Pindac
Func. class.:
Antihypertensive
Chem. class.:
Vasodilator—peripheral

Action: Directly relaxes arteriolar smooth muscle, causing vasodilation

Uses: Severe hypertension not responsive to other therapy; topically to treat alopecia

Dosage and routes:
■ *Adult:* PO 12.5-25 mg bid
Available forms: Tabs 12.5, 25 mg

Side effects/adverse reactions:

CV: Severe rebound hypertension, tachycardia, angina, increased T wave, *CHF,* pulmonary edema, edema, Na and water retention

CNS: Drowsiness, dizziness, sedation, headache, depression

GI: Nausea, vomiting, diarrhea, constipation, dry mouth

GU: Gynecomastia, breast tenderness

INTEG: Pruritus, *Stevens-Johnson syndrome,* rash, hirsutism

Contraindications: Acute myocardial infarction, dissecting aortic aneurysm, hypersensitivity, pheochromocytoma

Precautions: Pregnancy (C), lactation, children, renal disease, CAD, post MI

Pharmacokinetics: Peak 1 hr, 60% protein bound; metabolized in the liver, excreted in urine, feces (active metabolites); half-life 1½-3 hr

Interactions/ incompatibilities:
- Orthostatic hypotension: guanethidine
- Reduced effect of pinacidil: nonsteroidal antiinflammatory drugs

Lab test interferences:
Increase: Renal function studies
Decrease: Hgb/Hct/RBC

RESPIRATORY CARE CONSIDERATIONS:
Assess/evaluate:
- Evaluate BP and pulse for efficacy of hypertension treatment and to avoid hypotension.
- Evaluate BP with COPD or asthmatic subjects who require beta agonists for reversible airway obstruction.
- Assess for symptoms of CHF: edema, dyspnea, wet rales, BP.
- Assess BP if on mechanical ventilatory support to minimize mean airway pressures which can increase hypotensive effect through impeded venous return and decreased cardiac output; minimize inspiratory times and optimize flow patterns and avoid large tidal volumes.

Patient education:
- Do not use OTC products containing α-adrenergic stimulants (nasal decongestants, OTC cold preparations) unless directed by physician.
- Report symptoms of CHF: difficult breathing, especially on exertion or when lying down, night cough, swelling of extremities.
- It is necessary to quit smoking to prevent excessive vasoconstriction.
- Avoid hazardous activities until stabilized on medication; dizziness may occur.
- Make position changes slowly, or fainting will occur.

pindolol
(pin'doe-lole)
Visken
Func. class.: Antihypertensive
Chem. class.: Nonselective β-blocker

Action: Competitively blocks stimulation of β-adrenergic receptor within vascular smooth muscle; produces negative chronotropic, inotropic activity (decreases rate of

SA node discharge, increases recovery time), slows conduction of AV node, decreases heart rate, which decreases O_2 consumption in myocardium; also decreases renin-aldosterone-angiotensin system; at high doses inhibits β_2-receptors in bronchial system

Uses: Mild to moderate hypertension

Dosage and routes:
■ *Adult:* PO 5 mg bid, usual dose 15 mg/day (5 mg tid), may increase by 10 mg/day q3-4wk to a max of 60 mg/day
Available forms: Tabs 5, 10 mg

Side effects/adverse reactions:
CV: Hypotension, bradycardia, **CHF,** edema, chest pain, palpitation, claudication, tachycardia, *AV block*
CNS: Insomnia, dizziness, hallucinations, anxiety, fatigue
GI: Nausea, vomiting, *ischemic colitis,* diarrhea, *abdominal pain, mesenteric arterial thrombosis*
INTEG: Rash, alopecia, pruritus, fever
HEMA: **Agranulocytosis, thrombocytopenia, purpura**
EENT: Visual changes, sore throat, *double vision,* dry burning eyes
GU: Impotence, frequency
RESP: **Bronchospasm,** *dyspnea,* cough, rales
MISC: Joint pain, muscle pain

Contraindications: Hypersensitivity to β-blockers, cardiogenic shock, 2nd or 3rd degree heart block, sinus bradycardia, CHF, cardiac failure, bronchial asthma

Precautions: Major surgery, pregnancy (B), lactation, diabetes mellitus, renal disease, thyroid disease, COPD, well-compensated heart failure, CAD, nonallergic bronchospasm

Pharmacokinetics:
PO: Peak 2-4 hr, half-life 3-4 hr, excreted 30%-45% unchanged, 60%-65% metabolized by liver, excreted in breast milk

Interactions/ incompatibilities:
■ Increased hypotension, bradycardia: reserpine, hydralazine, methyldopa, prazosin, anticholinergics
■ Decreased antihypertensive effects: indomethacin, sympathomimetics
■ Increased hypoglycemic effect: insulin
■ Decreased bronchodilation: theophyllines, β_2-agonists

Lab test interferences:
Increase: Liver function tests, renal function tests

RESPIRATORY CARE CONSIDERATIONS:
Assess/evaluate:
■ Avoid use with reversible airway obstruction or bronchospastic disease such as asthma or chronic bronchitis due to potential for bronchospasm (wheezing, dyspnea, complaints of chest tightness) secondary to beta-blockade; consider use of other classes of antihypertensive agents for these patients.
■ Monitor all subjects for symptoms of increased airway resistance (wheezing, tightness in chest, difficulty breathing).
■ Monitor effect on BP and pulse, especially if on positive pressure ventilatory support.

italic = common side effects   **bold** = life-threatening reactions

- Assess effectiveness of beta-adrenergic bronchodilator therapy for possible antagonism and effect on BP to avoid increasing BP, if used.
- Consider use of nonadrenergic bronchodilator such as ipratropium bromide as alternative to beta-adrenergic agents for patients to avoid positive inotropic effect.

Patient education:
- Do not use OTC products containing α-adrenergic stimulants (nasal decongestants, OTC cold preparations) unless directed by physician.
- Report symptoms of CHF: difficult breathing, especially on exertion or when lying down, night cough, swelling of extremities
- Caution patient that orthostatic hypotension may occur.

pipecuronium bromide

(pi-pe-cure-ó-nee-um)
Arduan
Func. class.: Neuromuscular blocker (nondepolarizing)
Chem. class.: Modified steroid nucleus

Action: Inhibits transmission of nerve impulses at the neuromuscular junction by binding with cholinergic receptor sites, antagonizing action of acetylcholine, and causing muscle weakness or paralysis, depending on dose.

Uses: Facilitation of endotracheal intubation, skeletal muscle relaxation during mechanical ventilation, surgery, or general anesthesia

Dosage and routes: Dosage is individualized; in patients with normal renal function who are not obese, initial dose is 70-85 µg/kg; maintenance dose is 10-15 µg/kg
Available forms: Inj IV 10-mg vials

Side effects/adverse reactions:
CV: Bradycardia, tachycardia, increased or decreased BP, ventricular extrasystole, myocardial ischemia, cardiovascular accident, thrombosis, atrial fibrillation
RESP: Prolonged apnea, bronchospasm, cyanosis, respiratory depression
GU: Anuria
EENT: Increased secretions
CNS: Hypesthesia, CNS depression
MS: Weakness to prolonged skeletal muscle relaxation
INTEG: Rash, urticaria
META: Hypoglycemia, hyperkalemia, increased creatinine

Contraindications: Hypersensitivity to bromide ion

Precautions: Pregnancy (C), renal disease, cardiac disease, lactation, children < 3 mo, fluid and electrolyte imbalances, neuromuscular diseases, respiratory disease, obesity

Pharmacokinetics:
IV: Onset 30-45 sec, peak 3-5 min, metabolized (small amounts), excreted in urine (unchanged), crosses placenta

Interactions/incompatibilities:
- Increased neuromuscular blockade: aminoglycosides, quinidine, local anesthetics, polymyxin antibiotics, enflurane, isoflurane, tetracyclines, halothane, magnesium, colistin

RESPIRATORY CARE CONSIDERATIONS:
Assess/evaluate:
■ Provide airway and ventilatory support before administering drug.
■ Note possible interaction with the following antibiotics, which can increase neuromuscular blockade: the aminoglycosides, the polymyxins, clindamycin, and lincomycin.
■ Use with mechanical ventilation, assess patient for adequate and preferably optimal ventilator settings *before* paralyzing. If patient is "fighting" the ventilator, provide adequately high flow rates and tidal volumes, short inspiratory times, and reasonable I:E ratios, check the sensitivity in assist-control mode, provide sufficiently high rates to avoid patient fatigue; consider paralysis if these measures fail.
■ Assess ventilator patients for pain, hypoxemia, or ventilator malfunction, if restless and anxious, before instituting muscle paralysis.
■ Assess need of patient and provide for pain control and sedation during neuromuscular blockade; *neuromuscular blocking agents do not provide analgesia or sedation.*
■ Close eyelids and provide eye lubricant during prolonged paralysis.
■ Since usual signs of pain or anxiety (restlessness, tachynea, distress, thrashing) are blocked, monitor vital signs closely and overall patient appearance and state to detect problems (e.g., IV infiltration).
■ Check ventilator alarm settings for sufficient limits and sensitivity; a disconnect alarm is critical.
■ Assess reversal of drug before attempting to wean from mechanical ventilatory support.

Administer:
■ Administer by IV, not by IM, for more consistent absorption and distribution and to avoid the pain associated with IM injection of the drug.
■ Reversal: neostigmine or edrophonium, preceded by atropine to inhibit muscarinic response especially in upper airway.

pirbuterol acetate
(pur-byoo'-ter-ole)
Maxair
Func. class.: Beta₂-adrenergic bronchodilator
Chem. class.: Catecholamine derivative

See Section III: Aerosol Agents for Oral Inhalation

plasma protein fraction
Plasmanate, Plasma-Plex, Plasmatein, PPF Protenate
Func. class.: Blood derivative
Chem. class.: Human plasma in NaCl

Action: Exerts oncotic pressure similar to human plasma, expands blood volume

Uses: Hypovolemic shock, hypoproteinemia, ARDS, preoperative cardiopulmonary bypass, acute liver failure

Dosage and routes:
Shock
■ *Adult:* IV INF 250-500 ml (12.5-25 g protein), not to exceed 10 ml/min
■ *Child:* IV INF 22-33 ml/kg at 5-10 ml/min

italic = common side effects   **bold** = life-threatening reactions

Hypoproteinemia
- *Adult:* IV INF 1000-1500 ml qd, not to exceed 8 ml/min
Available forms: Inj IV 50 mg/ml

Side effects/adverse reactions:
GI: Nausea, vomiting, increased salivation
INTEG: Rash, urticaria, cyanosis
CNS: Fever, chills, headache, paresthesias, flushing
RESP: Altered respirations, dyspnea, pulmonary edema
CV: Fluid overload, hypotension, erratic pulse

Contraindications: Hypersensitivity, CHF, severe anemia, renal insufficiency

Precautions: Decreased salt intake, decreased cardiac reserve, lack of albumin deficiency, hepatic disease, renal disease, pregnancy (C)

Pharmacokinetics: Metabolized as a protein/energy source

Interactions/incompatibilities:
- Incompatible with sol containing alcohol or norepinephrine

Lab test interferences:
False increase: Alk phosphatase

RESPIRATORY CARE CONSIDERATIONS:
Assess/evaluate:
- Monitor ECG for tachycardia and blood pressure for hypertension, hypotension.
- Assess circulatory volume of patient: pulse pressure, capillary refill with skin pressure.
- Assess improvement in cardiac output and minimize airway pressures on mechanical ventilation, particularly mean airway pressure, by adjusting peak flows and I:E ratios and using modes such as pressure support if possible, especially while patient is being stabilized.
- Monitor blood pressure with concomitant administration of beta agonist bronchodilators to avoid hypertension.
- Auscultate breath sounds for rales, signs of pulmonary edema, or improvement and clearing of transudates.
- Inspect chest radiograph when available, for pulmonary clearing of infiltrates if previously present.
- Evaluate hematocrit and hemoglobin with administration to assess for adequate or improved oxygen transport to the tissues.

potassium bicarbonate/ potassium acetate/ potassium chloride/ potassium gluconate/ potassium phosphate
Effer-K, K-Lyte, K-Lyte DS, Klorvess, Tri-K, Twin-K, Cena-K, Gen-K, K⁺ 10, K-Tab, K-Norm, K-Dur 10, K-Dur 20, K-Lyte/Cl, K-Lease, K⁺ Care, Kaon-Cl, Kaon-Cl-10, Kaochlor, Kaochlor S-F, Kato, Kay Ciel, Klor, Klor-Con, Klor-Con 8, Klor-Con 10, Klor-Con/25, Klortrix, Klorvess, Micro-K, Micro KLS, Potachlor, Potage, Potasalan, Potassium Chloride, Rum-K, Slow-K, Ten-K, Urocit-K, Kao-Nor, Kaylixir, K-G Elixir, My-K Elixir, Potassium Gluconate
Func. class.: Electrolyte
Chem. class.: Potassium

Action: Needed for adequate transmission of nerve impulses and cardiac contraction, renal function, intracellular ion maintenance

Uses: Prevention and treatment of hypokalemia

Dosage and routes:
Potassium bicarbonate
▪ *Adult:* PO dissolve 25-50 mEq in water qd-qid
Potassium acetate—hypokalemia
▪ *Adult and child:* PO 40-100 mEq/day in divided doses 2-4 days
Hypokalemia (prevention)
▪ *Adult and child:* PO 20 mEq/day in 2-4 divided doses
Potassium chloride
▪ *Adult:* PO 40-100 mEq in divided doses tid-qid; IV 20 mEq/hr when diluted as 40 mEq/1000 ml, not to exceed 150 mEq/day
Potassium gluconate
▪ *Adult:* PO 40-100 mEq in divided doses tid-qid
Potassium phosphate
▪ *Adult:* IV 1 mEq/hr in sol of 60 mEq/L, not to exceed 150 mEq/day; PO 40-100 mEq/day in divided doses
Available forms: Tabs for sol 6.5, 25 mEq/inj for prep of IV 2, 4 mEq/caps ext rel 8, 10 mEq; powder for sol 3.3, 5, 6.7, 10, 13.3 mEq/5 ml; tabs 4, 13.4 mEq; tabs ext rel 6.7, 8, 10 mEq; inj for prep of IV 1.5, 2, 2.4, 3, 3.2 mEq/ml; elix 6.7 mEq/5 ml; tabs 2, 5 mEq; oral sol 2.375 mEq/5 ml; inj for prep of IV 4.4, 4.7 mEq/ml

Side effects/adverse reactions:
CNS: Confusion
CV: Bradycardia, *cardiac depression, dysrhythmias, arrest,* *peaking T waves, lowered R and depressed RST, prolonged P-R interval, widened QRS complex*
GI: Nausea, vomiting, cramps, pain, *diarrhea,* ulceration of small bowel
GU: Oliguria
INTEG: Cold extremities, rash

Contraindications: Renal disease (severe), severe hemolytic disease, Addison's disease, hyperkalemia, acute dehydration, extensive tissue breakdown

Precautions: Cardiac disease, K-sparing diuretic therapy, systemic acidosis, pregnancy (A)

Interactions/incompatibilities:
▪ Hyperkalemia: potassium phosphate IV and products containing Ca or Mg; K-sparing, diuretic, or other K products
▪ Incompatible with amikacin, amphotericin B, dobutamine, fat emulsion, penicillin G sodium

Pharmacokinetics:
PO: Excreted by kidneys and in feces; onset of action ≈ 30 min
IV: Immediate onset of action

RESPIRATORY CARE CONSIDERATIONS:
Assess/evaluate:
▪ Monitor ECG for peaking T waves, lowered R, depressed RST, prolonged P-R interval, widening QRS complex, hyperkalemia; drug should be reduced or discontinued.
▪ Evaluate K level during treatment (3.5-5.0 mg/dl is normal level).
▪ Monitor cardiac status: rate, rhythm, CVP, PWP, PAWP, if being monitored directly.

---

italic = common side effects   **bold** = life-threatening reactions

- Monitor acid-base balance; potassium-sparing diuretic therapy can result in hyperkalemia, acidosis. Thiazides and other diuretics may lower potassium, causing metabolic alkalosis.

potassium iodide (SSKI)
Pima, Iosat, Thyro-Block
Func. class.: Expectorant
Chem. class.: Iodine compound

Action: Increases respiratory tract fluid by incorporation in and stimulation of submucosal glands in the airway.

Uses: Bronchial asthma, emphysema, bronchitis, nuclear radiation protection

Dosage and routes:
- *Adult:* PO 0.3-0.6 ml q4-6h
- *Child:* PO 0.25-1 ml saturated sol bid-qid
Radiation protection:
- *Adult:* PO 0.13 ml SSKI before or after initial exposure
Infant <1 yr: Half adult dose
Available forms: Sol 1 g/ml

Side effects/adverse reactions:
EENT: Burning mouth, throat, eye irritation, swelling of eyelids
GI: Gastric irritation
ENDO: Iodism, goiter, myxedema
RESP: Pulmonary edema
INTEG: Angioedema, rash
CNS: Frontal headache, *CNS depression,* fever, parkinsonism

Contraindications: Hypersensitivity to iodides, pulmonary TB, pregnancy (D), hyperthyroidism, hyperkalemia

Precautions: Hypothyroidism, cystic fibrosis, lactation

Pharmacokinetics: Excreted in urine

Interactions/ incompatibilities:
- Increased hypothyroid effects: lithium, antithyroid drugs
- Dysrhythmias, hyperkalemia: K-sparing diuretics, K-containing medication

RESPIRATORY CARE CONSIDERATIONS:
Assess/evaluate:
- Therapeutic effect: improved clearance of secretions evidenced by patient report of sputum production, breath sounds.
- Monitor color, consistency, amount of sputum produced before and after treatment, using 24-hour collection system.
- In chronic bronchitis, monitor airflow changes for improvement; monitor improvement in number of respiratory infections.
- Assess respiratory status: breath sounds, breathing pattern.
- Assess patient's ability to clear and expectorate secretions, to determine need for adjunct bronchial hygiene such as postural drainage, percussion, PEP therapy, or autogenic drainage.

Patient education:
- Drink large amount of nondiuresing fluids such as water, milk, juice, Gatorade to aid mucus clearance and expectoration.
- Do not use if pregnant
- Watch for symptoms of iodism: eruptions, burning of oral cavity, eye irritation
Be aware of symptoms of hy-

perthyroidism: CNS depression, fever, glomerulonephritis.
- Discontinue and notify physician if fever, rash, metallic taste occur.

pralidoxime chloride
(pra-li-dox'eem)
Protopam chloride, 2-PAM
Func. class.: Cholinesterase reactivator
Chem. class.: Quaternary ammonium oxide

Action: Reactivated cholinesterase enzyme metabolizes and inactivates acetylcholine at both muscarinic and nicotinic sites in the periphery.

Uses: Cholinergic crisis in myasthenia gravis, organophosphate poisoning antidote, relief of paralysis of respiratory muscles, adjunct to systemic atropine administration

Dosage and routes:
Anticholinesterase overdose
- *Adult:* IV 1-2 g, then 250 mg q5min until desired response
Organophosphate poisoning
- *Adult:* IV INF 1-2 g/100 ml NS over 15-30 min; may repeat in 1 hr, PO 1-3 g q5h
- *Child:* IV INF 20-40 mg/kg/dose diluted in 100 ml NS over 15-30 min
Available forms: Inj IV 600 mg/2 ml; tabs 500 mg; emergency kit 1 g/20-ml vial

Side effects/adverse reactions:
CNS: Dizziness, headache, drowsiness, blurred vision, diplopia, impaired accommodation
GI: Nausea
MS: Weakness, muscle rigidity
CV: Tachycardia
RESP: Hyperventilation, *laryngospasm*

Contraindications: Hypersensitivity, carbamate insecticide poisoning

Precautions: Myasthenia gravis, pregnancy (C), renal insufficiency, children, lactation

Pharmacokinetics:
PO: Peak 2-3 hr
IV: Peak 5-15 min
IM: Peak 10-20 min
Half-life 1½ hr, metabolized in liver, excreted in urine (unchanged)

Interactions/incompatibilities:
- Avoid use with aminophylline, morphine, phenothiazines, reserpine, succinylcholine, theophylline in organophosphate poisoning
- Incompatible with any drug in sol or syringe

RESPIRATORY CARE CONSIDERATIONS:
Assess/evaluate:
- Therapeutic response: reversal of neuromuscular blockade or improved muscle function, especially diaphragmatic contractile force as evidenced by tidal volume, vital capacity, grip strength.
- In reversing neuromuscular blockade, maintain airway and ventilatory support until complete recovery of adequate ventilation is seen in spontaneous respiratory rate and pattern.
- Monitor for exacerbation of asthma or airway resistance in COPD subject, due to parasympathetic induced bronchoconstriction.
- Assess respiratory rate and pattern, breath sounds for wheezing.

italic = common side effects   **bold** = life-threatening reactions

- Assess subjective response of patient for difficulty in breathing, tightness in chest.
- Assess pulse for bradycardia and BP for decrease.

prazosin HCl
(pra′zoe-sin)
Minipress, Prazosin
Func. class.:
Antihypertensive
Chem. class.: α₁-adrenergic blocker

Action: Peripheral blood vessels dilate, peripheral resistance drops; reduction in blood pressure results from α-adrenergic receptors being blocked

Uses: Hypertension, refractory CHF, Raynaud's vasospasm

Dosage and routes:
- *Adult:* PO 1 mg bid or tid, increasing to 20 mg qd in divided doses if required, usual range 6-15 mg/day, not to exceed 1 mg initially
Available forms: Caps 1, 2, 5 mg

Side effects/adverse reactions:
CV: Palpitations, orthostatic hypotension, tachycardia, edema, rebound hypertension
CNS: Dizziness, headache, drowsiness, anxiety, depression, vertigo, weakness, fatigue
GI: Nausea, vomiting, diarrhea, constipation, abdominal pain
GU: Urinary frequency, incontinence, impotence, priapism, H₂O, Na retention
EENT: Blurred vision, epistaxis, tinnitus, dry mouth, red sclera

Contraindications: Hypersensitivity

Precautions: Pregnancy (C), children

Pharmacokinetics:
PO: Onset 2 hr, peak 1-3 hr, duration 6-12 hr, half-life 2-3 hr, metabolized in liver, excreted via bile, feces (>90%), in urine (<10%)

Interactions/incompatibilities:
- Increased hypotensive effects: β-blockers, nitroglycerin
- Decreased effect: indomethacin

Lab test interferences:
Increased: Urinary norepinephrine, VMA

RESPIRATORY CARE CONSIDERATIONS:
Assess/evaluate:
- Monitor for "first dose" effect: marked hypotension (especially postural), syncope with loss of consciousness with first few doses.
- Monitor effect on BP and pulse, especially if on positive pressure ventilatory support.
- Assess effectiveness of beta-adrenergic bronchodilator therapy for possible antagonistic effect on BP to avoid increasing BP, or decreasing BP due to beta receptor stimulation of vascular smooth muscle in the presence of blocked alpha receptors.
- Consider use of nonadrenergic bronchodilator such as ipratropium bromide as alternative to beta-adrenergic agents, for asthmatics, COPD patients.
- Note: since alpha-receptors are blocked, other adrenergic agents that stimulate both types of sympathetic

receptors or beta receptors, such as epinephrine, may cause exaggerated response of tachycardia and hypotension.
■ Treatment of overdose with epinephrine can cause worsening of hypotension, as outlined previously; use leg elevation, discontinue the drug, support circulation, use a "pure" alpha-agonist such as phenylephrine.

Patient education:
■ Do not use OTC products containing α-adrenergic stimulants (nasal decongestants, OTC cold preparations) or other sympathomimetics unless directed by physician.
■ Report symptoms of CHF: difficulty breathing, especially on exertion or when lying down, night cough, swelling of extremities

---

**prednisolone/
prednisolone
acetate/prednisolone
phosphate/
prednisolone
tebutate**

(pred-niss'oh-lone)
Delta-Cortef, Prednisolone, Prelone, Articulose-50, Key-Pred 25, Key-Pred 50, Predaject-50, Predalone 50, Predcor-25, Predcor-50, Prednisolone Acetate, Hydeltrasol, Key-Pred-SP, Pediapred, Hydeltra-T.B.A., Predalone-T.B.A., Prednisol TBA, Prednisolone Tebutate
Func. class.:
Corticosteroid
Chem. class.: Glucocorticoid, immediate acting

Action: Decreases inflammation by suppression of migration of polymorphonuclear leukocytes, fibroblasts; reversal to increase capillary permeability and lysosomal stabilization

Uses: Severe inflammation, immunosuppression, neoplasms

Dosage and routes:
■ *Adult:* PO 2.5-15 mg bid-qid; IM 2-30 mg (acetate, phosphate) q12h; IV 2-30 mg (phosphate) q12h, 2-30 mg in joint or soft tissue (phosphate), 4-40 mg in joint of lesion (tebutate), 0.25-1 ml qwk in joints (acetate-phosphate)
Available forms: Tabs 5 mg; inj 25, 50, 100 mg/ml acetate; inj 20 mg/ml tebutate; inj 20 mg/ml phosphate; inj 80 mg/ml acetate/phosphate

Side effects/adverse reactions:
INTEG: Acne, poor wound healing, ecchymosis, petechiae
CNS: Depression, flushing, sweating, headache, mood changes
CV: Hypertension, circulatory collapse, thrombophlebitis, embolism, tachycardia
HEMA: Thrombocytopenia
MS: Fractures, osteoporosis, weakness
GI: Diarrhea, nausea, abdominal distention, GI hemorrhage, increased appetite, *pancreatitis*
EENT: Fungal infections, increased intraocular pressure, blurred vision

Contraindications: Psychosis, hypersensitivity, idiopathic thrombocytopenia, acute glomerulonephritis, amebiasis, fungal infections,

---

italic = common side effects   **bold** = life-threatening reactions

nonasthmatic bronchial disease, child <2 yr

Precautions: Pregnancy (C), diabetes mellitus, glaucoma, osteoporosis, seizure disorders, ulcerative colitis, CHF, myasthenia gravis

Pharmacokinetics:
PO: Peak 1-2 hr, duration 2 days
IM: Peak 3-4 hr

Interactions/ incompatibilities:
■ Decreased action of prednisolone: cholestyramine, colestipol, barbiturates, rifampin, ephedrine, phenytoin, theophylline
■ Decreased effects of: anticoagulants, anticonvulsants, antidiabetics, ambenonium, neostigmine, isoniazid, toxoids, vaccines, anticholinesterases, salicylates, somatrem
■ Increased side effects: alcohol, salicylates, indomethacin, amphotericin B, digitalis, cyclosporine, diuretics
■ Increased action of prednisolone: salicylates, estrogens, indomethacin, oral contraceptives, ketoconazole, macrolide antibiotics
■ Incompatible with calcium gluconate/gluceptate, dimenhydrinate, metaraminol, methotrexate, polymyxin B, prochlorperazine, promazine, promethazine

Lab test interferences:
Increase: Cholesterol, Na, blood glucose, uric acid, Ca, urine glucose
Decrease: Ca, K, T_4, T_3, thyroid ^{131}I uptake test, urine 17-OHCS, 17-KS, PBI
False negative: Skin allergy tests

RESPIRATORY CARE CONSIDERATIONS:
Assess/evaluate:
■ Monitor for side effects of increased corticosteroid level: Cushingoid symptoms (moon face, peripheral wasting, central edema).
■ Monitor patients with latent tuberculosis or reactive skin tests for reactivation of the disease.
■ Evaluate muscle weakness and steroid myopathy, especially in chronic lung disease patients.
■ Evaluate cardiovascular system for hypertension, CHF.
■ Monitor electrolytes; potassium and calcium loss can occur with hypokalemic alkalosis.
■ Infection, including pneumonia, can occur.
■ Increased corticosteroid levels can mask symptoms of infection.
■ If asthma is present, monitor for breakthrough symptoms (bronchospasm, wheezing) if drug is discontinued.
■ Evaluate possible adrenal insufficiency when transferring from systemic to inhaled aerosol corticosteroids in asthma.
■ Monitor for symptoms of adrenal insufficiency: nausea, anorexia, fatigue, dizziness, dyspnea, weakness, joint pain.

prednisone
(pred'ni-sone)
Deltasone, Liquid Pred, Meticorten, Orasone, Panasol-S, Prednicen-M, Prednisone, Prednisone Intensol Concentrate, Sterapred, Sterapred OS
Func. class.: Corticosteroid
Chem. class.: Intermediate-acting glucocorticoid

Action: Decreases inflammation by suppression of migration of polymorphonuclear leukocytes, fibroblasts, reversal to increase capillary permeability, and lysosomal stabilization

Uses: Severe inflammation, immunosuppression, neoplasms, multiple sclerosis, collagen disorders, dermatologic disorders

Dosage and routes:
- *Adult:* PO 1.5-2.5 mg bid-qid, then qd or qod; maintenance up to 250 mg/day
Nephrosis
- *Child 18 mo-4 yr:* 7.5-10 mg qid initially
- *Child 4-10 yr:* 15 mg qid initially
- *Child >10 yr:* 20 mg qid initially
Multiple sclerosis
- *Adult:* PO 200 mg/day × 1 wk, then 80 mg qod × 1 mo
Available forms: Tabs 1, 2.5, 5, 10, 20, 25, 50 mg; oral sol 5 mg/5 ml; syr 5 mg/5 ml

Side effects/adverse reactions:
CNS: Depression, flushing, sweating, headache, mood changes
CV: Hypertension, *circulatory collapse, thrombophlebitis, embolism,* tachycardia
EENT: Fungal infections, increased intraocular pressure, blurred vision
GI: Diarrhea, nausea, abdominal distention, *GI hemorrhage,* increased appetite, pancreatitis
HEMA: Thrombocytopenia
INTEG: Acne, poor wound healing, ecchymosis, petechiae

MS: Fractures, osteoporosis, weakness

Contraindications:
Psychosis, hypersensitivity, idiopathic thrombocytopenia, acute glomerulonephritis, amebiasis, fungal infections, nonasthmatic bronchial disease, child <2 yr, AIDS, TB

Precautions: Pregnancy (C), diabetes mellitus, glaucoma, osteoporosis, seizure disorders, ulcerative colitis, CHF, myasthenia gravis, renal disease, esophagitis, peptic ulcer

Pharmacokinetics:
Well absorbed PO
PO: Peak 1-2 hr, duration 1-1½ days, half-life 3½-4 hr, crosses placenta, enters breast milk, metabolized by the liver after conversion

Interactions/ incompatibilities:
- Decreased action of prednisone: cholestyramine, colestipol, barbiturates, rifampin, ephedrine, phenytoin, theophylline
- Decreased effects of: anticoagulants, anticonvulsants, antidiabetics, ambenonium, neostigmine, isoniazid, toxoids, vaccines, anticholinesterases, salicylates, somatrem
- Increased side effects: alcohol, salicylates, indomethacin, amphotericin B, digitalis, cyclosporine, diuretics
- Increased action of prednisone: salicylates, estrogens, indomethacin, oral contraceptives, ketoconazole, macrolide antibiotics

italic = common side effects   **bold** = life-threatening reactions

Lab test interferences:

Increase: Cholesterol, Na, blood glucose, uric acid, Ca, urine glucose

Decrease: Ca, K, T_4, T_3, thyroid ^{131}I uptake test, urine 17-OHCS, 17-KS, PBI

False negative: Skin allergy tests

RESPIRATORY CARE CONSIDERATIONS:

Assess/evaluate:

- Monitor for side effects of increased corticosteroid level: Cushingoid symptoms (moon face, peripheral wasting, central edema).
- Monitor patients with latent tuberculosis or reactive skin tests for reactivation of the disease.
- Evaluate muscle weakness and steroid myopathy, especially in chronic lung disease patients.
- Evaluate cardiovascular system for hypertension, CHF.
- Monitor electrolytes; potassium and calcium loss can occur with hypokalemic alkalosis.
- Infection, including pneumonia, can occur.
- Increased corticosteroid levels can mask symptoms of infection.
- If asthma is present, monitor for breakthrough symptoms (bronchospasm, wheezing) if drug is discontinued.
- Evaluate possible adrenal insufficiency when transferring from systemic to inhaled aerosol corticosteroids in asthma.
- Monitor for symptoms of adrenal insufficiency: nausea, anorexia, fatigue, dizziness, dyspnea, weakness, joint pain.

procainamide HCI
(proe-kane-a'mide)
Procan SR, Promine, Procainamide, Pronestyl, Sub-Quin, Rhythmin
Func. class.: Antidysrhythmic (Class IA)
Chem. class.: Procaine HCl amide analog

Action: Depresses excitability of cardiac muscle to electrical stimulation and slows conduction in atrium, bundle of His, and ventricle

Uses: PVCs, atrial fibrillation, PAT, ventricular tachycardia, atrial dysrhythmias, ventricular tachycardia

Dosage and routes:
Atrial fibrillation/PAT
- *Adult:* PO 1-1.25 g, may give another 750 mg if needed; if no response, 500 mg-1g q2h until desired response; maintenance 50 mg/kg in divided doses q6h
Ventricular tachycardia
- *Adult:* PO 1g; maintenance 50 mg/kg/day given in 3 hr intervals; SUS REL TABS 500 mg-1.25 g q6h
Other dysrhythmias
- *Adult:* IV BOL 100 mg q5min, given 25-50 mg/min, not to exceed 500 mg; or 17 mg/kg total then IV INF 2-6 mg/min
Available forms: Caps 250, 375, 500 mg; tabs 250, 375, 500 mg; tabs sus rel 250, 500, 750, 1000 mg; inj IV 100, 500 mg/ml

Side effects/adverse reactions:
CNS: Headache, dizziness, confusion, psychosis, restlessness, irritability, weakness

GI: Nausea, vomiting, anorexia, diarrhea, hepatomegaly
*CV: Hypotension, **heart block, cardiovascular collapse, arrest***
HEMA: SLE syndrome, *agranulocytosis, thrombocytopenia, neutropenia, hemolytic anemia*
INTEG: Rash, urticaria, edema, swelling (rare),
pruritus

Contraindications: Hypersensitivity, myasthenia gravis, severe heart block

Precautions: Pregnancy (C), lactation, children, renal disease, liver disease, CHF, respiratory depression

Pharmacokinetics:
PO: Peak 1-2 hr, duration 3 hr (8 hr extended)
IM: Peak 10-60 min, duration 3 hr
Half-life 3 hr, metabolized in liver to active metabolites, excreted unchanged by kidneys (60%)

Interactions/ incompatibilities:
■ Increased effects of: neuromuscular blockers, anticholinergics, antihypertensives
■ Increased procainamide effects: cimetidine
■ Decreased effects of procainamide: barbiturates
■ Increased toxicity: other antidysrhythmics
■ Incompatible with phenytoin

RESPIRATORY CARE CONSIDERATIONS:
Assess/evaluate:
■ Monitor ECG; in case of increased QT and/or widening QRS, drug should be discontinued.
■ Monitor for dehydration or hypovolemia, I&O ratio, electrolytes (Na, K, Cl).

■ Monitor pulse rate and BP for hypotension.
■ Assess respiratory rate and pattern (labored, dyspnea).
■ Provide resuscitation support in the event of cardiac arrest, life-threatening dysrhythmias.
■ Evaluate therapeutic response: decreased dysrhythmias.

Patient education:
■ Make position change slowly to prevent orthostatic hypotension and fainting.
■ Avoid hazardous activities if dizziness or blurred vision occurs.

P

procaine HCl
(proe'-kane)
Novocain, Unicaine
Func. class.: Local anesthetic
Chem. class.: Ester

Action: Competes with calcium for sites in nerve membrane that control sodium transport across cell membrane; decreases rise of depolarization phase of action potential

Uses: Spinal anesthesia, epidural, peripheral nerve block, perineum, lower extremities, infiltration

Dosage and routes:
■ Varies by route of anesthesia
Available forms: Inj 1%, 2%, 10%

Side effects/adverse reactions:
CNS: Anxiety, restlessness, *convulsions, LOC,* drowsiness, disorientation, tremors, shivering
*CV: **Myocardial depression, cardiac arrest, dysrhythmias,***

italic = common side effects   **bold** = life-threatening reactions

bradycardia, hypotension, hypertension, fetal bradycardia
GI: Nausea, vomiting
EENT: Blurred vision, tinnitus, pupil constriction
INTEG: Rash, urticaria, allergic reactions, edema, burning, skin discoloration at injection site, tissue necrosis
RESP: Status asthmaticus, respiratory arrest, anaphylaxis

Contraindications: Hypersensitivity, child <12 yr, elderly, severe liver disease

Precautions: Elderly, severe drug allergies, pregnancy (C)

Pharmacokinetics: Onset 2-5 min, duration 1 hr, metabolized by liver, excreted in urine (metabolites)

Interactions/ incompatibilities:
- Dysrhythmias: epinephrine, halothane, enflurane
- Hypertension: MAOIs, tricyclic antidepressants, phenothiazines
- Decreased action of procaine: chloroprocaine

RESPIRATORY CARE CONSIDERATIONS:
Assess/evaluate:
- Monitor CV status and respiratory rate/pattern, level of consciousness.
- Twitching, drowsiness, dizziness, tremors, blurred vision can all indicate early signs of CNS toxicity.
- Toxicity or overdose can cause convulsions requiring airway and ventilatory support.
- Hypersensitivity can result in anaphylaxis, requiring airway/ventilatory support or resuscitation.

- Some solutions contain sulfites which may trigger asthmatic episodes.
- Assess control of pain in subject.

prochlorperazine edisylate/ prochlorperazine maleate
(proe-klor-per'a-zeen)
Compazine, Stemetil*
Func. class.: Antiemetic
Chem. class.: Phenothiazine, piperazine derivative

Action: Acts centrally by blocking chemoreceptor trigger zone, which in turn acts on vomiting center

Uses: Nausea, vomiting

Dosage and routes:
Postoperative nausea/vomiting
- *Adult:* IM 5-10 mg 1-2 hr before anesthesia; may repeat in 30 min; IV 5-10 mg 15-30 min before anesthesia; IV INF 20 mg/L D$_5$W or NS 15-30 min before anesthesia, not to exceed 40 mg/day
Severe nausea/vomiting
- *Adult:* PO 5-10 mg tid-qid; SUST REL 15 mg qd in AM or 10 mg q12h; REC 25 mg/ bid; IM 5-10 mg; may repeat q4h, not to exceed 40 mg/day
- *Child 18-39 kg:* PO 2.5 mg tid or 5 mg bid; do not exceed 15 mg/day; IM 0.132 mg/kg
- *Child 14-17 kg:* PO/REC 2.5 mg bid-tid, not to exceed 10 mg/day; IM 0.132 mg/kg
- *Child 9-13 kg:* PO/REC 2.5 mg qd-bid, not to exceed 7.5 mg/day; IM 0.132 mg/kg
Available forms: Oral sol 5 mg/ ml; inj 5 mg/ml; tabs 5, 10, 25 mg; caps ext rel 10, 15, 30 mg

Side effects/adverse reactions:

CNS: Euphoria, depression, extrapyramidal symptoms, restlessness, tremor, dizziness
GI: Nausea, vomiting, anorexia, dry mouth, diarrhea, constipation, weight loss, metallic taste, cramps
CV: Circulatory failure, tachycardia
RESP: Respiratory depression

Contraindications: Hypersensitivity to phenothiazines, coma, seizure, encephalopathy, bone marrow depression

Precautions: Children <2 yr, pregnancy (C), elderly

Pharmacokinetics:
PO: Onset 30-40 min, duration 3-4 hr
EX REL: Onset 30-40 min, duration 10-12 hr
REC: Onset 60 min, duration 3-4 hr
IM: Onset 10-20 min, duration 12 hr,
Metabolized by liver, excreted by kidneys, crosses placenta, excreted in breast milk

Interactions/incompatibilities:
■ Decreased effect of prochlorperazine: barbiturates, antacids
■ Increased anticholinergic action: anticholinergics, antiparkinson drugs, antidepressants
■ Incompatible with aminophylline, amobarbital, amphotericin B, ampicillin, calcium, cephalothin, chloramphenicol, chlorothiazide, dexamethasone, dimenhydrinate, epinephrine, erythromycin, heparin, hydrocortisone, hydromorphone, kanamycin, methicillin, methohexital, midazolam, penicillin G, pentobarbital, phenobarbital, phenytoin, prednisolone, secobarbital, tetracycline, thiopental, vancomycin
■ Do not mix with other drug in syringe or sol

RESPIRATORY CARE CONSIDERATIONS:
Assess/evaluate:
■ Monitor respiratory status before, during, after administration of drug; check rate, volume, character. Respiratory depression can occur rapidly with elderly, debilitated patients or those with COPD.
■ Assess VS, BP; check patients with cardiac disease more often.
■ Evaluate fluid replacement to avoid dehydration, especially in chronic bronchitis.

Patient education:
■ Avoid hazardous activities, activities requiring alertness; dizziness may occur.
■ Avoid alcohol while taking this drug.

promethazine HCl
(proe-meth′a-zeen)
Anergan 25, Anergan 50, Pentazine, Phenameth, Phenazine 25, Phenazine 50, Phenergan, Phenergan Fortis, Phenergan Plain, Phenoject-50, Pro 50, Prometh-50, Promethazine HCl, Prorex 25, Prorex 50, Prothazine, Prothazine Plain, V-Gan 25, V-Gan 50
Func. class.: Antihistamine, H₁-receptor antagonist
Chem. class.: Phenothiazine derivative

Action: Blocks the action of histamine at H₁-receptor sites

italic = common side effects   **bold** = life-threatening reactions

on blood vessels, GI, respiratory tract to decrease allergic inflammatory response and in general the pharmacologic effects of histamine. There is also an anticholinergic (drying) and sedative effect as well as an antiemetic effect.

Uses: Motion sickness, rhinitis, allergy symptoms, sedation, nausea, preoperative and postoperative sedation

Dosage and routes:
Nausea
- *Adult:* PO/IM 25 mg; may repeat 12.5-25 mg q4-6h
- *Child:* PO/IM 0.5 mg/lb q4-6h
Motion sickness
- *Adult:* PO 25 mg bid
- *Child:* PO/IM/REC 12.5-25 mg bid
Allergy/rhinitis
- *Adult:* PO 12.5 mg qid or 25 mg hs
- *Child:* PO 6.25-12.5 mg tid or 25 mg hs
Sedation
- *Adult:* PO/IM 25-50 mg hs
- *Child:* PO/IM/REC 12.5-25 mg hs
Sedation (preoperative/postoperative)
- *Adult:* PO/IM/IV 25-50 mg
- *Child:* PO/IM/IV 12.5-25 mg
Available forms: Tabs 12.5, 25, 50 mg; syr 6.25, 25 mg/5 ml; supp 12.5, 25, 50 mg; inj 25, 50 mg/ml

Side effects/adverse reactions:
CNS: Dizziness, drowsiness, poor coordination, fatigue, anxiety, euphoria, confusion, paresthesia, neuritis
CV: Hypotension, palpitations, tachycardia
RESP: Increased thick secretions, wheezing, chest tightness

HEMA: Thrombocytopenia, agranulocytosis, hemolytic anemia
GI: Constipation, dry mouth, nausea, vomiting, anorexia, diarrhea
INTEG: Rash, urticaria, photosensitivity
GU: Retention, dysuria, frequency
EENT: Blurred vision, dilated pupils, tinnitus, nasal stuffiness, dry nose, throat, mouth, photosensitivity

Contraindications: Hypersensitivity to H_1-receptor antagonist, acute asthma attack, lower respiratory tract disease

Precautions: Increased intraocular pressure, renal disease, cardiac disease, hypertension, bronchial asthma, seizure disorder, stenosed peptic ulcers, hyperthyroidism, prostatic hypertrophy, bladder neck obstruction, pregnancy (C)

Pharmacokinetics:
PO: Onset 20 min, duration 4-6 hr, metabolized in liver, excreted by kidneys, GI tract (inactive metabolites)

Interactions/incompatibilities:
- Increased CNS depression: barbiturates, narcotics, hypnotics, tricyclic antidepressants, alcohol
- Decreased effect of: oral anticoagulants, heparin
- Increased effect of promethazine: MAOIs
- Incompatible with aminophylline, calcium gluconate, carbenicillin, chloramphenicol, chlordiazepoxide, chlorothiazide, codeine, dextran, dimenhydrinate, heparin, hy-

drocortisone, methicillin, methohexital, methylprednisolone, morphine, penicillin G, pentobarbital, phenobarbital, phenytoin, secobarbital, thiopental, Vit B with C

Lab test interferences:
False negative: Skin allergy test
False positive: Urine pregnancy test

RESPIRATORY CARE CONSIDERATIONS:
Assess/evaluate:
- Note drying of the upper airway.
- Caution is suggested if used in asthma, although thickening of lower respiratory tract secretions has not been established.
- Drowsiness may be a risk factor in subjects with sleep apnea.
- Assess nasal passages during long-term treatment for changes in mucus.
- Therapeutic response: decrease in runny nose.

Patient education:
- Avoid hazardous activities or use caution while drug action persists.
- Additional CNS depression may occur with concomitant use of CNS depressants (tranquilizers, sedatives, or alcohol).

propafenone
(proe-pa-fen'one)
Rythmol
Func. class.: Antidysrhythmic (Class IC)
Chem. class.: Structurally similar to propranolol

Action: Slows conduction velocity; reduces membrane responsiveness; inhibits automaticity; increases ratio of effective refractory period to action potential duration; β-blocking activity

Uses: Life-threatening dysrhythmias, sustained ventricular tachycardia

Dosage and routes:
- *Adult:* PO 300-900 mg/day in divided doses, 150 mg q8h; allow a 3-4 day interval before increasing dose
Available forms: Tabs 150, 300 mg

Side effects/adverse reactions:
INTEG: Rash
CV: Dysrhythmias, palpitations, AV block, intraventricular conduction delay, AV dissociation, CHF, *sudden death,* atrial flutter
HEMA: Leukopenia, agranulocytosis, granulocytopenia, thrombocytopenia, anemia
CNS: Headache, dizziness, abnormal dreams, syncope, confusion, *seizures*
GI: Nausea, vomiting, constipation, dyspepsia, cholestasis, *hepatitis,* abnormal liver function studies, dry mouth
RESP: Dyspnea
EENT: Blurred vision, altered taste, tinnitus

Contraindications: 2nd or 3rd degree AV block, right bundle branch block, cardiogenic shock, hypersensitivity, bradycardia, uncontrolled CHF, sick-sinus node syndrome, marked hypotension, bronchospastic disorders

Precautions: CHF, hypokalemia, hyperkalemia, recent MI, nonallergic bronchospasm, pregnancy (C), lactation, children, hepatic or renal disease

italic = common side effects   **bold** = life-threatening reactions

Pharmacokinetics: Peak 3-5 hr, half-life 2-10 hr, metabolized in liver, excreted in urine (metabolite)

Interactions/ incompatibilities:
- Increased effect of propafenone: cimetidine, quinidine
- Increased anticoagulation: warfarin
- Increased digoxin level: digoxin
- Increased β-blocker effect: propranolol, metoprolol

Lab test interferences:
Increase: CPK

RESPIRATORY CARE CONSIDERATIONS:
Assess/evaluate:
- Avoid use in patients with bronchospasm or reversible airway obstruction: beta-adrenergic blocking effect can worsen obstruction.
- Assess cardiac status for CHF prior to use: negative inotropic effect can worsen CHF.
- Monitor ECG; in case of increased QT and/or widening QRS; drug should be discontinued.
- Assess for dehydration or hypovolemia, I&O ratio, electrolytes (Na, K, Cl).
- Monitor BP for hypotension, hypertension and pulse rate.
- Assess respiratory rate and pattern (labored, dyspnea); differentiate causes other than drug side effect.
- Provide resuscitation support in the event of cardiac arrest, life-threatening arrhythmias.
- Evaluate therapeutic response: decreased dysrhythmias.

Patient education:
- Make position change slowly to prevent orthostatic hypotension and fainting.
- Avoid hazardous activities if dizziness or blurred vision occurs.

propofol
(proe-po'foel)
Diprivan
Func. class.: General anesthetic
Controlled Substance Schedule II
Chem. class.: 2,6-diisopropylphenol

Action: Produces dose-dependent CNS depression

Uses: Induction or maintenance of anesthesia as part of balanced anesthetic technique

Dosage and routes:
Induction
- *Adult:* IV 2-2.5 mg/kg, approximately 40 mg q10sec until induction onset
- *Elderly:* 1-1.5 mg/kg, approximately 20 mg q10sec until induction onset
Maintenance
- *Adult:* 0.1-0.2 mg/kg/min (6-12 mg/kg/hr)
- *Elderly:* 0.05-0.1 mg/kg/min (3-6 mg/kg/hr)
Intermittent bolus
- *Adult:* Increments of 25-50 mg as needed
Available forms: Inj 10 mg/ml in 20 ml amp

Side effects/adverse reactions:
CNS: Movement, headache, jerking, fever, dizziness, shivering, tremor, confusion, somnolence, paresthesia, agitation, abnormal dreams, euphoria, fatigue

GI: Nausea, vomiting, abdominal cramping, dry mouth, swallowing, hypersalivation
MS: Myalgia
GU: Urine retention, green urine
EENT: Blurred vision, tinnitus, eye pain, strange taste
CV: Bradycardia, hypotension, hypertension, PVC, PAC, tachycardia, abnormal ECG, ST segment depression, *asystole*
RESP: Apnea, cough, hiccups, dyspnea, hypoventilation, sneezing, wheezing, tachypnea, hypoxia
INTEG: Flushing, phlebitis, hives, burning/stinging at injection site

Contraindications: Hypersensitivity, hyperlipidemia

Precautions: Elderly, respiratory depression, severe respiratory disorders, cardiac dysrhythmias, pregnancy (B), labor and delivery, lactation, children

Pharmacokinetics: Onset 40 sec, rapid distribution, half-life 1-8 min, terminal elimination half-life 5-10 hr, 70% excreted in urine, metabolized in liver by conjugation to inactivate metabolites

Interactions/ incompatibilities:
■ Increased CNS depression: alcohol, narcotics, sedative/hypnotics, antipsychotics, skeletal muscle relaxants, inhalational anesthetics

RESPIRATORY CARE CONSIDERATIONS:
Assess/evaluate:
■ Assess degree of respiratory depression; provide airway control/protection, oxygenation, and ventilatory support until recovery from drug.

Assess degree of recovery before instituting weaning or removing patient from mechanical ventilation.
■ Monitor cardiovascular status for circulatory depression: BP, pulse.
■ Propofol does not provide analgesia, provide suitable pain control.
■ Note that concomitant administration of narcotic analgesics, antidepressants, or barbiturates will increase sedative effect and CNS depression, including respiratory depression, apnea, and muscle rigidity; assess sensorium, respiratory rate and pattern.

Patient education:
■ Use deep breathing, turning, coughing after surgery to prevent increased secretions in lungs.

propranolol HCl
(proe-pran'oh-lole)
Betachron, Inderal, Inderal LA, Inderal 10, Inderal 20, Inderal 40, Inderal 60, Inderal 80, Ipran, Propranolol HCl, Propranolol Intensol
Func. class.: Antihypertensive, antianginal
Chem. class.: β-adrenergic blocker

Action: Nonselective β-blocker with negative inotropic, chronotropic, dromotropic properties

Uses: Chronic stable angina pectoris, hypertension, supraventricular dysrhythmias, migraine, prophylaxis, MI, pheochromocytoma, essential tremor, tetralogy of Fallot, cyanotic spells

italic = common side effects   **bold** = life-threatening reactions

Dosage and routes:

Dysrhythmias
- *Adult:* PO 10-30 mg tid-qid; IV BOL 0.5-3 mg over 1 mg/min may repeat in 2 min

Hypertension
- *Adult:* PO 40 mg bid or 80 mg qd (sus rel) initially; usual dose 120-240 mg/day bid-tid or 120-160 mg qd (sus rel)

Angina
- *Adult:* PO 80-320 mg in divided doses bid-qid or 80 mg qd (sus rel); usual dose 160 mg qd (sus rel)

MI
- *Adult:* PO 180-240 mg/day tid-qid

Pheochromocytoma
- *Adult:* PO 60 mg/day × 3 days preoperatively in divided doses or 30 mg/day in divided doses (inoperable tumor)

Migraine
- *Adult:* PO 80 mg/day (sus rel) or in divided doses; may increase to 160-240 mg/day in divided doses

Essential tremor
- *Adult:* PO 40 mg bid; usual dose 120 mg/day

Available forms: Caps ext rel 80, 120, 160 mg; tabs 10, 20, 40, 60, 80, 90 mg; inj 1 mg/ml; oral sol 4 mg, 8 mg/ml; conc oral sol 80 mg/ml; ext rel cap 60 mg

Side effects/adverse reactions:

RESP: Dyspnea, respiratory dysfunction, *bronchospasm*
CV: Bradycardia, hypotension, CHF, palpitations, AV block, peripheral vascular insufficiency, vasodilation
HEMA: Agranulocytosis, thrombocytopenia
GI: Nausea, vomiting, diarrhea, colitis, constipation, cramps, dry mouth, hepatomegaly, gastric pain, acute pancreatitis
GU: Impotence, decreased libido, urinary tract infections
MS: Joint pain, arthralgia, muscle cramps, pain
MISC: Facial swelling, weight change, Raynaud's phenomenon
INTEG: Rash, pruritus, fever
CNS: Depression, hallucinations, dizziness, fatigue, lethargy, paresthesias, bizarre dreams, disorientation
EENT: Sore throat, *laryngospasm*, blurred vision, dry eyes
META: Hyperglycemia, hypoglycemia

Contraindications: Hypersensitivity to this drug, cardiac failure, cardiogenic shock, 2nd or 3rd degree heart block, bronchospastic disease, sinus bradycardia, CHF

Precautions: Diabetes mellitus, pregnancy (C), renal disease, lactation, hyperthyroidism, COPD, hepatic disease, children, myasthenia gravis, peripheral vascular disease, hypotension, CHF

Pharmacokinetics:
PO: Onset 30 min, peak 1-1½ hr
IV: Onset 2 min, peak 15 min, duration 3-6 hr, immediate rel half-life 3-5 hr, sus rel half-life 8-11 hr, metabolized by liver, crosses placenta, blood-brain barrier, excreted in breast milk

Interactions/incompatibilities:
- AV block: digitalis, calcium channel blockers
- Increased negative inotropic effects: verapamil, disopyramide

- Increased effects of: reserpine, digitalis, neuromuscular blocking agents
- Decreased β-blocking effects: norepinephrine, isoproterenol, barbiturates, rifampin, dopamine, dobutamine, smoking
- Increased β-blocking effect: cimetidine
- Increased hypotension: quinidine, haloperidol, hydralazine
- Incompatible with any drug in sol or syringe

Lab test interferences:
Increase: Serum K, serum uric acid, ALT/AST, alk phosphatase, LDH
Decrease: Blood glucose

RESPIRATORY CARE CONSIDERATIONS:
Assess/evaluate:
- Avoid use with reversible airway obstruction or bronchospastic disease such as asthma or chronic bronchitis due to potential for bronchospasm (wheezing, dyspnea, complaints of chest tightness) secondary to beta-blockade; consider use of other classes of antihypertensive agents for these patients.
- Monitor all subjects for symptoms of increased airway resistance (wheezing, tightness in chest, difficulty breathing).
- Monitor effect on BP and pulse, especially if on positive pressure ventilatory support.
- Assess effectiveness of beta-adrenergic bronchodilator therapy for possible antagonism and effect on BP to avoid increasing BP, if used.

Patient education:
- Do not use OTC products containing α-adrenergic

stimulants (nasal decongestants, OTC cold preparations) unless directed by physician
- Caution patient that orthostatic hypotension may occur.
- Report symptoms of CHF: difficulty breathing, especially on exertion or when lying down, night cough, swelling of extremities.

protamine sulfate
(proe'ta-meen)
Func. class.: Heparin antagonist
Chem. class.: Low-molecular-weight protein

Action: Binds heparin, making it ineffective
Uses: Heparin overdose
Dosage and routes:
- *Adult:* IV 1 mg of protamine/90-115 U heparin given; administer slowly 1-3 min; give undiluted to 1%, not to exceed 50 mg/10 min
Available forms: Inj IV 10 mg/ml
Side effects/adverse reactions:
CV: Hypotension, bradycardia, *circulatory collapse*
GI: Nausea, vomiting, anorexia
INTEG: Rash, dermatitis, urticaria
CNS: Lassitude
HEMA: Bleeding, *anaphylaxis*
RESP: Dyspnea, pulmonary edema, severe respiratory distress
Contraindications: Hypersensitivity
Precautions: Pregnancy (C), lactation, children, allergy to fish
Pharmacokinetics:
IV: Onset 5 min, duration 2 hr

italic = common side effects   **bold** = life-threatening reactions

Interactions/ incompatibilities:
- Considered incompatible with any drug in sol or syringe

RESPIRATORY CARE CONSIDERATIONS:

Assess/evaluate:
- Therapeutic response: reversal of heparin-induced bleeding.
- Assess blood studies, especially hematocrit, hemoglobin, for decreases or improvements.
- Note: protamine alone is an anticoagulant and can cause bleeding; when given with heparin, a stable salt forms, inactivating both agents.
- Noncardiogenic pulmonary edema of uncertain origin has occurred with protamine during cardiopulmonary bypass.
- Circulatory collapse with reduced cardiac output has occurred; assess blood pressure.

pseudoephedrine HCl/ pseudoephedrine sulfate

(soo-doe-e-fed′rin)

Afrinol Repetabs, Allerid, Cenafed, Cenafed Syrup, Children's Sudafed, Decofed Syrup, DeFed-60, Dorcol Children's Decongestant, Drixoral Non-Drowsy Formula, Eltor,* Efidac/24, Genaphed, Halofed, Myfedrine, Novafed, PediaCare Infant's Decongestant, Pseudoephedrine HCl, Pseudogest Decongestant, Pseudo Syrup, Sinustat, Sudafed, Sudafed 12 hour, Sudrin

Func. class.: Adrenergic
Chem. class.: Substituted phenylethylamine

Action: Primary activity through α-effects on respiratory mucosal membranes reducing congestion, hyperemia, edema; minimal bronchodilation secondary to β-effects

Uses: Nasal decongestant

Dosage and routes:
- *Adult:* PO 60 mg q6h; EXT REL 60-120 mg q12h or q24h
- *Child 6-12 yr:* PO 30 mg q6h, not to exceed 120 mg/day
- *Child 2-6 yr:* PO 15 mg q6h, not to exceed 60 mg/day
Available forms: Caps ext rel 120 mg; sol 15 mg, 30 mg/5 ml, 7.5 mg/0.8 ml; tabs 30, 60, 120 mg

Side effects/adverse reactions:
CNS: Tremors, anxiety, insomnia, headache, dizziness, anxiety, hallucinations, *seizures*
EENT: Dry nose, irritation of nose and throat
CV: Palpitations, tachycardia, hypertension, chest pain, *dysrhythmias*
GI: Anorexia, nausea, vomiting, dry mouth
GU: Dysuria

Contraindications: Hypersensitivity to sympathomimetics, narrow-angle glaucoma

Precautions: Pregnancy (C), cardiac disorders, hyperthyroidism, diabetes mellitus, prostatic hypertrophy

Pharmacokinetics:
PO: Onset 15-30 min, duration 4-6 hr, 8-12 hr (extended release), metabolized in liver, excreted in feces and breast milk

Interactions/ incompatibilities:
- Do not use with MAOIs or tricyclic antidepressants; hypertensive crisis may occur
- Decreased effect of this drug: methyldopa, urinary acidifiers, rauwolfia alkaloids
- Increased effect of this drug: urinary alkalizers

RESPIRATORY CARE CONSIDERATIONS:
Assess/evaluate:
- Therapeutic response: decreased nasal congestion.
- Avoid use with hypertensive patients or those on beta agonists due to additive effect increasing BP.
- Assess BP prior to use.
- Consider use of antihistamine cold remedies to dry secretions, if BP is difficult to control.

Patient/family education:
- Do not use continuously, or more than recommended dose, or rebound congestion may occur.
- Check with physician before using other drugs, as drug interactions may occur.
- Insomnia can occur if taken at night due to sympathomimetic effect on CNS.
- Stimulation, restlessness, or tremors can occur.

pyrazinamide
(peer-a-zin′a-mide)
Pyrazinamide, Tebrazid*
Func. class.: Antitubercular agent
Chem. class.: Pyrazinoic acid amine/nicoturimide analog

Action: Bactericidal interference with lipid, nucleic acid biosynthesis

Uses: Tuberculosis, as an adjunct when other drugs are not feasible

Dosage and routes:
- *Adult:* PO 20-35 mg/kg/day in 3-4 divided doses, not to exceed 3 g/day
Available forms: Tabs 500 mg

Side effects/adverse reactions:
INTEG: Photosensitivity, urticaria
CNS: Headache
GI: Hepatotoxicity, abnormal liver function tests, peptic ulcer
GU: Urinary difficulty, increased uric acid
HEMA: Hemolytic anemia

Contraindications: Hypersensitivity

Precautions: Pregnancy (C), child < 13 yr

Pharmacokinetics:
PO: Peak 2 hr, half-life 9-10 hr, metabolized in liver, excreted in urine (metabolites/ unchanged drug)

Lab test interferences:
Increase: PBI
Decrease: 17-KS

RESPIRATORY CARE CONSIDERATIONS:
Assess/evaluate:
- Monitor bacteriologic response to therapy using drug-susceptibility testing.
- Assess subject for adverse reactions to drug therapy for mycobacteria such as hyperuricemia, hepatotoxicity; evaluate liver enzymes.
- Monitor signs of anemia: hematocrit, hemoglobin, fatigue.
- Respiratory care practitioners and other health care personnel should self-screen for

infection with TB routinely and following exposure.
- Proper environmental and personnel protection programs should be implemented when treating subjects with TB.
- Consider the possibility of HIV infection in individuals with confirmed or suspected TB.

Patient education:
- Compliance with dosage schedule, duration is necessary.
- Scheduled appointments must be kept or relapse may occur.

pyridostigmine bromide

(peer-id-oh-stig′meen)
Mestinon, Regonol
Func. class.: Cholinergic
Chem. class.: Tertiary amine carbamate

Action: Prevents destruction of acetylcholine by inhibiting cholinesterase enzymes, which increases concentration at sites where acetylcholine is released; this facilitates transmission of impulses across myoneural junction

Uses: Nondepolarizing muscle relaxant antagonist, myasthenia gravis

Dosage and routes:
Myasthenia gravis
- *Adult:* PO 60-180 mg bid-qid, not to exceed 1.5 g/day; IM/IV ⅟₃₀ of PO dose, sus rel 180-540 mg qd or bid at intervals of at least 6 hr
Tubocurare antagonist
- *Adult:* 0.6-1.2 mg IV atropine, then 10-30 mg
Available forms: Tabs 60 mg; tabs sus rel 180 mg; syr 60 mg/5 ml; inj IM/IV 5 mg/ml

Side effects/adverse reactions:
INTEG: Rash, urticaria, flushing
CNS: Dizziness, headache, sweating, weakness, *convulsions*, incoordination, paralysis, drowsiness, LOC
GI: Nausea, diarrhea, vomiting, cramps, increased salivary and gastric secretions, peristalsis
CV: Tachycardia, dysrhythmias, bradycardia, AV block, hypotension, ECG changes, *cardiac arrest*, syncope
GU: Frequency, incontinence, urgency
RESP: Respiratory depression, bronchospasm, constriction, laryngospasm, respiratory arrest
EENT: Miosis, blurred vision, lacrimation, visual changes

Contraindications: Bradycardia hypotension obstruction of intestine or renal system bromide sensitivity

Precautions: Seizure disorders, bronchial asthma, coronary occlusion, hyperthyroidism, dysrhythmias, peptic ulcer, megacolon, poor GI motility, pregnancy (C)

Pharmacokinetics:
PO: Onset 20-30 min, duration 3-6 hr
IM/IV/SC: Onset 2-15 min, duration 2½-4 hr, metabolized in liver, excreted in urine

Interactions/ incompatibilities:
- Decreased action: gallamine, metocurine, pancuronium, tubocurarine, atropine
- Increased action: decamethonium, succinylcholine
- Decreased action of pyridostigmine: aminoglycosides, anesthetics, procainamide, quinidine, mecamylamine,

polymyxin, magnesium, corticosteroids, antidysrhythmics
- Considered incompatible with any drug in sol or syringe

RESPIRATORY CARE CONSIDERATIONS:
Assess/evaluate:
- Therapeutic response: reversal of neuromuscular blockade or improved muscle function, especially diaphragmatic contractile force as evidenced by tidal volume, vital capacity, grip strength.
- In reversing neuromuscular blockade, maintain airway and ventilatory support until complete recovery of adequate ventilation is seen in spontaneous respiratory rate and pattern.
- Monitor for exacerbation of asthma or airway resistance in COPD subject, due to parasympathetic induced bronchoconstriction.
- Assess respiratory rate and pattern, breath sounds for wheezing.
- Assess subjective response of patient for difficulty in breathing, tightness in chest.
- Assess pulse for bradycardia and BP for decrease.
- Note: use of a cholinergic agent can intensify and prolong a depolarizing blockade induced by succinylcholine, due to the inactivation of acetylcholine needed for neuromuscular transmission.

quinapril
(kwye'na-preel)
Accupril
Func. class.:
Antihypertensive
Chem. class.: Angiotensin-converting enzyme (ACE) inhibitor

Action: Selectively suppresses renin-angiotensin-aldosterone system; inhibits ACE, prevents conversion of angiotensin I to angiotensin II; results in dilation of arterial, venous vessels

Uses: Hypertension, alone or in combination with thiazide diuretics

Dosage and routes:
- *Adult:* PO 10 mg qd initially, then 20-80 mg/day divided bid or qd
Available forms: Tabs 5, 10, 20, 40 mg

Side effects/adverse reactions:
CV: Hypotension, postural hypotension, syncope, palpitations, angina pectoris, MI, tachycardia, vasodilation
GU: Increased BUN, creatinine, decreased libido, impotence, urinary tract infection
HEMA: **Thrombocytopenia, agranulocytosis**
INTEG: **Angioedema,** rash, sweating, photosensitivity, pruritus
RESP: Cough, bronchitis
META: Hyperkalemia
GI: Nausea, constipation, vomiting, gastritis, GI hemorrhage, dry mouth
CNS: Headache, dizziness, fatigue, somnolence, depression, malaise, nervousness, vertigo
MISC: Back pain, amblyopia, pharyngitis
MS: Arthralgia, arthritis, myalgia

Contraindications: Hypersensitivity to ACE inhibitors, pregnancy (D), children

Precautions: Impaired renal, liver function, dialysis

---

patients, hypovolemia, blood dyscrasias, COPD, asthma, elderly, lactation

Pharmacokinetics:
PO: Peak ½-1 hr, serum protein binding 97%, half-life 2 hr, metabolized by liver (metabolites), metabolities excreted in urine

Interactions/ incompatibilities:
■ Increased hypotension: diuretics, other antihypertensives, ganglionic blockers, adrenergic blockers, phenothiazines
■ Use caution with vasodilators, hydralazine, prazosin, potassium-sparing diuretics, sympathomimetics, K supplements
■ Decreased absorption of: tetracycline
■ Reduced hypotensive effect of quinipril: indomethacin
■ Increased toxicity: lithium, digoxin

Lab test interferences:
False positive: Urine acetone

RESPIRATORY CARE CONSIDERATIONS:
Assess/evaluate:
■ Therapeutic response: decrease in BP.
■ Persistent cough and fever are common side effects of the ACE inhibitors, which should be differentiated from other possible causes, such as respiratory infection.
■ Monitor for possible hypotension.
■ Evaluate BP with COPD or asthmatic subjects who require beta agonists for reversible airway obstruction.
■ Assess for symptoms of CHF: edema, dyspnea, wet rales, BP.

quinidine gluconate/ quinidine polygalacturonate/ quinidine sulfate
(kwin'i-deen)
Quinaglute Dura-Tabs, Quinalan, Quinidine Gluconate, Cardioquin, Quinidex Extentabs, Quinidine Sulfate, Quinora
Func. class.: Antidysrhythmic (Class IA)
Chem. class.: Quinine dextro isomer

Action: Prolongs action, potential duration, and effective refractory period, thus decreasing myocardial excitability; anticholinergic properties

Uses: PVCs, atrial fibrillation, PAT, ventricular tachycardia, atrial dysrhythmias

Dosage and routes:
Atrial fibrillation/flutter
■ *Adult:* PO 200 mg q2-3h × 5-8 doses; may increase qd until sinus rhythm is restored; max 4 g/day given only after digitalization
Paroxysmal supraventricular tachycardia
■ *Adult:* PO 400-600 mg q2-3h
All other dysrhythmias
■ *Adult:* PO 50-200 mg as a test dose, then 200-400 mg q4-6h; IM 600 mg, then 400 mg q2h, after test dose (gluconate); IV INF 800 mg in 40 ml D_5W run at 16 mg/min
Available forms: (Gluconate) tabs sus rel 324, 330 mg; inj IM gluconate 80 mg/ml; (sulfate) tabs 100, 200, 300 mg; caps 200, 300 mg; tabs sus rel 300 mg; inj IV (polygalacturonate) tabs 275 mg, sulfate 200 mg/ml

Side effects/adverse reactions:
CNS: Headache, dizziness, involuntary movement, confusion, psychosis, restlessness, irritability, syncope, excitement
EENT: Cinchonism: tinnitus, blurred vision, hearing loss, mydriasis, disturbed color vision
GI: Nausea, vomiting, anorexia, *diarrhea,* **hepatotoxicity**
CV: Hypotension, bradycardia, PVCs, *heart block,* **cardiovascular collapse, arrest**
HEMA: **Thrombocytopenia,** hemolytic anemia, agranulocytosis, hypoprothrombinemia
RESP: Dyspnea, *respiratory depression*
INTEG: Rash, urticaria, angioedema, swelling, photosensitivity

Contraindications: Hypersensitivity, blood dyscrasias, severe heart block, myasthenia gravis

Precautions: Pregnancy (C), lactation, children, renal disease, K imbalance, liver disease, CHF, respiratory depression

Pharmacokinetics:
PO: Peak ½-6 hr, duration 6-8 hr, half-life 6-7 hr, metabolized in liver, excreted unchanged by kidneys

Interactions/ incompatibilities:
■ Increased effects of: neuromuscular blockers, digoxin, coumadin
■ Increased effects of quinidine: cimetidine, propranolol, thiazides, sodium bicarbonate, carbonic anhydrase inhibitors, antacids, hydroxide suspensions
■ May decrease effects of quinidine: barbiturates, phenytoin, rifampin, nifedipine

■ Additive vagolytic effect: anticholinergic blockers
■ Additive cardiac depression: other antidysrhythmics, phenothiazines, reserpine
■ Considered incompatible with any drug in sol or syringe

Lab test interferences:
Increase: CPK

RESPIRATORY CARE CONSIDERATIONS:
Assess/evaluate:
■ Monitor ECG; in case of increased QT and/or widening QRS, drug should be discontinued.
■ Assess for dehydration or hypovolemia, I&O ratio, electrolytes (Na, K, Cl).
■ Monitor BP for hypotension, hypertension and pulse rate.
■ Monitor respiratory rate and pattern (labored, dyspnea, depression/hypoventilation).
■ Note: quinidine may intensify neuromuscular blockade with nondepolarizing agents and prolong a depolarizing block with succinylcholine; monitor paralyzed ventilator patients for adequate ventilatory support or ability to wean.
■ Assess for cinchonism: tinnitus, headache, nausea, dizziness, fever, vertigo, tremor; may lead to hearing loss.
■ Evaluate therapeutic response: decreased dysrhythmias.
■ Quinidine intoxication can result in lethargy, coma, and respiratory arrest; support airway and ventilation until drug effect is reversed or subsides.
■ Provide resuscitation support in the event of cardiac

Q

---

italic = common side effects   **bold** = life-threatening reactions

arrest, life-threatening arrhythmias.

Patient education:
- Avoid hazardous activities if dizziness or blurred vision occurs.

---

ramipril
(ra-mi′pril)
Altace
Func. class.:
Antihypertensive
Chem. class.: Angiotensin-converting enzyme (ACE) inhibitor

Action: Selectively suppresses renin-angiotensin-aldosterone system; inhibits ACE, prevents conversion of angiotensin I to angiotensin II; results in dilation of arterial, venous vessels

Uses: Hypertension, alone or in combination with thiazide diuretics

Dosage and routes:
- *Adult:* PO 2.5 mg qd initially, then 2.5-20 mg/day divided bid or qd; renal impairment: 1.25 mg qd with CrCl < 4 0 ml/min/1.73 m^2, increase as needed to maximum or 5 mg/day
Available forms: Caps 1.25, 2.5, 5, 10 mg

Side effects/adverse reactions:
CV: Hypotension, chest pain, palpitations, angina, syncope, dysrhythmia
GU: Proteinuria, increased BUN, creatinine, impotence
HEMA: Decreased Hct, Hgb, *eosinophilia, leukopenia*
INTEG: Angioedema, rash, sweating, photosensitivity, pruritus

RESP: Cough, dyspnea
META: Hyperkalemia
GI: Nausea, constipation, vomiting, dyspepsia, dysphagia, anorexia, diarrhea, abdominal pain
CNS: Headache, dizziness, anxiety, insomnia, paresthesia, fatigue, depression, malaise, vertigo, *convulsions,* hearing loss
MS: Arthralgia, arthritis, myalgia

Contraindications: Hypersensitivity to ACE inhibitors, pregnancy (D), lactation, children

Precautions: Impaired renal, liver function, dialysis patients, hypovolemia, blood dyscrasias, CHF, COPD, asthma, elderly

Pharmacokinetics:
PO: Peak ½-1 hr, serum protein binding 97%, half-life 1-2 hr, metabolized by liver (metabolites excreted in urine, feces)

Interactions/incompatibilities:
- Increased hypotension: diuretics, other antihypertensives, ganglionic blockers, adrenergic blockers
- Increased toxicity: vasodilators, hydralazine, prazosin, K-sparing diuretics, sympathomimetics, K supplements
- Decreased absorption: antacids
- Decreased antihypertensive effect: indomethacin
- Increased serum levels of: digoxin, lithium
- Increased hypersensitivity: allopurinol

Lab test interferences:
False positive: Urine acetone

RESPIRATORY CARE CONSIDERATIONS:
Assess/evaluate:
- Therapeutic response: decrease in BP.
- Persistent cough and fever are common side effects of the ACE inhibitors, which should be differentiated from other possible causes, such as respiratory infection.
- Monitor for possible hypotension.
- Evaluate BP with COPD or asthmatic subjects who require beta agonists for reversible airway obstruction.
- Assess for symptoms of CHF: edema, dyspnea, wet rales, BP.

reserpine
(re-ser'peen)
Novoreserpine,* Serpalan
Func. class.: Antihypertensive
Chem. class.: Antiadrenergic agent

Action: Inhibits norepinephrine release, depleting norepinephrine stores in adrenergic nerve endings

Uses: Hypertension; relief in agitated psychotic states unable to tolerate phenothiazines or requiring antihypertensive medication

Dosage and routes:
Hypertension
- *Adult:* PO 0.25-0.5 mg qd × 1-2 wk, then 0.1-0.25 mg qd maintenance
- *Child:* PO 0.07 mg/kg or 2 mg/m³ given with hydralzine IM q12-24h
Pyschiatric disorders
- *Adult:* 0.5 mg/day (range 0.1-1 mg)

Available forms: Tabs 0.2, 0.1, 0.25, 1 mg; time rel caps 0.5 mg; inj 2.5 mg/ml

Side effects/adverse reactions:
CV: Bradycardia, chest pain, dysrhythmias, prolonged bleeding time, ***thrombocytopenia,*** purpura
CNS: Drowsiness, fatigue, lethargy, dizziness, depression, anxiety, headache, increased dreaming, nightmares, convulsions, parkinsonism, EPS (high doses)
GI: Nausea, vomiting, cramps, peptic ulcer, dry mouth, increased appetite, anorexia
INTEG: Rash, purpura, alopecia, flushing, warm feeling, pruritus, ecchymosis
EENT: Lacrimation, miosis, blurred vision, ptosis, dry mouth, epistaxis
GU: Impotence, dysuria, nocturia, Na and H_2O retention, edema, breast engorgement, galactorrhea, gynecomastia
RESP: Bronchospasm, dyspnea, cough, rales

Contraindications: Hypersensitivity, depression, suicidal patients, active peptic ulcer disease, ulcerative colitis, pregnancy (D), Parkinson's disease

Precautions: Lactation, seizure disorders, renal disease

Pharmacokinetics:
PO: Peak 4 hr, duration 2-6 wk; half-life 50-100 hr; metabolized by liver; excreted in urine, feces; crosses placenta, blood-brain barrier; excreted in breast milk

Interactions/incompatibilities:
- Increased hypotension: diuretics, hypotension,

---
italic = common side effects   **bold** = life-threatening reactions

β-blockers, methotri-
meprazine
- Dysrhythmias: cardiac
glycosides
- Increased cardiac depression: quinidine, procainamide
- Excitation, hypertension:
MAOIs
- Increased CNS depression:
barbiturates, alcohol, narcotics
- Increased pressor effects:
epinephrine, isoproterenol,
norepinephrine
- Decreased pressor effects:
ephedrine, amphetamine

Lab test interferences:
Increase: VMA excretion,
5-HIAA excretion
Interferences: 17-OHCS, 17-KS

**RESPIRATORY CARE
CONSIDERATIONS:
Assess/evaluate:**
- Monitor patients with reversible airway obstruction or
bronchospastic disease such as
asthma or chronic bronchitis
for presence of bronchospasm
(wheezing, dyspnea, com-
plaints of chest tightness) due
to depletion of catecholamines.
- Monitor effect on BP and
pulse, especially if on positive
pressure ventilatory support.
- Assess effectiveness of beta-
adrenergic bronchodilator
therapy for possible antagonism and effect on BP to
avoid increasing BP.
- Consider use of nonadrenergic bronchodilator such as ipratropium bromide as alternative to beta-adrenergic agents
for asthmatics, COPD patients.

Patient education:
- Do not use OTC products
containing α-adrenergic
stimulants (nasal deconges-

tants, OTC cold preparations)
unless directed by physician.
- Caution patient that orthostatic hypotension may occur.
- Report symptoms of CHF:
difficulty breathing, especially
on exertion or when lying
down, night cough, swelling
of extremities
- Avoid hazardous activities
(driving, power saws, etc) if
drowsiness occurs.

rifampin
(rif'am-pin)
Rifadin, Rimactane, Rofact*
Func. class.:
Antitubercular
Chem. class.: Rifamycin B
derivative

Action: Inhibits DNA-
dependent polymerase, de-
creases tubercle bacilli replication

Uses: Pulmonary tuberculosis, meningococcal carriers
(prevention)

Dosage and routes:
- *Adult:* PO/IV 600 mg/day as
single dose 1 hr ac or 2 hr pc
- *Child >5 yr:* PO/IV 10-20
mg/kg/day as single dose 1 hr
ac or 2 hr pc, not to exceed
600 mg/day, with other anti-
tuberculars
Meningococcal carriers
- *Adult:* PO/IV 600 mg bid × 2
days
- *Child >5 yr:* PO/IV 10 mg/kg
bid × 2 days, not to exceed
600 mg/dose
- *Infant 3 mo-1 yr:* 5 mg/kg PO
bid for 2 days
Available forms: Caps 150, 300
mg

Side effects/adverse reactions:
INTEG: Rash, pruritus, urticaria

EENT: Visual disturbances
MS: Atoxia, weakness
MISC: Flulike syndrome, menstrual disturbances, edema, shortness of breath
GI: Nausea, vomiting, anorexia, diarrhea, *pseudomembranous colitis,* heartburn, sore mouth and tongue, pancreatitis
GU: Hematuria, acute renal failure, hemoglobinuria
CNS: Headache, fatigue, anxiety, drowsiness, confusion
HEMA: Hemolytic anemia, eosinophilia, thrombocytopenia, leukopenia

Contraindications: Hypersensitivity

Precautions: Pregnancy (C), lactation, hepatic disease, blood dyscrasias

Pharmacokinetics:
PO: Peak 2-3 hr, duration >24 hr, half-life 3 hr, metabolized in liver (active/inactive metabolites), excreted in urine as free drug (30% crosses placenta), excreted in breast milk

Interactions/ incompatibilities:
■ Decreased action: barbiturates, clofibrate, corticosteroids, dapsone, anticoagulants, antidiabetics, hormones, digoxin, PAS, alcohol, oral contraceptives
■ Hepatotoxicity: INH
■ Incompatible with sodium lactate

Lab test interferences:
Interference: Folate level, vit B_{12}, BSP, gallbladder studies

RESPIRATORY CARE CONSIDERATIONS:
Assess/evaluate:
■ Monitor bacteriologic response to therapy using drug-susceptibility testing.

■ Assess subject for adverse reactions to drug therapy for mycobacteria: hepatotoxicity (liver enzymes), febrile reaction, and rarely purpura.
■ Monitor for signs of anemia: Hct, Hgb, fatigue.
■ Respiratory care practitioners and other health care personnel should self-screen for infection with TB routinely and following exposure.
■ Proper environmental and personnel protection programs should be implemented when treating subjects with TB.
■ Consider the possibility of HIV infection in individuals with confirmed or suspected TB.

Patient education:
■ That compliance with dosage schedule, duration is necessary.
■ Scheduled appointments must be kept or relapse may occur.
■ Urine, feces, saliva, sputum, sweat, tears may be colored red-orange; soft contact lenses may be permanently stained.
■ Report flulike symptoms: excessive fatigue, anorexia, vomiting, sore throat unusual bleeding, yellowish discoloration of skin, eyes.

R

ritodrine HCl
(ri'toe-dreen)
Yutopar
Func. class.: Tocolytic, uterine relaxant
Chem. class.: β_2-adrenergic agonist

Action: Reduces frequency, intensity of uterine contractions by stimulation of the β_2-receptors in uterine smooth muscle

---

italic = common side effects   **bold** = life-threatening reactions

Uses: Management of pre-term labor

Dosage and routes:
- Adult: IV INF 150 mg/500 ml (0.3 mg/ml) given 0.1 mg/min, increased gradually by 0.05 mg/min q10min until desired response; PO 10 mg given ½ hr before termination of IV, then 10 mg q2h × 24 hr, then 10-20 mg q4-6h, not to exceed 120 mg/day
Available forms: Tabs 10 mg; inj 10 mg/ml, 15 mg/ml

Side effects/adverse reactions:
MISC: Erythema, rash, dyspnea, hyperventilation, glycosuria, lactic acidosis
META: Hyperglycemia, hypokalemia
CNS: Headache, restlessness, anxiety, nervousness, sweating, chills, drowsiness, tremor
GI: Nausea, vomiting, anorexia, malaise, bloating, constipation, diarrhea
CV: Altered maternal, fetal heart rate, BP, dysrhythmias, palpitation, chest pain

Contraindications: Hypersensitivity, eclampsia, hypertension, dysrhythmias, thyrotoxicosis, before 20th wk of pregnancy, antepartum hemorrhage, intrauterine fetal death, maternal cardiac disease, pulmonary hypertension, uncontrolled diabetes, pheochromocytoma, bronchial asthma

Precautions: Migraine, sulfite sensitivity, pregnancy-induced hypertension, hypertension, diabetes

Pharmacokinetics:
PO: Peak ½-1 hr
IV: Immediate, distribution half-life 6 min, 2nd phase 1½-2½ hr, elimination phase >10 hr, metabolized in liver, 90% excreted in urine, crosses placenta

Interactions/incompatibilities:
- Pulmonary edema: corticosteroids
- Increased CV effects of ritodrine: magnesium sulfate, diazoxide, meperidine, potent general anesthetics
- Increased effects of: sympathomimetic amines
- Systemic hypertension: atropine
- Decreased action of ritodrine: β-blockers
- Considered incompatible with any drug in sol or syringe

Lab test interferences:
Increase: Blood glucose, free fatty acids, insulin, GTT
Decrease: K

RESPIRATORY CARE CONSIDERATIONS:
Assess/evaluate:
- Therapeutic response: decreased intensity, length of contraction, absence of preterm labor, decreased BP
- Evaluate breath sounds, and overall respiratory status for occurrence of maternal pulmonary edema following drug administration, especially if patient was concomitantly treated with corticosteroids.
- Assess patient medical history: preexisting maternal asthma *already treated by beta agonists or corticosteroids* is considered a contraindication to use of the drug; additive effects on blood pressure, heart rate, increased myocardial oxygen consumption may occur.

salsalate **281**

- Note: presence of sulfites in solution may precipitate an asthmatic reaction of increased airway resistance, wheezing, difficulty in breathing.

salsalate
(sal-sa'late)
Amigesic, Argesic-SA, Arthra-G, Disalcid, Mono-Gesic, Salflex, Salsalate, Salsitab
Func. class.: Nonnarcotic analgesic
Chem. class.: Salicylate

Action: Blocks formation of peripheral prostaglandins, which cause pain and inflammation; antipyretic action results from inhibition of hypothalamic heat-regulating center; does not inhibit platelet aggregation

Uses: Mild to moderate pain or fever, including arthritis, juvenile rheumatoid arthritis

Dosage and routes:
- *Adult:* PO 3 g/day in divided doses
Available forms: Caps 500 mg; tabs 500, 750 mg

Side effects/adverse reactions:
HEMA: Thrombocytopenia, agranulocytosis, leukopenia, neutropenia, hemolytic anemia, increased pro-time
CNS: Stimulation, drowsiness, dizziness, confusion, *convulsions,* headache, flushing, hallucinations, coma
GI: Nausea, vomiting, GI bleeding, diarrhea, heartburn, anorexia, *hepatotoxicity*
INTEG: Rash, urticaria, bruising
EENT: Tinnitus, hearing loss
CV: Rapid pulse, *pulmonary edema*
RESP: Wheezing, hyperpnea

ENDO: Hypoglycemia, hyponatremia, hypokalemia, alteration in acid-base balance

Contraindications: Hypersensitivity to salicylates, NSAIDs, GI bleeding, bleeding disorders, children < 3 yr, Vit K deficiency

Precautions: Anemia, hepatic disease, renal disease, Hodgkin's disease, pregnancy (C), lactation

Pharmacokinetics: Metabolized by liver, excreted by kidneys, half-life 1 hr, highly protein bound, crosses blood-brain barrier and placenta slowly

Interactions/ incompatibilities:
- Decreased effects of salsalate: antacids, steroids, urinary alkalizers
- Increased blood loss: alcohol, heparin, ibuprofen, warfarin
- Increased effects of: anticoagulants, insulin, methotrexate, probenecid
- Decreased effects of: spironolactone, sulfinpyrazone, sulfonylmides, loop diuretics
- Toxic effects: PABA
- Decreased blood sugar levels: salicylates

Lab test interferences:
Increase: Coagulation studies, liver function studies, serum uric acid, amylase, CO_2, urinary protein
Decrease: Serum K, PBI, cholesterol, blood glucose
Interfere: Urine catecholamines, pregnancy test

RESPIRATORY CARE CONSIDERATIONS:
Assess/evaluate:
- Avoid or use with caution in subjects with asthma, nasal

italic = common side effects   **bold** = life-threatening reactions

polyps, or rhinitis, evaluate respiratory status (rate, pattern) for bronchospasm, and for exacerbation of rhinitis.
- Overdose will result in hyperpnea and tachypnea (Kussmaul breathing) due to metabolic acidosis.
- Monitor acid-base status, and treat metabolic acidosis appropriately with buffering agent; ventilatory status will normalize with correction of metabolic acidosis.
- Avoid use in subjects with severe anemia or history of blood coagulation defects.

scopolamine hydrobromide

(skoe-pol′a-meen)
Atrohist, Bellatal, Donatal, Ru-Tuss, Rextal
Func. class.: Cholinergic blocker
Chem. class.: Belladonna alkaloid

Action: Blocks acetylcholine at receptor sites in autonomic nervous system, which controls secretions, free acids in stomach; blocks central muscarinic receptors, which decreases involuntary movements

Uses: Reduction of secretions before surgery, calm delirium, motion sickness

Dosage and routes:
Parkinson symptoms
- *Adult:* IM/SC/IV 0.3-0.6 mg tid-qid diluted using dilution provided
- *Child:* SC 0.006 mg/kg tid-qid or 0.2 mg/m²
Preoperatively
- *Adult:* SC 0.4-0.6 mg

Available forms: Inj 0.3, 0.4, 0.86, 1 mg/ml

Side effects/adverse reactions:
CNS: Confusion, anxiety, restlessness, irritability, delusions, hallucinations, headache, sedation, depression, incoherence, dizziness, excitement, delirium, flushing, weakness
INTEG: Urticaria
MISC: Suppression of lactation, nasal congestion, decreased sweating
EENT: Blurred vision, photophobia, dilated pupils, difficulty swallowing, mydriasis, cycloplegia
CV: Palpitations, tachycardia, postural hypotension, paradoxical bradycardia
GI: Dryness of mouth, constipation, nausea, vomiting, abdominal distress, *paralytic ileus*
GU: Hesitancy, retention

Contraindications: Hypersensitivity, narrow-angle glaucoma, myasthenia gravis, GI/GU obstruction, hypersensitivity to belladonna, barbiturates

Precautions: Pregnancy (C), elderly, lactation, prostatic hypertrophy, CHF, hypertension, dysrhythmia, children, gastric ulcer

Pharmacokinetics:
SC/IM: Peak 30-45 min, duration 7 hr
IV: Peak 10-15 min, duration 4 hr
Excreted in urine, bile, feces (unchanged)

Interactions/ incompatibilities:
- Increased anticholinergic effect: alcohol, narcotics, antihistamines, phenothiazines, tricyclics

- Do not mix with diazepam, chloramphenicol, pentobarbital, sodium bicarbonate in syringe or sol

RESPIRATORY CARE CONSIDERATIONS:
Assess/evaluate:
- Consider use of anticholinergic agents for bronchodilation, such as ipratropium bromide, which are quaternary compounds, to avoid compounding side effects due to wide absorption and distribution throughout the body.
- Monitor heart rate for tachycardia.
- Monitor ECG if available with patient.
- Assess respiratory status: rate, rhythm, cyanosis, wheezing, dyspnea.

Patient education:
- Blurred vision may occur, and reading may not be possible; this will subside.
- Avoid activities that are hazardous or require alertness if drowsiness occurs.
- A dry mouth is likely to occur.
- If difficulty in urination or constipation occurs, check with physician.

selegiline HCl (L-Deprenyl)
(sel-ee-gill'ene)
Eldepryl
Func. class.: Antiparkinson agent
Chem. class.: Levorotatory acetylenic derivative of phenethylamine

Action: Increased dopaminergic activity by inhibition of MAO type B activity; not fully understood

Uses: Adjunct management of Parkinson's disease in patients being treated with levodopa/carbidopa who have had a poor response to therapy

Dosage and routes:
- *Adult:* PO 10 mg/day in divided doses 5 mg at breakfast and lunch, after 2-3 days begin to reduce the dose of levodopa/carbidopa 10%-30%
Available forms: Tabs 5 mg

Side effects/adverse reactions:
CNS: Increased tremors, chorea, restlessness, blepharospasm, increased bradykinesia, grimacing, tardive dyskinesia, dystonic symptoms, involuntary movements, increased apraxia, hallucinations, dizziness, mood changes, nightmares, delusions, lethargy, apathy, overstimulation, sleep disturbances, headache, migraine, numbness, muscle cramps, confusion, anxiety, tiredness, vertigo, personality change, back/leg pain
CV: Orthostatic hypotension, hypertension, dysrhythmia, palpitations, angina pectoris, hypotension, tachycardia, edema, sinus bradycardia, syncope
GI: Nausea, vomiting, constipation, weight loss, anorexia, diarrhea, heartburn, rectal bleeding, poor appetite, dysphagia
GU: Slow urination, nocturia, prostatic hypertrophy, hesitation, retention, frequency, sexual dysfunction
INTEG: Increased sweating, alopecia, hematoma, rash, photosensitivity, facial hair
RESP: Asthma, shortness of breath

italic = common side effects   **bold** = life-threatening reactions

EENT: Diplopia, dry mouth, blurred vision, tinnitus

Contraindications: Hypersensitivity

Precautions: Pregnancy (C), lactation, children

Pharmacokinetics: Rapidly absorbed, peak ½-2 hr, rapidly metabolized (active metabolites: N-desmethyldeprenyl, amphetamine, methamphetamine), metabolites excreted in urine

Interactions/ incompatibilities:
▪ **Fatal interaction:** opioids (especially meperidine); do not administer together

Lab test interferences:
False positive: urine ketones, urine glucose
False negative: urine glucose (glucose oxidase)
False increase: uric acid, urine protein
Decrease: VMA

RESPIRATORY CARE CONSIDERATIONS:
Assess/evaluate:
▪ Monitor BP for increase if placing on beta-adrenergic bronchodilator therapy.
▪ Monitor for side effects affecting the respiratory system: shortness of breath, wheezing, and asthma reaction.
▪ Differentiate respiratory symptoms from other possible causes, including pulmonary embolism, spontaneous pneumothorax, MI, respiratory infection.
▪ Dry mouth may be further exacerbated by use of anticholinergic bronchodilators such as ipratropium bromide.

Patient education:
▪ Avoid hazardous activity if dizziness or blurred vision, diplopia occur.
▪ Note that use of beta agonists may increase peripheral tremor; consider use of anticholinergic bronchodilator if dry mouth is not a problem.
Avoid foods high in tyramine: cheese, pickled products, wine, beer, large amounts of caffeine.

sodium bicarbonate
Func. class.: Alkalinizer
Chem. class.: $NaHCO_3$

Action: neutralizes acid, which forms water, NaCl, CO_2; increases plasma bicarbonate, which buffers H^+ ion concentration; reverses acidosis

Uses: Acidosis (metabolic), cardiac arrest, alkalinization (systemic/urinary) antacid

Dosage and routes:
Acidosis
Adult and child: IV INF 2-5 mEq/kg over 4-8 hr depending on CO_2, pH
Cardiac arrest
▪ *Adult and child:* IV BOL 1 mEq/kg, then 0.5 mEq/kg q10 min, then doses based an ABGs
▪ *Infant:* IV INF not to exceed 8 mEq/kg/day based on ABGs (4.2% sol)
Alkalinization
▪ *Adult:* PO 325 mg-2 g qid
▪ *Child:* PO 12-120 mg/kg/day
Antacid
▪ *Adult:* PO 300 mg-2 g chewed, taken with H_2O qd-qid
Available forms: Tabs 325, 520, 650 mg; powder; inj 4%, 4.2%, 5%, 7.5%, 8.4%

Side effects/adverse reactions:

CNS: Irritability, headache, confusion, stimulation, trem-ors, *twitching, hyperreflexia, tetany,* weakness, *convulsions* caused by alkalosis

CV: Irregular pulse, *cardiac arrest,* water retention, edema, weight gain

GI: Flatulence, *belching, distention, paralytic ileus,* acid rebound

META: Alkalosis

GU: Calculi

RESP: Shallow, slow respira-tions, cyanosis, *apnea*

Contraindications: Hyper-tension, peptic ulcer, renal disease, hypocalcemia

Precautions: CHF, cirrhosis, toxemia, renal disease, preg-nancy (C)

Pharmacokinetics:

PO: Onset 2 min, duration 10 min

IV: Onset 15 min, duration 1-2 hr, excreted in urine

Interactions/ incompatibilities:

■ Increases effects: amphet-amines, mecamylamine, qui-nine, quinidine, pseudoephe-drine, flecainide, anorexants

■ Decreases effects: lithium, chlorpropamide, barbiturates, salicylates, benzodiazepines

■ Increased Na and decreased K: corticosteroids

■ Incompatible with atropine, Ca, carmustine, cefotaxime, chlorpromazine, cisplatin, co-deine, corticotropin, dobu-tamine, dopamine, epinephrine, glycopyrrolate, hydromorphone, insulin, isoproterenol, labetalol, levarterenol, levorphanol, linco-mycin, magnesium sulfate, me-peridine, methadone, methicil-lin, morphine, penicillin G, pentobarbital, pentazocine, phe-nobarbital, procaine, promazine, secobarbital, streptomycin, suc-cinylcholine, tetracycline, thio-pental, vancomycin

Lab test interferences:

Increase: Urinary urobilinogen

False positive: Urinary protein, blood lactate

RESPIRATORY CARE CONSIDERATIONS:
Assess/evaluate:

■ Therapeutic response: ABGs, electrolytes: arterial pH, HCO_3 WNL; potassium depletion may lead to meta-bolic alkalosis and overcorrec-tion of acidosis.

■ Note: bicarbonate is not rou-tinely recommended in cardiac arrest as it was previously; re-view existing American Heart Association guidelines on re-suscitation protocols.

■ Ventilatory correction of metabolic acidosis is not rec-ommended; maintain level of ventilation as indicated by arterial PCO_2 and PO2.

■ Monitor fluid balance (I&O, weight qd, edema); sodium may lead to further fluid retention in CHF or overloaded patients.

■ Assess for alkalosis: irrita-bility, confusion, twitching, hyperreflexia stimulation, slow respirations, cyanosis, irregular pulse

sodium thiosalicylate
(thye-o-sa-li′-sa-late)
Rexolate, Tusal
Func. class.: Nonnarcotic analgesic
Chem. class.: Salicylate

Action: Salicylates have analgesic, antipyretic, and

---

italic = common side effects   **bold** = life-threatening reactions

antiinflammatory activity. Body temperature is lowered through vasodilation of peripheral vessels, facilitating heat dissipation. The antiinflammatory and analgesic effect seems to be mediated through inhibition of the prostaglandin synthetase enzyme complex.

Uses: Mild to moderate pain (rheumatic fever, acute gout)

Dosage and routes:
Pain
■ *Adult:* IM 50-100 mg qd or qod
Rheumatic fever
■ *Adult:* IM 100-150 mg q4-6h × 3 days, then 100 mg bid
Arthritis
■ *Adult:* IM 100 mg/day
Available forms: Inj IM 50 mg/ml

Side effects/adverse reactions:
HEMA: Thrombocytopenia, agranulocytosis, leukopenia, neutropenia, hemolytic anemia, increased pro-time
CNS: Stimulation, drowsiness, dizziness, confusion, *convulsions,* headache, flushing, hallucinations, coma
GI: Nausea, vomiting, GI bleeding, diarrhea, heartburn, anorexia, *hepatitis*
INTEG: Rash, urticaria, bruising
EENT: Tinnitus, hearing loss
CV: Rapid pulse, *pulmonary edema*
RESP: Wheezing, hyperpnea
ENDO: Hypoglycemia, hyponatremia, hypokalemia

Contraindications: Hypersensitivity to salicylates, GI bleeding, bleeding disorders, children < 3 yr, Vit K deficiency, peptic ulcer

Precautions: Anemia, hepatic disease, renal disease, Hodgkin's disease, pregnancy (C), lactation

Pharmacokinetics:
PO: Onset 15-30 min, peak 1-2 hr, duration 4-6 hr
REC: Onset slow, duration 4-6 hr, half-life 1-3½ hr, metabolized by liver, excreted by kidneys, crosses placenta, excreted in breast milk

Interactions/ incompatibilities:
■ Decreased effects of sodium thiosalicylate: antacids, steroids, urinary alkalizers
■ Increased blood loss: alcohol, heparin
■ Increased effects of: anticoagulants, insulin, methotrexate
■ Decreased effects of: probenecid, spironolactone, sulfinpyrazone, sulfonylmides
■ Toxic effects: PABA

Lab test interferences:
Increase: Coagulation studies, liver function studies, serum uric acid, amylase, CO_2, urinary protein
Decrease: Serum K, PBI, cholesterol, blood glucose
Interfere: Urine catecholamines, pregnancy test

RESPIRATORY CARE CONSIDERATIONS:
Assess/evaluate:
■ Avoid or use with caution in subjects with asthma, nasal polyps or rhinitis, evaluate respiratory status (rate, pattern) for bronchospasm and for exacerbation of rhinitis; consider use of non-salicylate analgesic instead.
■ Salicylates cause increased risk of bleeding during endoscopic procedures, such as

bronchoscopy patients should be advised to avoid this type of analgesic use prior to such procedures.
- Perform arterial blood sampling with caution, and use adequate compression of artery to avoid hematoma.
- Salicylate overdose can cause hyperpnea (Kussmaul breathing), due to resulting metabolic acidosis.
- Monitor acid-base status, and treat metabolic acidosis appropriately with buffering agent; ventilatory status will normalize with correction of metabolic acidosis.
- Avoid use in subjects with severe anemia or history of blood coagulation defects.

Patient education:
- Advise patients, especially asthmatics, to use alternative analgesic preparations such as acetaminophen.

---

sotalol hydrochloride
(soe-ta'-lole)
Betapace
Func. class.:
Antidysrhythmic
Chem. class.: Nonselective
beta-blocker

Action: Blockade of B$_1$- and B$_2$-receptors leads to antidysrhythmic effect; also has Class III effects

Uses: Life-threatening ventricular dysrhythmias

Dosage and routes:
- *Adult:* PO initial 80 mg bid, may increase to a total of 240-320 mg/day
Available forms: Tabs 80, 160, 240 mg

Side effects/adverse reactions:
CV: Orthostatic hypotension, bradycardia, CHF, chest pain, ventricular dysrhythmias, AV block, peripheral vascular insufficiency, palpitations
CNS: Dizziness, mental changes, drowsiness, fatigue, headache, catatonia, depression, anxiety, nightmares, paresthesia, lethargy, insomnia, decreased concentration
GI: Nausea, vomiting, diarrhea, dry mouth, flatulence, constipation, anorexia
INTEG: Rash, alopecia, urticaria, pruritus, fever
HEMA: **Agranulocytosis, thrombocytopenic purpura (rare), thrombocytopenia, leukopenia**
EENT: Tinnitus, visual changes, sore throat, double vision, dry burning eyes
GU: Impotence, dysuria, ejaculatory failure, urinary retention
RESP: **Bronchospasm,** dyspnea, wheezing, nasal stuffiness, pharyngitis
MS: Joint pain, arthralgia, muscle cramps, pain
OTHER: Facial swelling, decreased exercise tolerance, weight change, Raynaud's disease

Contraindications: Hypersensitivity to β-blockers, cardiogenic shock, heart block (2nd or 3rd degree), sinus bradycardia, CHF, bronchial asthma, congenital or acquired long QT syndrome

Precautions: Major surgery, pregnancy (B), lactation, diabetes mellitus, renal disease, thyroid disease, COPD, well-compensated heart failure, CAD, nonallergic bronchospasm, electrolyte disturbances, bradycardia, cardiac

S

---

italic = common side effects   **bold** = life-threatening reactions

dysrhythmias, peripheral vascular disease

Pharmacokinetics:
PO: Onset 1-2 hr, peak 2-4 hr, duration 8-12 hr, half-life 12 hr, metabolized by liver (metabolites inactive), excreted unchanged in urine, crosses placenta, excreted in breast milk

Interactions/ incompatibilities:
■ Increased hypotension: diuretics, other antihypertensives, nitroglycerin, prazosin
■ Decreased β-blocker effects: sympathomimetics, nonsteroidal antiinflammatory agents, salicylates
■ Increased hypoglycemia effect: insulin
■ Increased effects of: lidocaine
■ Decreased bronchodilating effects of: theophylline
■ Decreased hypoglycemic effects of: sulfonylureas

Lab test interferences:
False increase: Urinary catecholamines
Interference: Glucose, insulin tolerance tests

RESPIRATORY CARE CONSIDERATIONS
Assess/evaluate:
■ Avoid use with reversible airway obstruction or bronchospastic disease such as asthma or chronic bronchitis due to potential for bronchospasm (wheezing, dyspnea, complaints of chest tightness) secondary to beta-blockade; consider use of other classes of antihypertensive agents for these patients.
■ Monitor all subjects for symptoms of increased airway resistance (wheezing, tightness in chest, difficulty breathing).
■ Monitor effect on BP and pulse, especially if on positive pressure ventilatory support.
■ Assess effectiveness of beta-adrenergic bronchodilator therapy for possible antagonism and effect on BP to avoid increasing BP.
■ Consider use of nonadrenergic bronchodilator such as ipratropium bromide as alternative to beta-adrenergic agents for patients to avoid positive inotropic effect.

Patient education:
■ Do not use OTC products containing α-adrenergic stimulants (nasal decongestants, OTC cold preparations) unless directed by physician.
■ Caution patient that orthostatic hypotension may occur.
■ Report symptoms of CHF: difficulty breathing, especially on exertion or when lying down, night cough, swelling of extremities.

spironolactone
(speer'on-oh-lak'tone)
Alatone, Aldactone, Novospiroton, Sincomen
Func. class.: Potassium-sparing diuretic
Chem. class.: Aldosterone antagonist

Action: Competes with aldosterone at receptor sites in distal tubule, resulting in excretion of sodium chloride, water, retention of potassium, phosphate

Uses: Edema, hypertension, diuretic-induced hypokalemia, primary hyperaldosteronism (diagnosis, short-term treatment, long-term treatment), nephrotic syndrome, cirrhosis of the liver with ascites

Dosage and routes:
Edema/hypertension
■ *Adult:* PO 25-200 mg/qd in single or divided doses
■ *Child:* PO 3.3 mg/kg/day in single or divided doses
Hypokalemia
■ *Adult:* PO 25-100 mg/day; if PO, K supplements cannot be used
Primary hyperaldosteronism diagnosis
■ *Adult:* PO 400 mg/day × 4 days or 4 wk depending on test, then 100-400 mg/day maintenance
Available forms: Tab 25, 50, 100 mg

Side effects/adverse reactions:
CNS: Headache, confusion, drowsiness, lethargy, ataxia
GI: Diarrhea, cramps, *bleeding,* gastritis, *vomiting,* anorexia, nausea
CV: dysrythmias
INTEG: Rash, pruritus, urticaria
ENDO: Impotence, gynecomastia, irregular menses, amenorrhea, postmenopausal bleeding, hirsutism, deepening voice
HEMA: Decreased WBCs, platelets
ELECT: Hyperchloremic metabolic acidosis, *hyperkalemia,* hyponatremia

Contraindications: Hypersensitivity, anuria, severe renal disease, hyperkalemia, pregnancy (D)

Precautions: Dehydration, hepatic disease, lactation

Pharmacokinetics:
PO: Onset 24-48 hr, peak 48-72 hr, metabolized in liver, excreted in urine, crosses placenta

Interactions/ incompatibilities:
■ Increased action of: antihypertensives, digitalis, lithium
■ Increased hyperkalemia: K-sparing diuretics, K products, ACE inhibitors, salt substitutes
■ Decreased effect of spironolactone: ASA

Lab test interferences:
Interference: 17-OHCS, 17-KS, radioimmunoassay, digoxin assay

RESPIRATORY CARE CONSIDERATIONS:
Assess/evaluate:
■ Monitor serum electrolytes; spironolactone produces an increase in sodium excretion and decrease in potassium excretion, leading to possible hyponatremia and hyperkalemia.
■ Evaluate for dehydration, especially in COPD subjects or those with excess respiratory tract secretions.
■ Monitor color, consistency of sputum.
■ Monitor BP.
■ Evaluate breath sounds and respiratory pattern for pulmonary congestion.

streptokinase
(strep-toe-kye'nase)
Kabikinase, Streptase
Func. class.: Thrombolytic enzyme
Chem. class.: β-hemolytic streptococcus filtrate (purified)

Action: Acts with plasminogen to produce an "activator

italic = common side effects   **bold** = life-threatening reactions

complex" that converts plasminogen to the proteolytic enzyme plasmin; plasmin breaks down fibrin clots, and is then inactivated by circulating inhibitors such as alpha-2-macroglobulin

Uses: Deep vein thrombosis, pulmonary embolism, arterial thrombosis, arterial embolism, arteriovenous cannula occlusion, lysis of coronary artery thrombi after MI, acute evolving transmural MI

Dosage and routes:
Lysis of coronary artery thrombi
■ *Adult:* CC 20,000 IU, then 2000 IU/min over 1 hr as IV INF
Arteriovenous cannula occlusion
■ *Adult:* IV INF 250,000 IU/2 ml sol into occluded limb of cannula run over ½ hr; clamp for 2 hr; aspirate contents; flush with NaCl sol and reconnect
Thrombosis/embolism
■ *Adult:* IV INF 250,000 IU over ½ hr, then 100,000 IU/hr for 72 hr for deep thrombosis; 100,000 IU/hr over 24-72 hr for pulmonary embolism
Acute evolving transmural MI
■ *Adult:* IV INF 1,500,000 IU diluted to a volume of 45 ml; give within 1 hr
Available forms: Inj IV 250,000, 600,000, 750,000 IU

Side effects/adverse reactions:
CNS: Headache, fever
EENT: Periorbital edema
GI: Nausea
HEMA: Decreased Hct, *bleeding*
INTEG: Rash, urticaria, phlebitis at IV inj site, itching, flushing
MS: Low back pain

RESP: Altered respirations, SOB, *bronchospasm*
SYST: GI, GU, *intracranial retroperitoneal bleeding, surface bleeding, anaphylaxis*

Contraindications: Hypersensitivity, active bleeding, intraspinal surgery, neoplasms of the CNS, ulcerative colitis, enteritis, severe hypertension, severe renal disease, hepatic disease, hypocoagulation, COPD, subacute bacterial endocarditis, rheumatic valvular disease, cerebral embolism/thrombosis/hemorrhage, intraarterial diagnostic procedure or surgery (10 days), recent major surgery

Precautions: Arterial emboli from left side of heart, pregnancy (C)

Pharmacokinetics:
IV: Onset immediate, duration <12 hr, half-life <20 min, excreted in bile, urine

Interactions/incompatibilities:
■ Bleeding potential: aspirin, indomethacin, phenylbutazone, anticoagulants
■ Considered incompatible with any drug in sol or syringe

Lab test interferences:
Increase: PT, APTT, TT

RESPIRATORY CARE CONSIDERATIONS:
Assess/evaluate:
■ Bleeding from invasive procedures, such as cutdowns, catheter insertions, or arterial punctures, is an increased risk with fibrinolytic therapy and is common.
■ Minimize arterial or venous punctures.

*Available in Canada only

- Use sites accessible to manual compression for arterial punctures.
- Use pressure dressings for arterial puncture after prolonged manual compression.
- Monitor for bleeding from any puncture sites.
- Risk of fibrinolytic therapy is increased with hypertension, hemostatic defects, or treatment with anticoagulant agents.

Patient education:
- Instruct patient to notify health care personnel of any swelling, hematoma, or bleeding at a puncture site.

succinylcholine chloride

(suk-sin-ill-koéleen)

Anectine, Anectine Flo-Pack, Brevidil M* (Bromide Salt), Min-I-Mix, Quelicin, Scaline,* Succinylcholine Chloride Min-I-Mix, Sucostrin, Sux-Cert*

Func. class.: Neuromuscular blocker (depolarizing-ultrashort)
Chem. class.: Diacetylcholine

Action: Inhibits transmission of nerve impulses by binding to and depolarizing cholinergic receptor sites at the neuromuscular junction; muscle cells are held in a depolarized, refractory state, preventing repolarization and subsequent depolarization, causing paralysis if given in sufficient dose. Cholinergic agonists such as neostigmine prolong and intensify the resulting neuromuscular blockade. Succinylcholine is metabolized by plasma pseudocholinesterase enzymes. Occasional genetic variation of these enzymes can lead to prolonged paralysis requiring supported ventilation.

Uses: Facilitation of endotracheal intubation, skeletal muscle relaxation during orthopedic manipulations

Dosage and routes:
- *Adult:* IV 25-75 mg, then 2.5 mg/min as needed; IM 2.5 mg/kg, not to exceed 150 mg
- *Child:* IV/IM 1-2 mg/kg, not to exceed 150 mg IM
Available forms:
Inj IM, IV 20, 50, 100 mg/ml; powder for inj 100, 500 mg/vial, 1 g/vial

Side effects/adverse reactions:
CV: Bradycardia, tachycardia; increased, decreased BP, *sinus arrest, dysrhythmias*
RESP: Prolonged apnea, bronchospasm, cyanosis, respiratory depression
EENT: Increased secretions, increased intraocular pressure
MS: Weakness, muscle pain, fasciculations, prolonged relaxation
HEMA: Myoglobulinemia
INTEG: Rash, flushing, pruritus, urticaria

Contraindications: Hypersensitivity, malignant hyperthermia, decreased plasma pseudocholinesterase, penetrating eye injuries, acute narrow-angle glaucoma

Precautions: Pregnancy (C), cardiac disease, severe burns, fractures (fasciculations may increase damage), lactation, children <2 yr, electrolyte imbalances, dehydration, neuromuscular disease, respiratory disease, collagen diseases,

italic = common side effects

bold = life-threatening reactions

glaucoma, eye surgery, penetrating eye wounds, elderly or debilitated patients

Pharmacokinetics:
IV: Onset 1 min, peak 2-3 min, duration 6-10 min
IM: Onset 2-3 min
Hydrolyzed in urine (active/inactive metabolites)

Interactions/incompatibilities:
■ Increased neuromuscular blockade: aminoglycosides, clindamycin, lincomycin, quinidine, local anesthetics, polymyxin antibiotics, lithium, narcotic analgesics, thiazides, enflurane, isoflurane, Mg salts, oxytocin
■ Dysrhythmias: theophylline
■ Incompatible with barbiturates, chlorpromazine, nafcillin, alkaline sol

RESPIRATORY CARE CONSIDERATIONS:
Assess/evaluate:
■ Note: use of a depolarizing agent for prolonged periods of time with ventilator patients can lead to a combined nondepolarizing and depolarizing neuromuscular blockade; if recovery is delayed, consider use of reversing agent such as neostigmine.
■ Provide airway and ventilatory support before administering drug.
■ Note possible interaction with the following antibiotics, which can increase neuromuscular blockade: the aminoglycosides, the polymyxins, clindamycin, and lincomycin.
■ Succinylcholine is not an optimal agent to use for prolonged paralysis with mechanical ventilation; nondepolarizing agents with longer duration of action and reversibility (e.g., atracurium, vecuronium, doxacurium) are preferred.
■ In paralysis with mechanical ventilation assess patient for adequate and preferably optimal ventilator settings *before* paralyzing. If patient is "fighting" the ventilator, provide adequately high flow rates and tidal volumes, short inspiratory times, and reasonable I:E ratios, check the sensitivity in assist-control mode, provide sufficiently high rates to avoid patient fatigue; consider paralysis if these measures fail.
■ Assess ventilator patients for pain, hypoxemia, or ventilator malfunction, if restless and anxious, before instituting muscle paralysis.
■ Assess need of patient and provide for pain control and sedation during neuromuscular blockade; *neuromuscular blocking agents do not provide analgesia or sedation.*
■ Close eyelids and provide eye lubricant during prolonged paralysis.
■ Since usual signs of pain or anxiety (restlessness, tachypnea, distress, thrashing) are blocked, monitor vital signs closely and overall patient appearance and state to detect problems (e.g., IV infiltration).
■ Check ventilator alarm settings for sufficient limits and sensitivity; a disconnect alarm is critical.
■ Assess reversal of drug before attempting to wean from mechanical ventilatory support.

Administer:
- Administer by IV, not by IM, for more consistent absorption and distribution.
- Reversal: none; use of an anticholinergic drug such as neostigmine will normally cause intensified blockade unless a dual block has occurred.

terazosin HCl
(ter-ay′zoe-sin)
Hytrin
Func. class.: antihypertensive
Chem. class.: α_1-adrenergic blocker

Action: Decreases total vascular resistance, which leads to a decrease in BP; this occurs by blockade of α_1-adrenoreceptors

Uses: Hypertension, as a single agent or in combination with diuretics or β-blockers, BPH

Dosage and routes:
- *Adult:* PO 1 mg hs, may increase dose slowly to desired response; not to exceed 20 mg/day
Available forms: Tabs 1, 2, 5 mg

Side effects/adverse reactions:
CV: Palpitations, orthostatic hypotension, tachycardia, edema, rebound hypertension
CNS: Dizziness, headache, drowsiness, anxiety, depression, vertigo, weakness, fatigue
GI: Nausea, vomiting, diarrhea, constipation, abdominal pain
GU: Urinary frequency, incontinence, impotence, priapism
EENT: Blurred vision, epistaxis, tinnitus, dry mouth, red sclera, nasal congestion, sinusitis

RESP: Dyspnea

Contraindications: Hypersensitivity

Precautions: Pregnancy (C), children, lactation

Pharmacokinetics: Peak 1 hr, half-life 9-12 hr, highly bound to plasma proteins metabolized in liver, excreted in urine, feces

Interactions/ incompatibilities:
- Increased hypotensive effects: β-blockers, nitroglycerin, verapamil, nifedipine

RESPIRATORY CARE CONSIDERATIONS:
Assess/evaluate:
- Monitor for "first dose" effect: marked hypotension (especially postural), syncope with loss of consciousness with first few doses.
- Monitor effect on BP and pulse, especially if on positive pressure ventilatory support.
- Assess effectiveness of beta-adrenergic bronchodilator therapy for possible antagonistic effect on BP to avoid increasing BP or decreasing BP due to beta receptor stimulation of vascular smooth muscle in the presence of blocked alpha receptors.
- Consider use of nonadrenergic bronchodilator such as ipratropium bromide as alternative to beta-adrenergic agents, for asthmatics, COPD patients.
- Note: since alpha receptors are blocked, other adrenergic agents that stimulate both types of sympathetic receptors or beta receptors, such as epinephrine, may cause exaggerated response of tachycardia and hypotension.

italic = common side effects   **bold** = life-threatening reactions

- Treatment of overdose with epinephrine can cause worsening of hypotension, as outlined previously; use leg elevation, discontinue the drug, support circulation.

Patient education:
- Do not use OTC products containing α-adrenergic stimulants (nasal decongestants, OTC cold preparations) or other sympathomimetics unless directed by physician.
- Report symptoms of CHF: difficulty breathing, especially on exertion or when lying down, night cough, swelling of extremities.

terbutaline sulfate
(ter-byoo'te-leen)
Brethaire, Brethine, Bricanyl
Func. class.: Selective β₂-agonist
Chem. class.: Catecholamine derivative (a resorcinol)

See also Section III: Aerosol Agents for Oral Inhalation

Action: Relaxes bronchial smooth muscle by direct action on β₂-adrenergic receptors through accumulation of cAMP at β-adrenergic receptor sites

Uses: Bronchospasm, premature labor

Dosage and routes:
Bronchospasm
- *Adult and child >15 yr:* MDI 2 puffs q4-6h; PO 5.0 mg q6h, or tid; SC 0.25 mg not to exceed 0.5 mg in 4 hrs
Premature labor
- *Adult:* IV INF 0.01 mg/min, increased by 0.005 mg q10min, not to exceed 0.025 mg/min; SC 0.25 mg q1h; PO 5 mg q4h × 48 hr, then 5 mg q6h as maintenance for above doses

Available forms:
Tabs 2.5, 5 mg; MDI 0.2 mg/actuation; inj 1.0 mg/ml

Side effects/adverse reactions:
CNS: Tremors, anxiety, insomnia, headache, dizziness, stimulation
CV: Palpitations, tachycardia, hypertension, dysrhythmias, *cardiac arrest*
GI: Nausea, vomiting

Contraindications: Hypersensitivity to sympathomimetics, narrow-angle glaucoma, tachydysrhythmias

Precautions: Pregnancy (B), cardiac disorders, hyperthyroidism, diabetes mellitus, prostatic hypertension, lactation, elderly, hypertension, glaucoma

Pharmacokinetics:
PO: Onset ½ hr, peak 1-2 hr, duration 4-8 hr
SC: Onset 6-15 min, peak ½-1 hr, duration 1½-4 hr
INH: Onset 5-30 min, peak 1-2 hr, duration 3-6 hr

Interactions/incompatibilities:
- Increased effects of both drugs: other sympathomimetics
- Decreased action: β-blockers
- Hypertensive crisis: MAOIs
- Incompatible with bleomycin
- Considered incompatible in sol or syringe with any other drug

RESPIRATORY CARE CONSIDERATIONS:
Assess/evaluate:
- Assess effectiveness of drug therapy based on the indica-

tion(s) for the aerosol agent: presence of reversible airflow due to primary bronchospasm or other obstruction secondary to an inflammatory response and/or secretions, either acute or chronic.
■ Monitor flow rates using office or bedside peak flow meters or laboratory reports of pulmonary function, especially before and after bronchodilator studies, to assess reversibility of airflow obstruction.
■ Instruct and then verify correct use of aerosol delivery device (SVN, MDI, reservoir, DPI). See Section I: Methods and Devices for Aerosol Delivery of Drugs.
■ Assess breathing rate and pattern.
■ Assess breath sounds by auscultation before and after treatment.
■ Assess pulse before and after treatment.
■ Assess patient's subjective reaction to treatment for any change in breathing effort or pattern.
■ Assess arterial blood gases or pulse oximeter saturation, as needed, for acute states with asthma or COPD to monitor changes in ventilation and gas exchange (oxygenation).
■ Note effect of beta agonists on blood glucose (increase) and K^+ (decrease) laboratory values, if these are available.
■ Monitor BP and pulse rate if subject is on other adrenergic agents or tricyclic antidepressants.
■ Long-term: monitor pulmonary function studies of lung

volumes, capacities, and flows.

Patient education:
■ Instruct asthmatic patients in use and interpretation of disposable peak flow meters to assess severity of asthmatic episodes.
■ Instruct patients in use, assembly, and especially cleaning of aerosol inhalation devices.
■ Note: death has been associated with excessive use of inhaled adrenergic agents in severe acute asthma crises; individuals using such drugs should be instructed to contact a physician or an emergency room if there is no response to the usual dose of the inhaled agent.

terfenadine
(ter-fen'-a-deen)
Seldane
Func. class.: Antihistamine
Chem. class.: Butyrophenone derivative

Action: Blocks the action of histamine at H_1-receptor sites on blood vessels, GI, respiratory tract to decrease allergic inflammatory response and in general the pharmacologic effects of histamine. Terfenadine has little or no anticholinergic and sedative effect.

Uses: Rhinitis, allergy symptoms

Dosage and routes:
■ *Adult and child >12 yr:* PO 60 mg bid
■ *Child <12 yr:* PO 15-30 mg bid
Available forms: Tabs 60 mg

italic = common side effects   **bold** = life-threatening reactions

Side effects/adverse reactions:
CV: Life-threatening dysrhythmias (rare)
CNS: Dizziness, poor coordination
RESP: Increased thick secretions
GI: Anorexia, increased liver function tests, dry mouth
GU: Retention

Contraindications: Hypersensitivity, severe hepatic disease; concomitant therapy with erythromycin, ketoconazole, or itraconazole

Precautions: Pregnancy (C)

Pharmacokinetics:
PO: Peak 1-2 hr, 97% bound to plasma proteins half-life biphasic 3½ hr, 16-23 hr

Interactions/incompatibilities:
■ Not to be taken with ketoconazole, erythromycin

Lab test interferences:
False negative: Skin allergy tests

RESPIRATORY CARE CONSIDERATIONS:
Assess/evaluate:
■ Note drying of the upper airway.
■ Note that terfenadine is longer acting and less sedating than many antihistamines.
■ Caution is suggested if used in asthma, although thickening of lower respiratory tract secretions has not been established.
■ Assess nasal passages during long-term treatment for changes in mucus.
■ Therapeutic response: decrease in runny nose, eye inflammation.

Patient education:
■ Avoid hazardous activities or use caution while drug action persists if drowsiness does occur.
■ Additional CNS depression may occur with concomitant use of CNS depressants (tranquilizers, sedatives, or alcohol).

terpin hydrate
(ter'pin)
Func. class.: Expectorant

Action: Direct action on respiratory tract, probably through vagally mediated stomach reflexes when taken orally; increased mucus secretion allows for mucociliary clearance and expectoration

Uses: Bronchial secretions

Dosage and routes:
■ *Adult:* ELIX 5-10 ml q4-6h
Available forms: Elix terpin hydrate codeine 10 mg codeine/85 mg terpin hydrate; elix, plain 85 mg/5 ml

Side effects/adverse reactions:
GI: Nausea, vomiting, anorexia

Contraindications: Hypersensitivity, child <12 yr

Precautions: Pregnancy (C)

RESPIRATORY CARE CONSIDERATIONS:
Assess/evaluate:
■ Assess cough: type, frequency, character, including sputum production, with color, consistency, and amount.
■ If respiratory infection is present, evaluate respiratory

status: rate and pattern; auscultate breath sounds and assess chest radiograph when available and needed.
■ Evaluate WBC, temperature if infection present, along with sputum culture to identify organism(s).
■ Evaluate ability of patient to clear secretions prior to therapy; are tidal volume, expiratory force adequate?
■ Assess need for concomitant bronchial hygiene techniques such as postural drainage, chest percussion.

Patient education:
■ Drink large amount of non-diuresing fluids (e.g., water, juice, Gatorade) to facilitate mucociliary clearance.
■ Avoid hazardous activities if drowsiness occurs (alcohol content).

tetrahydrozoline HCl
(tet-ra-hi-drozz'o-leen)
Tyzine HCl, Tyzine Pediatric
Func. class.: Nasal decongestant
Chem. class.: Sympathomimetic amine

Action: Produces vasoconstriction (rapid, long-acting) of arterioles by alpha-adrenergic stimulation, thereby decreasing fluid exudation, mucosal engorgement

Uses: Nasal congestion

Dosage and routes:
■ *Adult and child >6 yr:* INSTILL 2-4 gtts or sprays q4-6h prn (0.1%)
■ *Child 2-6 yr:* INSTILL 2-3 gtts q4-6h prn (0.05%)

Available forms: Sol 0.05%, 0.1%

Side effects/adverse reactions:
GI: Nausea, vomiting, anorexia
EENT: Irritation, burning, sneezing, stinging, dryness, rebound congestion
INTEG: Contact dermatitis
CNS: Anxiety, restlessness, tremors, weakness, insomnia, dizziness, fever, headache

Contraindications: Hypersensitivity to sympathomimetic amines

Precautions: Child <6 yr, elderly, diabetes, cardiovascular disease, hypertension, hyperthyroidism, increased ICP, prostatic hypertrophy, pregnancy (C), glaucoma

Interactions/ incompatibilities:
■ Hypertension: MAOIs, β-adrenergic blockers
■ Hypotension: methyldopa, mecamylamine, reserpine

RESPIRATORY CARE CONSIDERATIONS:
Assess/evaluate:
■ Therapeutic response: decreased nasal congestion.
■ Assess subject's BP for possible increases if using beta agonist bronchodilator simultaneously.

Patient education:
■ Environmental humidification may help to decrease nasal congestion, dryness.
■ Warn patient that rebound nasal congestion can occur.
■ Use for short-term symptoms only; prolonged rhinitis should be evaluated by physician, ENT specialist, or allergist.

---

italic = common side effects   **bold** = life-threatening reactions

theophylline, theophylline sodium glycinate
(thee-off'i-lin)
Accurbron, Aerolate III, Aerolate Jr., Aerolate Slo-Phyllin, Aerolate Sr., Aquaphyllin, Asmalix, Bronkodyl, Constant-T, Elixomin, Elixophyllin, Elixophyllin SR, Lanophyllin, Quibron-T Dividose, Quibron-T/SR Dividose, Respbid, Slo-Bid Gyrocaps, Slo-Phyllin Gyrocaps, Sustaire, Theolair-SR, Theo-24, Theobid Duracaps, Theobid Jr. Duracaps, Theochron, Theoclear-80, Theoclear L.A., Theo-Dur, Theo-Dur Sprinkle, Theolair, Theolair-SR, Theophylline, Theophylline and 5% Dextrose, Theophylline Extended Release, Theophylline Oral, Theophylline S.R., Theo-Sav, Theospan-SR, Theostat 80, Theovent, Theo-X, T-Phyl, Uniphyl
Func. class.: Bronchodilator
Chem. class.: Xanthine

Action: Exact mode of action not understood; may block adenosine receptors to reduce or inhibit bronchoconstriction mediated by those receptors. Drug is a weak bronchodilator and may improve ventilatory flow rates by central respiratory stimulation and by strengthened diaphragmatic contraction.

Uses: Bronchial asthma, bronchospasm of COPD, chronic bronchitis

Dosage and routes:
Bronchospasm, bronchial asthma

- *Adult:* PO 100-200 mg q6h; dosage must be individualized; REC 250-500 mg q8-12h
- *Child:* PO 50-100 mg q6h, not to exceed 12 mg/kg/24 hr
COPD, chronic bronchitis
- *Adult:* PO 330-660 mg q6-8h pc (sodium glycinate)
- *Child >12 yr:* PO 220-330 mg q6-8h pc (sodium glycinate)
- *Child 6-12 yr:* PO 330 mg q6-8h pc (sodium glycinate)
- *Child 3-6 yr:* PO 110-165 mg q6-8h pc (sodium glycinate)
- *Child 1-3 yr:* PO 55-110 mg q6-8h pc (sodium glycinate)
Available forms: Caps 50, 100, 200, 250 mg; tabs 100, 125, 200, 225, 250, 300 mg; tabs time-release 100, 200, 250, 300, 400, 500 mg; caps time-release 50, 65, 100, 125, 130, 200, 250, 260, 300, 400, 500 mg; elix 80, 11.25 mg/15 ml; sol 80 mg/15 ml; liq 80, 150, 160 mg/15 ml; susp 300 mg/15 ml

Side effects/adverse reactions:
CNS: Anxiety, restlessness, insomnia, dizziness, convulsions, headache, lightheadedness, muscle twitching
CV: Palpitations, sinus tachycardia, hypotension, other dysrhythmias, fluid retention with tachycardia
GI: Nausea, vomiting, anorexia, diarrhea, bitter taste, dyspepsia, gastric distress
RESP: Increased rate
INTEG: Flushing, urticaria

Contraindications: Hypersensitivity to xanthines, tachydysrhythmias

Precautions: Elderly, CHF, cor pulmonale, hepatic disease, active peptic ulcer disease, diabetes mellitus, hyperthyroidism, hypertension, children, pregnancy (C)

Pharmacokinetics:
SOL: Peak 1 hr, metabolized in liver, excreted in urine and breast milk, crosses placenta

Interactions/ incompatibilities:
■ Increased action of theophylline: cimetidine, propranolol, erythromycin, troleandomycin
■ May increase effects of: anticoagulants
■ Cardiotoxicity: β-blockers
■ Decreased effect of: lithium

RESPIRATORY CARE CONSIDERATIONS:
Assess/evaluate:
■ Therapeutic response: decreased dyspnea, respiratory rate and pattern; respiratory stimulation in infancy.
■ Assess theophylline blood levels (therapeutic level is 10-20 µg/ml); toxicity may occur with small increase above 20 µg/ml, especially elderly; 10-12 µg/ml may be optimal in COPD or asthma patients.
■ Monitor fluid intake for onset of diuresis; dehydration may result in elderly or children.
■ Monitor respiratory rate, rhythm, depth; auscultate lung fields bilaterally; notify physician of abnormalities.
■ Assess for allergic reactions: rash, urticaria. If these occur, drug should be discontinued.
■ Assess side effects reported, and evaluate blood level for toxic range.

Patient education:
■ Take doses as prescribed, do not skip dose.

■ Check OTC medications, current prescription medications for ephedrine, which will increase CNS stimulation. Do not drink alcohol or caffeine products (tea, coffee, chocolate, colas) which will increase diuresis or add to the xanthine level (caffeine).
■ Avoid hazardous activities; dizziness may occur.
■ If GI upset occurs, take drug with 8 oz water; avoid food, since absorption may be decreased.
■ Notify physician of toxicity: insomnia, anxiety, nausea, vomiting, rapid pulse, convulsions.
■ Cigarette smoking will increase metabolism of the drug, lowering blood levels.
■ Increase fluid intake if sputum becomes thicker when taking drug.
■ Use nondiuresing liquids, such as water, juice, Gatorade, and milk, rather than diuretic products such as caffeinated coffee, tea, or colas.

timolol maleate
(tye'moe-lole)
Blocadren, Timolol maleate
Func. class.: Antihypertensive
Chem. class.: Nonselective β-blocker

Action: Competitively blocks stimulation of β-adrenergic receptor within vascular smooth muscle; produces negative chronotropic, inotropic activity (decreases rate of SA node discharge, increases recovery time), slows conduction of AV node, decreases heart rate, which decreases O_2 consumption in myocardium; also decreases reninaldosterone-angiotensin system, at high doses inhibits β-2 receptors in bronchial system

Uses: Mild to moderate hypertension, sinus tachycardia, persistent atrial extrasystoles, tachydysrhythmias, prophylaxis of angina pectoris, reduction of mortality after MI

Dosage and routes:
Hypertension
- *Adult:* PO 10 mg bid, or 20 mg qd, may increase by 10 mg q2-3d, not to exceed 60 mg/day
Myocardial infarction
- *Adult:* 10 mg bid
Available forms: Tabs 5, 10, 20 mg

Side effects/adverse reactions:
CV: Hypotension, bradycardia, *CHF,* edema, chest pain, bradycardia, claudication
CNS: Insomnia, dizziness, hallucinations, anxiety
GI: Nausea, vomiting, *ischemic colitis,* diarrhea, *abdominal pain, mesenteric arterial thrombosis*
INTEG: Rash, alopecia, pruritus, fever
HEMA: Agranulocytosis, thrombocytopenia, purpura
EENT: Visual changes, sore throat, *double vision,* dry burning eyes
GU: Impotence, frequency
RESP: Bronchospasm, dyspnea, cough, rales
META: Hypoglycemia
MS: Joint pain, muscle pain

Contraindications: Hypersensitivity to β-blockers, cardiogenic shock, heart block (2nd, 3rd degree), sinus bradycardia, CHF, cardiac failure

Precautions: Major surgery, pregnancy (C), lactation, diabetes mellitus, renal disease, thyroid disease, COPD, well-compensated heart failure, CAD, nonallergic bronchospasm

Pharmacokinetics:
PO: Peak 2-4 hr, half-life 3-4 hr, excreted 30%-45% unchanged, 60%-65% metabolized by liver, excreted in breast milk

Interactions/ incompatibilities:
- Increased hypotension, bradycardia: reserpine, hydralazine, methyldopa, prazosin, anticholinergics
- Decreased antihypertensive effects: indomethacin
- Increased hypoglycemic effects: insulin
- Decreased bronchodilation: theophyllines

Lab test interferences:
Increase: Liver function tests, renal function tests, K, uric acid
Decrease: Hct, Hgb, HDL

RESPIRATORY CARE CONSIDERATIONS:
Assess/evaluate:
- Avoid use with reversible airway obstruction or bronchospastic disease such as asthma or chronic bronchitis due to potential for bronchospasm (wheezing, dyspnea, complaints of chest tightness) secondary to beta-blockade; consider use of other classes of antihypertensive agents for these patients.
- Monitor all subjects for symptoms of increased airway resistance (wheezing, tightness in chest, difficulty breathing).

---

*Available in Canada only

- Monitor effect on BP and pulse, especially if on positive pressure ventilatory support.
- Assess effectiveness of beta-adrenergic bronchodilator therapy for possible antagonism and effect on BP to avoid increasing BP, if used.

Patient education:
- Do not use OTC products containing α-adrenergic stimulants (nasal decongestants, OTC cold preparations) unless directed by physician.
- Caution patient that orthostatic hypotension may occur.
- Report symptoms of CHF: difficulty breathing, especially on exertion or when lying down, night cough, swelling of extremities.

tocainide HCl
(toe-kay′nide)
Tonocard
Func. class.: Antidysrhythmic (Class IB)
Chem. class.: Lidocaine analog

Action: Decreases sodium and potassium influx in myocardial cells, resulting in decreased excitability

Uses: PVCs, ventricular tachycardia

Dosage and routes:
- *Adult:* PO 600 mg loading dose, then 400 mg q8h
Available forms: Tabs 400, 600 mg

Side effects/adverse reactions:
CNS: Headache, dizziness, involuntary movement, confusion, psychosis, restlessness, irritability, paresthesias, tremors, *seizures*

EENT: Tinnitus, blurred vision, hearing loss
GI: Nausea, vomiting, anorexia, diarrhea, hepatitis
CV: Hypotension, bradycardia, angina, PVCs, *heart block, cardiovascular collapse, arrest, CHF,* chest pain, tachycardia
RESP: Dyspnea, *respiratory depression, pulmonary fibrosis*
INTEG: Rash, urticaria, edema, swelling
HEMA: Blood dyscrasias: leukopenia, agranulocytosis, hypoplastic anemia, thrombocytopenia

Contraindications: Hypersensitivity to amides, severe heart block

Precautions: Pregnancy (C), lactation, children, renal disease, liver disease, CHF, respiratory depression, myasthenia gravis, blood dyscrasias

Pharmacokinetics:
PO: Peak ½-3 hr, half-life 10-17 hr, metabolized by liver, excreted in urine

Interactions/ incompatibilities:
- Increased effects: propranolol, quinidine, and all other antidysrhythmics

Lab test interferences:
Increase: CPK
Positive: ANA titer

RESPIRATORY CARE CONSIDERATIONS:
Assess/evaluate:
- Monitor for anemia and fall in hematocrit, adversely affecting oxygen tissue transport.
- Assess respiratory status with both physical exam (inspection of rate and pattern, auscultation of breath sounds) and chest radiograph for

italic = common side effects   **bold** = life-threatening reactions

pulmonary fibrosis or other pulmonary side effects, including pulmonary edema, interstitial pneumonitis, pleurisy.

- Assess blood pressure for fluctuations.
- Monitor ECG for cardiac rhythm.
- Provide resuscitation support in the event of cardiac arrest, life-threatening arrhythmias.
- Evaluate therapeutic response: decreased dysrhythmias.

Patient education:

- Notify physician if exertional dyspnea, cough, wheezing, tremor, or palpitations occur.
- Avoid hazardous activities if dizziness or blurred vision occurs.

---

tolazoline HCl

(toe-laz'a-leen)
Priscoline
Func. class.: Peripheral vasodilator
Chem. class.: Imidazoline derivative

Action: Peripheral vasodilation occurs by direct relaxation on vascular smooth muscle; also has weak α- and β-adrenergic properties

Uses: Persistent pulmonary hypertension of newborn, hypoxic pulmonary hypertension

Dosage and routes:

- *Newborn:* IV 1-2 mg/kg via scalp vein; IV INF 1-2 mg/kg/hr
Available forms: Inj SC, IM, IV 25 mg/ml

Side effects/adverse reactions:

CV: Orthostatic hypotension, tachycardia, dysrhythmias, hypertension, *cardiovascular collapse*
RESP: Pulmonary hemorrhage
GU: Edema, oliguria, hematuria
GI: Nausea, vomiting, diarrhea, peptic ulcer, *GI hemorrhage, hepatitis*
INTEG: Flushing, tingling, rash, chills, sweating, increased pilomotor activity
HEMA: Thrombocytopenia, leukopenia

Contraindications: Hypersensitivity, CVA, CAD

Precautions: Pregnancy (C), active peptic ulcer, lactation, mitral stenosis

Pharmacokinetics:

IM/SC: Peak 30-60 min, duration 3-4 hr, excreted in urine, half-life 3-10 hr

Interactions/ incompatibilities:

- Increased effects with alcohol, β-blockers, antihypertensive
- Decrease BP, rebound hypertension: epinephrine
- Incompatible with ethacrynic acid, hydrocortisone, methylprednisolone

RESPIRATORY CARE CONSIDERATIONS:
Assess/evaluate:

- Monitor ABGs, electrolytes, VS in newborn.
- Monitor BP, pulse during treatment until stable.
- Assess respiratory status for possible side effect: rate, pattern, breath sounds.
- Assess BP if on mechanical ventilatory support to minimize mean airway pressures which can increase hypotensive effect through impeded

venous return and decreased cardiac output; minimize inspiratory times and optimal flow patterns and avoid large tidal volumes.
■ Therapeutic response: decrease in pulmonary hypertension or pulse volume.

Patient education:
■ Do not use OTC products containing α-adrenergic stimulants (nasal decongestants, OTC cold preparations) unless directed by physician.
■ Report symptoms of CHF: difficulty breathing, especially on exertion or when lying down, night cough, swelling of extremities.
■ It is necessary to quit smoking to prevent excessive vasoconstriction.
■ Avoid hazardous activities until stabilized on medication; dizziness may occur.
■ Make position changes slowly, or fainting will occur.

torsemide
(tore-sa′mide)
Demadox
Func. class.: Loop diuretic
Chem. class.: Sulfonamide derivative

Action: Acts on loop of Henle by increasing excretion of chloride, sodium, water

Uses: Treatment of hypertension and edema in CHF, hepatic disease, renal disease

Dosage and routes:
■ *Adult:* PO 2.5-5 mg qd; may gradually increase dose as needed
Available forms: Tabs 5, 10, 20, 100 mg; 10 mg/ml vials of 2, 5 ml

Side effects/adverse reactions:
CNS: Headache, fatigue, weakness, vertigo, paresthesias
CV: Orthostatic hypotension, chest pain, ECG changes, *circulatory collapse*
EENT: Loss of hearing, ear pain, tinnitus, blurred vision
ENDO: Hyperglycemia
ELECT: Hypokalemia, hypochloremic alkalosis, hypomagnesemia, hyperuricemia, hypocalcemia, hyponatremia, metabolic alkalosis
GI: Nausea, diarrhea, dry mouth, vomiting, anorexia, cramps, oral and gastric irritations, pancreatitis
*GU: Polyuria, **renal failure,*** glycosuria
*HEMA: **Thrombocytopenia, agranulocytosis, leukopenia, neutropenia, anemia***
INTEG: Rash, pruritus, purpura, ***Stevens-Johnson syndrome,*** sweating, photosensitivity, urticaria
MS: Cramps, stiffness

Contraindications: Hypersensitivity to sulfonamides, anuria, hypovolemia, infants, lactation, electrolyte depletion

Precautions: Diabetes mellitus, dehydration, severe renal disease, pregnancy (C)

Pharmacokinetics:
PO: Rapidly absorbed, duration 6 hr, excreted in urine and feces, crosses placenta, excreted in breast milk, half-life 2-4 hr, plasma protein binding 97%-99%

Interactions/ incompatibilities:
■ Increased toxicity: lithium, nondepolarizing skeletal muscle relaxants, digitalis

italic = common side effects   **bold** = life-threatening reactions

- Increased action of: antihypertensives, oral anticoagulants, nitrates
- Increased ototoxicity: aminoglycosides, cisplatin, vancomycin
- Decreased antihypertensive effect of torsemide: indomethacin, metolazone
- Incompatible with acidic sol, Vit C, corticosteroids, diphenhydramine, dobutamine, esmolol, epinephrine, gentamicin, levarterenol, meperidine, milrione, netilmicin, reserpine, spironolactone, tetracyclines in sol
- Incompatible with any drug in syringe

Lab test interferences:
Interference: GTT

RESPIRATORY CARE CONSIDERATIONS:
Assess/evaluate:
- Monitor serum electrolytes for hyponatremia and hypokalemia, with resulting acid-base abnormalities such as metabolic alkalosis.
- Overdose can cause reduction in blood volume and hypotension.
- Hypokalemia can also cause muscular weakness, possibly complicating weaning from mechanical ventilation.
- Monitor ECG for cardiac arrhythmias.
- Evaluate for dehydration, especially in COPD subjects or those with excess respiratory tract secretions.
- Monitor color, consistency of sputum.
- Evaluate breath sounds and respiratory pattern for pulmonary congestion.
- Evaluate chest radiograph if used in CHF to assess clearing of infiltrates and pulmonary edema.

triamcinolone/ triamcinolone acetonide/ triamcinolone diacetate/ triamcinolone hexacetonide

(trye-am-sin'oh-lone)
Aristocort, Atolone, Kenacort, Azmacort, Cenocort A-40, Kenaject-40, Kenalog, Kenalog-10, Kenalog-40, Tac-3, Tac-40, Triam-A, Triamcinolone Acetonide, Triamonide 40, Amcort, Aristocort Forte, Aristocort Intralesional, Articulose L.A., Cenocort Forte, Triamcinolone, Triam Forte, Triamolone 40, Trilone, Trisoject, Aristospan Intra-Articular, Aristospan Intralesional, Tri-Kort, Trilog
Func. class.: Corticosteroid
Chem. class.: Glucocorticoid, intermediate-acting

See also Section III: Aerosol Agents for Oral Inhalation

Action: Decreases inflammation by suppression of migration of polymorphonuclear leukocytes, fibroblasts, reversal to increase capillary permeability and lysosomal stabilization

Uses: Severe inflammation, immunosuppression, neoplasms, asthma (steroid dependent), collagen, respiratory, dermatologic disorders

Dosage and routes:
- *Adult:* PO 4-48 mg/day in divided doses qd-qid; IM 40

mg qwk (acetonide or diacetate), 5-48 mg into neoplasms (diacetate, acetonide), 2-40 mg into joint or soft tissue (diacetate, acetonide), 0.5 mg/sq in of affected intralesional skin (hexacetonide), 2-20 mg into joint or soft tissue (hexacetonide)

Asthma
- *Adult:* 2 inhalations tid-qid, not to exceed 16 inhalations/day
- *Child 6-12 yr:* 1-2 inhalations tid-qid, not to exceed 12 inhalations/day

Available forms: Tabs 1, 2, 4, 8, 16 mg; syr 2 mg/5 ml, 4.85 mg/5 ml; inj 25, 40 mg/ml diacetate; inj 3, 10, 40 mg/ml acetonide; inj 20, 5 mg/ml hexacetonide; MDI 200 mcg released per actuation delivers approximately 100 mcg at the mouthpiece

Side effects/adverse reactions:
INTEG: Acne, poor wound healing, ecchymosis, petechiae
CNS: Depression, flushing, sweating, headache, mood changes
CV: Hypertension, *circulatory collapse, thrombophlebitis, embolism,* tachycardia, edema
HEMA: Thrombocytopenia
MS: Fractures, osteoporosis, weakness
GI: Diarrhea, nausea, abdominal distention, GI hemorrhage, increased appetite, pancreatitis
EENT: Fungal infections, increased intraocular pressure, blurred vision

Contraindications: Psychosis, hypersensitivity, idiopathic thrombocytopenia, acute glomerulonephritis, amebiasis, fungal infections, nonasthmatic bronchial disease, child <2 yr, AIDS, TB

Precautions: Pregnancy (C), diabetes mellitus, glaucoma, osteoporosis, seizure disorders, ulcerative colitis, CHF, myasthenia gravis, renal disease, esophagitis, peptic ulcer

Pharmacokinetics:
PO/IM: Peak 1-2 hr, 2 days, 1-6 wk (IM), half-life 2-5 hr

Interactions/ incompatibilities:
- Decreased action of triamcinolone: cholestyramine, colestipol, barbiturates, rifampin, ephedrine, phenytoin, theophylline
- Decreased effects of: anticoagulants, anticonvulsants, antidiabetics, ambenonium, neostigmine, isoniazid, toxoids, vaccines, anticholinesterases, salicylates, somatrem
- Increased side effects: alcohol, salicylates, indomethacin, amphotericin B, digitalis, cyclosporine, diuretics
- Increased action of triamcinolone: salicylates, estrogens, indomethacin, oral contraceptives, ketoconazole, macrolide antibiotics

Lab test interferences:
Increase: Cholesterol, Na, blood glucose, uric acid, Ca, urine glucose
Decrease: Ca, K, T_4, T_3, thyroid ^{131}I uptake test, urine 17-OHCS, 17-KS, PBI
False negative: Skin allergy tests

RESPIRATORY CARE CONSIDERATIONS:
Note: for detailed evaluation of aerosol use, see Section III: Aerosol Agents for Oral Inhalation. Listed here are general guidelines for noninhaled use of triamcinolone.

---

italic = common side effects   **bold** = life-threatening reactions

T

Assess/evaluate:

- Monitor for side effects of increased corticosteroid level: Cushingoid symptoms (moon face, peripheral wasting, central edema).
- Monitor patients with latent tuberculosis or reactive skin tests for reactivation of the disease.
- Evaluate muscle weakness and steroid myopathy, especially in chronic lung disease patients.
- Evaluate cardiovascular system for hypertension, CHF.
- Monitor electrolytes: potassium and calcium loss can occur, with hypokalemic alkalosis.
- Infection, including pneumonia, can occur.
- Increased corticosteroid levels can mask symptoms of infection.
- If asthma is present, monitor for breakthrough symptoms (bronchospasm, wheezing) if drug is discontinued.
- Evaluate possible adrenal insufficiency when transferring from systemic to inhaled aerosol corticosteroids in asthma.
- Assess for symptoms of adrenal insufficiency: nausea, anorexia, fatigue, dizziness, dyspnea, weakness, joint pain.

triamterene
(trye-am′ter-een)
Dyrenium
Func. class.: Potassium-sparing diuretic
Chem. class.: Pteridine derivative

Action: Acts on distal tubule to inhibit reabsorption of sodium, chloride; increases potassium retention

Uses: Edema; may be used with other diuretics, hypertension

Dosage and routes:
- *Adults:* PO 100 mg bid pc, not to exceed 300 mg
Available forms: Cap 50, 100 mg

Side effects/adverse reactions:
GI: Nausea, diarrhea, vomiting, dry mouth, jaundice, liver disease
ELECT: Hyperkalemia, hyponatremia, hypochloremia
CNS: Weakness, headache, dizziness
INTEG: Photosensitivity, rash
HEMA: Thrombocytopenia, megaloblastic anemia, low folic acid levels
GU: Azotemia, interstitial nephritis, increased BUN, creatinine, renal stones, bluish discoloration of urine

Contraindications: Hypersensitivity, anuria, severe renal disease, severe hepatic disease, hyperkalemia, pregnancy (D), lactation

Precautions: Dehydration, hepatic disease, lactation, CHF, renal disease, cirrhosis

Pharmacokinetics:
PO: Onset 2 hr, peak 6-8 hr, duration 12-16 hr, half-life 3 hr, metabolized in liver, excreted in bile and urine

Interactions/ incompatibilities:
- Nephrotoxicity: indomethacin
- Enhanced action of: antihypertensives, lithium, amantadine

- Increased hyperkalemia: other K-sparing diuretics, K products, ACE inhibitors, salt substitutes

Lab test interferences:
Interference: quinidine serum levels, LDH

RESPIRATORY CARE CONSIDERATIONS:
Assess/evaluate:
- Monitor serum electrolytes; triamterene produces an increase in sodium excretion and decrease in potassium excretion, leading to possible hyponatremia and hyperkalemia.
- Evaluate for dehydration, especially in COPD subjects or those with excess respiratory tract secretions.
- Monitor color, consistency of sputum.
- Monitor BP.
- Evaluate breath sounds and respiratory pattern for pulmonary congestion.

trimeprazine tartrate
(trye-mep′ra-zeen)
Panectyl,* Temaril
Func. class.: Antihistamine
Chem. class.: Phenothiazine analog, H_1-receptor antagonist

Action: Blocks the action of histamine at H_1-receptor sites on blood vessels, GI, respiratory tract to decrease allergic inflammatory response and in general the pharmacologic effects of histamine. There is also an anticholinergic (drying) and sedative effect.

Uses: Pruritus

Dosage and routes:
- *Adult:* PO 2.5 mg qid; TIME-REL 5 mg bid
- *Child 3-12 yr:* PO 2.5 mg tid or hs
- *Child 6 mo-1 yr:* PO 1.25 mg tid or hs
Available forms: Tabs 2.5 mg; spans 5 mg; syr 2.5 mg/5 ml

Side effects/adverse reactions:
CNS: Dizziness, drowsiness, poor condition, fatigue, anxiety, euphoria, confusion, paresthesia, neuritis
CV: Hypotension, palpitations, tachycardia
RESP: Increased thick secretions, wheezing, chest tightness
HEMA: Thrombocytopenia, agranulocytosis, hemolytic anemia
GI: Dry mouth, nausea, vomiting, anorexia, constipation, diarrhea
INTEG: Rash, urticaria, photosensitivity
GU: Retention, dysuria, frequency
EENT: Blurred vision, dilated pupils, tinnitus, nasal stuffiness, dry nose, throat, mouth

Contraindications: Hypersensitivity to H_1-receptor antagonist, acute asthma attack, lower respiratory tract disease

Precautions: Increased intraocular pressure, renal disease, cardiac disease, hypertension, bronchial asthma, seizure disorder, stenosed peptic ulcers, hyperthyroidism, prostatic hypertrophy, bladder neck obstruction, pregnancy (C)

Interactions/ incompatibilities:
- Increased CNS depression: barbiturates, narcotics,

hypnotics, tricyclic antidepressants, alcohol
- Decreased effect of: oral anticoagulants, heparin
- Increased effect of trimeprazine: MAOIs

Lab test interferences:
False negative: Skin allergy tests

RESPIRATORY CARE CONSIDERATIONS
Assess/evaluate:
- Note drying of the upper airway.
- Caution is suggested if used in asthma, although thickening of lower respiratory tract secretions has not been established.
- Drowsiness may be a risk factor in subjects with sleep apnea.
- Therapeutic response: decreased itching associated with pruritus.

Patient education:
- Avoid hazardous activities or use caution while drug action persists.
- Additional CNS depression may occur with concomitant use of CNS depressants (tranquilizers, sedatives, or alcohol).

trimetrexate glucuronate
(try-me-treks'-ate gloo-coo-ro'-nate)
Neutrexin
Func. class.: Antineoplastic antimetabolite
Chem. class.: Nonclassical folic acid antagonist

Action: Inhibits an enzyme that reduces folic acid, which is needed for purine biosynthesis in all cells; result is disruption of RNA, DNA, cell

*Available in Canada only

death; leucovorin usually transported into cells by active, carrier-mediated process; however, *Pneumocystis carinii* organisms lack carrier system; trimetrexate must be given with leucovorin to protect normal cells

Uses: Moderate to severe *P. carinii* pneumonia as an alternative to TMP/SMZ; may be useful in treating non-small cell lung, prostate, colorectal cancer

Dosage and routes:
Leucovorin must be given concurrently and for 72 hr past last trimetrexate dose.
- *Adult:* IV 45 mg/m² qd over 60-90 min; with leucovorin IV 20 mg/m² over 5-10 min q 6 hr for a daily dose of 80 mg/m² or PO qid 20 mg/m² evenly spaced during the day; PO dose should be rounded to the next higher 25 mg; course is trimetrexate 21 days, leucovorin 24 days; modifications in dose must be based on hematologic toxicity
Available forms: Powder for inj lyophilized 25 mg

Side effects/adverse reactions:
CNS: Confusion, fatigue, fever
GI: Nausea, vomiting, *hepatotoxicity*, ulcer, stomatitis
GU: Increased serum creatinine
HEMA: Thrombocytopenia, anemia
INTEG: Rash, pruritus
META: Hyponatremia, hypocalcemia

Contraindications: Hypersensitivity to trimetrexate, leucovorin, methotrexate; thrombocytopenia (<25,000/mm³), severe anemia, neutropenia (<500 mm³), pregnancy (D)

Precautions: Renal disease, hepatic disease, lactation, children, seizures

Pharmacokinetics: Terminal half-life 7-15 hr, may be 95%-98% protein bound

Interactions/ incompatibilities:
Specific interactions not known; these interactions may occur:
■ Increased toxicity: aspirin, sulfa drugs, other antineoplastics, radiation
■ Decreased effect of trimetrexate. erythromycin, ketoconazole, fluconazole, rifampin, rifabutin, cimetidine

RESPIRATORY CARE CONSIDERATIONS:
Assess/evaluate:
■ Monitor for anemia and decreased tissue oxygen transport.
■ If used in patients with PCP, monitor respiratory status to evaluate efficacy: CXR, WBC, temperature, breath sounds, respiratory rate and pattern.
■ Verify that leucovorin is being given concomitantly to protect host cells from toxicity.
■ Practice infection control to prevent opportunistic infection in subjects.
■ Monitor subject for respiratory infections, especially *P. carinii* pneumonia (PCP).
■ Assess and screen for concomitant TB infection with all HIV positive subjects.
■ Use isolation techniques (e.g., negative pressure booth or hood) for all concomitant aerosol treatments.

tripelennamine HCl
(tri-pel-enn′a-meen)
PBZ, PBZ-SR, Pelamine, Tripelennamine HCl
Func. class.: Antihistamine
Chem. class.: Ethylenediamine derivative

Action: Blocks the action of histamine at H_1-receptor sites on blood vessels, GI, respiratory tract to decrease allergic inflammatory response and in general the pharmacologic effects of histamine. There is also an anticholinergic (drying) and sedative effect.

Uses: Rhinitis, allergy symptoms

Dosage and routes:
■ *Adult:* PO 25-50 mg q4-6h, not to exceed 600 mg/day; TIME-REL 100 mg bid-tid, not to exceed 600 mg/day
■ *Child >5 yr:* TIME-REL 50 mg q8-12hr, not to exceed 300 mg/day
■ *Child < 5 yr:* PO 5 mg/kg/day in 4-6 divided doses, not to exceed 300 mg/day
Available forms: Tabs 25, 50 mg; time-rel tabs 100 mg; elix 37.5 mg/5 ml

Side effects/adverse reactions:
CNS: Dizziness, drowsiness, poor coordination, fatigue, anxiety, euphoria, confusion, paresthesia, neuritis
CV: Hypotension, palpitations, tachycardia
RESP: Increased thick secretions, wheezing, chest tightness
HEMA: **Thrombocytopenia, agranulocytosis, hemolytic anemia**

italic = common side effects   **bold** = life-threatening reactions

GI: Constipation, dry mouth, nausea, vomiting, anorexia, diarrhea
INTEG: Rash, urticaria, photosensitivity
GU: Retention, dysuria, frequency
EENT: Blurred vision, dilated pupils, tinnitus, nasal stuffiness, dry nose, throat, mouth

Contraindications: Hypersensitivity to H_1-receptor antagonist, acute asthma attack, lower respiratory tract disease

Precautions: Increased intraocular pressure, renal disease, cardiac disease, hypertension, bronchial asthma, seizure disorder, stenosed peptic ulcers, hyperthyroidism, prostatic hypertrophy, bladder neck obstruction, pregnancy (C)

Pharmacokinetics:
PO: Onset 15-30 min, duration 4-6 hr, detoxified in liver, excreted by kidneys

Interactions/ incompatibilities:
■ Increased CNS depressants: barbiturates, narcotics, hypnotics, tricyclic antidepressants, alcohol
■ Decreased effect of: oral anticoagulants, heparin
■ Increased effect of tripelennamine: MAOIs

Lab test interferences:
False negative: Skin allergy test
False positive: Urine pregnancy tests

RESPIRATORY CARE CONSIDERATIONS:
Assess/evaluate:
■ Note drying of the upper airway.
■ Caution is suggested if used in asthma, although thickening of lower respiratory tract secretions has not been established.
■ Drowsiness may be a risk factor in subjects with sleep apnea.
■ Assess nasal passages during long-term treatment for changes in mucus.
■ Therapeutic response: decrease in runny nose or pruritis.

Patient education:
■ Avoid hazardous activities or use caution while drug action persists.
■ Additional CNS depression may occur with concomitant use of CNS depressants (tranquilizers, sedatives, or alcohol).

triprolidine HCl
(trye-proe'li-deen)
Actidil, Actifed Myidil, Triprolidine HCl
Func. class.: Antihistamine
Chem. class.: Alkylamine, H_1-receptor antagonist

Action: Blocks the action of histamine at H_1-receptor sites on blood vessels, GI, respiratory tract to decrease allergic inflammatory response and in general the pharmacologic effects of histamine. There is also an anticholinergic (drying) and sedative effect.

Uses: Rhinitis, allergy symptoms

Dosage and routes:
■ *Adult:* PO 2.5 mg tid-qid
■ *Child >6 yr:* PO 1.25 mg tid-qid
■ *Child 4-6 yr:* PO 0.9 mg tid-qid
■ *Child 2-4 yr:* PO 0.6 mg tid-qid
■ *Child 4 mo-2 yr:* 0.3 mg tid-qid

Available forms: Tab 2.5 mg; syr 1.25 mg/5 ml

Side effects/adverse reactions:

CNS: Dizziness, drowsiness, poor coordination, fatigue, anxiety, euphoria, confusion, paresthesia, neuritis

CV: Hypotension, palpitations, tachycardia

RESP: Increased thick secretions, wheezing, chest tightness

HEMA: Thrombocytopenia, agranulocytosis, hemolytic anemia

GI: Constipation, dry mouth, nausea, vomiting, anorexia, diarrhea

INTEG: Rash, urticaria, photosensitivity

GU: Retention, dysuria, frequency

EENT: Blurred vision, dilated pupils, tinnitus, nasal stuffiness, dry nose, throat, mouth

Contraindications: Hypersensitivity to H_1-receptor antagonist, acute asthma attack, lower respiratory tract disease

Precautions: Increased intraocular pressure, renal disease, cardiac disease, hypertension, bronchial asthma, seizure disorder, stenosed peptic ulcers, hyperthyroidism, prostatic hypertrophy, bladder neck obstruction, pregnancy (C)

Pharmacokinetics:
PO: Onset 20-60 min, duration 8-12 hr, half-life 20-24 hr, detoxified in liver, excreted by kidneys (metabolites/free drug)

Interactions/ incompatibilities:
- Increased CNS depression: barbiturates, narcotics, hypnotics, tricyclic antidepressants, alcohol
- Decreased effect of: oral anticoagulants, heparin
- Increased effect of triprolidine: MAOIs

Lab test interferences:
False negative: Skin allergy tests

RESPIRATORY CARE CONSIDERATIONS:
Assess/evaluate:
- Note drying of the upper airway.
- Caution is suggested if used in asthma, although thickening of lower respiratory tract secretions has not been established.
- Drowsiness may be a risk factor in subjects with sleep apnea.
- Assess nasal passages during long-term treatment for changes in mucus.
- Therapeutic response: decrease in runny nose, pruritis.

Patient education:
- Avoid hazardous activities or use caution while drug action persists.
- Additional CNS depression may occur with concomitant use of CNS depressants (tranquilizers, sedatives, or alcohol).

tromethamine
(troe-meth'a-meen)
Tham, Tham-E
Func. class.: Alkalinizer
Chem. class.: Amine

Action: Proton acceptor that corrects acidosis by combining with hydrogen ions to form bicarbonate and buffer; acts as diuretic (osmotic)

Uses: Acidosis (metabolic) associated with cardiac bypass surgery, cardiac arrest

Dosage and routes:
- *Adult:* 0.3 M required = kg of weight × HCO_3 deficit (mEq/L)
- *Child:* Same as above given over 3-6 hr, not to exceed 40 ml/kg

Available forms: Inj IV 36 mg/ml, powd for inj IV 36 g

Side effects/adverse reactions:
CV: Irregular pulse, *cardiac arrest*
META: Alkalosis, hypoglycemia
RESP: Shallow, slow respirations, cyanosis, *apnea*
GI: Hepatic necrosis
INTEG: Infection at injection site, extravasation, phlebitis

Contraindications: Hypersensitivity, anuria, uremia

Precautions: Severe respiratory disease/respiratory depression, pregnancy (C), cardiac edema, renal disease, infants

Pharmacokinetics:
IV: Excreted in urine

RESPIRATORY CARE CONSIDERATIONS:
Assess/evaluate:
- Therapeutic response: increase in pH.
- Assess acid-base status (PCO_2, pH, HCO_3) to guide therapy, and avoid overcorrection or undercorrection of pH.
- Monitor electrolyte levels.
- Note: it is not advisable to correct respiratory acidosis with a buffering agent or to correct metabolic acidosis with ventilatory adjustments.
- Monitor patients with chronic hypoventilation (COPD) or those treated with respiratory depressant drugs for decreases in ventilation level.

tubocurarine chloride
(too-boe-kyoo-ar'een)
Tubarine,* Tubocuraine
Func. class.: Neuromuscular blocker
Chem. class.: Curare alkaloid, an isoquinoline

Action: Inhibits transmission of nerve impulses at the neuromuscular junction by binding with cholinergic receptor sites, antagonizing action of acetylcholine, and causing muscle weakness or paralysis, depending on dose.

Uses: Facilitation of endotracheal intubation, skeletal muscle relaxation during mechanical ventilation, surgery, or general anesthesia

Dosage and routes:
- *Adult:* IV BOL 0.4-0.5 mg/kg, then 0.08-0.10 mg/kg 20-45 min after 1st dose if needed for prolonged procedures

Available forms: Inj IV 3 mg/ml, 20 U/ml

Side effects/adverse reactions:
CV: Bradycardia, tachycardia, increased, decreased BP
RESP: Prolonged apnea, bronchospasm, cyanosis, respiratory depression
EENT: Increased secretions
INTEG: Rash, flushing, pruritus, urticaria

Contraindications: Hypersensitivity

Precautions: Pregnancy (C), cardiac disease, lactation, children <2 yr, electrolyte imbalances, dehydration, neuromuscular disease, respiratory disease

Pharmacokinetics:
IV: Onset 15 sec, peak 2-3 min, duration ½-1½ hr, half-life 1-3 hr, degraded in liver, kidney (minimally), excreted in urine (unchanged), crosses placenta

Interactions/ incompatibilities:
■ Increased neuromuscular blockade: aminoglycosides, clindamycin, lincomycin, quinidine, local anesthetics, polymyxin antibiotics, lithium, narcotic analgesics, thiazides, enflurane, isoflurane, trimethophan, Mg salts
■ Dysrhythmias: theophylline
■ Incompatible with barbiturates in solution or syringe; do not mix with any other drug in syringe

RESPIRATORY CARE CONSIDERATIONS:
Assess/evaluate:
■ Provide airway and ventilatory support before administering drug.
■ Note possible interaction with the following antibiotics, which can increase neuromuscular blockade: the aminoglycosides, the polymyxins, clindamycin, and lincomycin.
■ Use with mechanical ventilation, assess patient for adequate and preferably optimal ventilator settings *before* paralyzing. If patient is "fighting" the ventilator, provide adequately high flow rates and tidal volumes, short inspiratory times, and reasonable I:E ratios, check the sensitivity in assist-control mode, and provide sufficiently high rates to avoid patient fatigue;

consider paralysis if these measures fail.
■ Assess ventilator patients for pain, hypoxemia, or ventilator malfunction, if restless and anxious, before instituting muscle paralysis.
■ Assess need of patient and provide for pain control and sedation during neuromuscular blockade; *neuromuscular blocking agents do not provide analgesia or sedation*
■ Monitor airway resistance for increases due to histamine release. wheezing or ventilator airway pressures (peak, plateau pressures).
■ Close eyelids and provide eye lubricant during prolonged paralysis.
■ Since usual signs of pain or anxiety (restlessness, tachypnea, distress, thrashing) are blocked, monitor vital signs closely, overall patient appearance and state to detect problems, (e.g., IV infiltration).
■ Check ventilator alarm settings for sufficient limits and sensitivity; a disconnect alarm is critical.
■ Assess reversal of drug before attempting to wean from mechanical ventilatory support.

Administer:
■ Administer by IV, not by IM, for more consistent absorption and distribution and to avoid the pain associated with IM injection of the drug.
■ Reversal: neostigmine or edrophonium, preceded by atropine to inhibit muscarinic response especially in upper airway.

italic = common side effects   **bold** = life-threatening reactions

urea

(yoor-ee'a)
Ureaphil, Carbamex*
Func. class.: Diuretic, osmotic
Chem. class.: Carbonic acid
diamide salt

Action: Elevates plasma
osmolality, increasing flow of
water into the extracellular
compartment

Uses: To decrease intracranial
pressure, intraocular pressure

Dosage and routes:
- *Adult:* IV 1-1.5 g/kg of a
30% sol over 1-3 hr; do not
exceed 120 g/day
- *Child >2 yr:* IV 0.5-1.5 g/kg,
not to exceed 4 ml/min
- *Child <2 yr:* IV 0.1 g/kg, not
to exceed 4 ml/min
Available forms: Inj IV 40
g/150 ml

**Side effects/adverse
reactions:**
CNS: Dizziness, headache, disorientation, fever, syncope,
headache
GI: Nausea, vomiting
INTEG: Venous thrombosis,
phlebitis, extravasation
CV: Postural hypotension, tachycardia

Contraindications: Severe
renal disease, active intracranial bleeding, marked dehydration, liver failure

Precautions: Hepatic disease,
renal disease, pregnancy (C),
electrolyte imbalances, lactation

Pharmacokinetics:
IV: Onset ½-1 hr, peak 1 hr,
duration 3-10 hr (diuresis),
5-6 hr (intraocular pressure)
half-life 1 hr, excreted in
urine, crosses placenta, excreted in breast milk

**Interactions/
incompatibilities:**
- Incompatible with whole
blood, alkalines in sol or
syringe
Increased renal excretion of:
lithium

**RESPIRATORY CARE
CONSIDERATIONS:**
Assess/evaluate:
- Monitor serum electrolytes
to detect hyponatremia or
hypokalemia; such agents are
generally free of pharmacologic effects due to their mode
of action (osmosis).
- Evaluate for dehydration,
especially in COPD subjects
or those with excess respiratory tract secretions.
- Monitor color, consistency
of sputum.
- Evaluate breath sounds and
respiratory pattern for pulmonary congestion.

urokinase

(yoor-oh-kin'ase)
Abbokinase, Abbokinase
Open-Cath
Func. class.: Thrombolytic
enzyme
Chem. class.: β-hemolytic
streptococcus filtrate
(purified)

Action: Promotes thrombolysis by directly converting
plasminogen to the enzyme
plasmin, which breaks down
fibrin clots and degrades
fibrinogen

Uses: Venous thrombosis,
pulmonary embolism, arterial
thrombosis, arterial embolism,
arteriovenous cannula occlusion,
lysis of coronary artery thrombi
after myocardial infarction

Dosage and routes:
Lysis of pulmonary emboli
- *Adult:* IV 4400 IU/kg/hr ×
12-24 hr, not to exceed 200
ml; then IV heparin, then
anticoagulants
Coronary artery thrombosis
- *Adult:* INSTILL 6000 IU/min
into occluded artery for 1-2
hr after giving IV bol of
heparin 2500-10,000 U
- May also give as IV infusion of 2-3 million U over
45-90 min
Venous catheter occlusion
- *Adult:* INSTILL 5000 IU into
line, wait 5 min, then aspirate, repeat aspiration attempts q5min × ½ hr; if occlusion has not been removed,
cap line and wait ½-1 hr then
aspirate; may need 2nd dose
if still occluded
Available forms: Inj

**Side effects/adverse
reactions:**
HEMA: Decreased Hct, bleeding
INTEG: Rash, urticaria, phlebi-
tis at IV infusion site, itching,
flushing
CNS: Headache, fever
GI: Nausea
RESP: Altered respirations,
SOB, *bronchospasm*
MS: Low back pain
CV: Hypertension, dysrhyth-
mias
EENT: Periorbital edema
*SYST: GI, GU, intracranial,
retroperitoneal bleeding,* sur-
face bleeding, *anaphylaxis*

Contraindications: Hypersensitivity, active bleeding,
intraspinal surgery, neoplasms
of CNS, ulcerative colitis/
enteritis, severe hypertension,
renal disease, hepatic disease,
hypocoagulation, COPD, subacute bacterial endocarditis,
rheumatic valvular disease,
cerebral embolism/
thrombosis/hemorrhage, intraarterial diagnostic procedure or surgery (10 days),
recent major surgery

Precautions: Arterial emboli
from left side of heart, pregnancy (B)

Pharmacokinetics:
IV: Half-life 10-20 min; small
amounts excreted in urine

**Interactions/
incompatibilities:**
- Bleeding potential: aspirin,
indomethacin, phenylbuta-
zone, anticoagulants
- Considered incompatible
with any drug in sol or syringe

**RESPIRATORY CARE
CONSIDERATIONS:**
Assess/evaluate:
- Bleeding from invasive procedures, such as cutdowns,
catheter insertions, or arterial
punctures, is an increased risk
with fibrinolytic therapy and
is common.
- Minimize arterial or venous
punctures.
- Use sites accessible to
manual compression for arterial punctures.
- Use pressure dressings for
arterial puncture after prolonged manual compression.
- Monitor for bleeding from
any puncture sites.
- Risk of fibrinolytic therapy
is increased with hypertension, hemostatic defects, or
treatment with anticoagulant
agents.

Patient education:
- Instruct patient to notify
health care personnel of any
swelling, hematoma, or bleeding at a puncture site.

italic = common side effects   **bold** = life-threatening reactions

vecuronium bromide

(vek-yoo-roe'nee-um)

Norcuron

Func. class.: Neuromuscular blocker (nondepolarizing)

Chem. class.: Monoquaternary analog of pancuronium

Action: Inhibits transmission of nerve impulses at the neuromuscular junction, by binding with cholinergic receptor sites, antagonizing action of acetylcholine, and causing muscle weakness or paralysis, depending on dose

Uses: Facilitation of endotracheal intubation, skeletal muscle relaxation during mechanical ventilation, surgery, general anesthesia

Dosage and routes:
▪ *Adult and child >9 yr:* IV BOL 0.08-0.10 mg/kg, then 0.010-0.015 mg/kg for prolonged procedures
Available forms: IV 10 mg/5 ml

Side effects/adverse reactions:
CNS: Skeletal muscle weakness or paralysis, rarely
RESP: Prolonged apnea, possible respiratory paralysis

Contraindications: Hypersensitivity

Precautions: Pregnancy (C), cardiac disease, lactation, children <2 yr, electrolyte imbalances, dehydration, neuromuscular disease, respiratory disease

Pharmacokinetics:
IV: Onset 15 min, peak 3-5 min, duration 45-60 min half-life 65-75 min, not metabo-

lized, excreted in feces, crosses placenta

Interactions/ incompatibilities:
▪ Increased neuromuscular blockade: aminoglycosides, clindamycin, lincomycin, quinidine, local anesthetics, polymyxin antibiotics, lithium, narcotic analgesics, thiazides, enflurane, isoflurane, succinylcholine
▪ Dysrhythmias: theophylline
▪ Incompatibility unknown

RESPIRATORY CARE CONSIDERATIONS:
Assess/evaluate:
▪ Provide airway and ventilatory support before administering drug.
▪ Note possible interaction with the following antibiotics, which can increase neuromuscular blockade: the aminoglycosides, the polymyxins, clindamycin, and lincomycin.
▪ Use with mechanical ventilation, assess patient for adequate and preferably optimal ventilator settings *before* paralyzing. If patient is "fighting" the ventilator, provide adequately high flow rates and tidal volumes, short inspiratory times, and reasonable I:E ratios, check the sensitivity in assist-control mode, and provide sufficiently high rates to avoid patient fatigue; consider paralysis if these measures fail.
▪ Assess ventilator patients for pain, hypoxemia, or ventilator malfunction, if restless and anxious, before instituting muscle paralysis.
▪ Assess need of patient and provide for pain control and sedation during neuromuscu-

lar blockade, *neuromuscular blocking agents do not provide analgesia or sedation.*
- Close eyelids and provide eye lubricant during prolonged paralysis.
- Since usual signs of pain or anxiety (restlessness, tachynea, distress, thrashing) are blocked, monitor vital signs closely and overall patient appearance and state to detect problems (e.g., IV infiltration).
- Check ventilator alarm settings for sufficient limits and sensitivity; a disconnect alarm is critical.
- Assess reversal of drug before attempting to wean from mechanical ventilatory support.

Administer:
- Administer by IV, not by IM, for more consistent absorption and distribution and to avoid the pain associated with IM injection of the drug.
- Reversal: neostigmine or edrophonium, preceded by atropine to inhibit muscarinic response especially in upper airway.

verapamil HCl
(ver-ap′-a-mill)
Calan, Calan SR, Isoptin, Isoptin SR, Verapamil HCl, Verelan
Func. class.: Calcium channel blocker
Chem. class.: Phenylalkylamine

Action: Inhibits calcium ion influx across cell membrane during cardiac depolarization produces relaxation of coronary vascular smooth muscle dilates coronary arteries de-

creases SA/AV node conduction dilates peripheral arteries

Uses: Chronic stable angina pectoris, vasospastic angina, dysrhythmias, hypertension

Dosage and routes:
- *Adult:* PO 80 mg tid or qid, increase qwk; IV BOL 5-10 mg > 2 min, repeat if necessary in 30 min
- *Child 0-1 yr:* IV BOL 0.1-0.2 mg/kg > 2 min with ECG monitoring, repeat if necessary in 30 min
- *Child 1-15 yr:* IV BOL 0.1-0.3 mg/kg over > 2 min, repeat in 30 min, not to exceed 10 mg in a single dose
Available forms: Tabs 40, 80, 120 mg; sus rel tabs, 240 mg; inj 2.5 mg/ml

Side effects/adverse reactions:
CV: Edema, CHF, bradycardia, hypotension, palpitations, AV block
GI: Nausea, diarrhea, gastric upset, constipation, increased liver function studies
GU: Nocturia, polyuria
CNS: Headache, drowsiness, dizziness, anxiety, depression, weakness, insomnia, confusion, lightheadedness

Contraindications: Sick sinus syndrome, 2nd or 3rd degree heart block, hypotension less than 90 mm Hg systolic, cardiogenic shock, severe CHF

Precautions: CHF, hypotension, hepatic injury, pregnancy (C), lactation, children, renal disease, concomitant β-blocker therapy

Pharmacokinetics:
IV: Onset 3 min, peak 3-5min, duration 10-20 min

V

PO: Onset variable, peak 3-4 hr, duration 17-24 hr, half-life (biphasic) 4 min, 3-7 hr (terminal), metabolized by liver, excreted in urine (96% as metabolites)

Interactions/ incompatibilities:

- Increased hypotension: prazosin, quinidine
- Increased effects: β-blockers, antihypertensives, cimetidine
- Decreased effects of: lithium
- Increased levels of: digoxin, theophylline, cyclosporine, carbamazepine, nondepolarizing muscle relaxants
- Incompatible with albumin, amphotericin B, ampicillin, dobutamine, hydralazine, mezlocillin, nafcillin, oxacillin, $NaCO_3$

Lab test interferences:
Increase: Liver function tests

RESPIRATORY CARE CONSIDERATIONS:
Assess/evaluate:

- Therapeutic response: decreased anginal pain, decreased BP, stabilized cardiac rhythm.
- Monitor cardiovascular status: BP, pulse, respiration, ECG.
- Assess for presence of adverse effects, especially dizziness or other signs of hypotension, bradycardia.
- If on positive pressure ventilatory support, monitor cardiac output and/or BP, and adjust level of positive pressure to extent possible, if necessary to maintain adequate cardiac output.
- Monitor BP if beta agonists are required to treat airway obstruction.
- Consider use of anticholinergic agent such as ipratro-

pium bromide as an alternative to beta agonists, if bronchodilator therapy is needed; aerosol inhalation (MDI, SVN, DPI) of adrenergic bronchodilators will generally give lower systemic levels and fewer cardiovascular effects.

Patient education:

- Note: hand tremor can occur, such as seen with beta agonist bronchodilators.
- Change position slowly to avoid orthostatic hypotension.

warfarin sodium
(war′far-in)
Carfin, Coumadin, Panwarfin, Sofarin, Warfarin Sodium, Warfilone Sodium,* Warnerin*
Func. class.:
Anticoagulant
Chem. class.: Congener of bishydroxycoumarin

Action: Interferes with blood clotting by indirect means; depresses hepatic synthesis of Vit K-dependent coagulation factors (II, VII, IX, X)

Uses: Pulmonary emboli, deep vein thrombosis, myocardial infarction, atrial dysrhythmias, postcardiac valve replacement

Dosage and routes:

- *Adult:* PO/IV 10-15 mg × 3 days, then titrated to INR qd
Available forms: Tabs 1 mg, 2, 2.5, 5, 7.5, 10 mg; inj 50 mg/ 2 ml

Side effects/adverse reactions:
GI: Diarrhea, nausea, vomiting, anorexia, stomatitis, cramps, *hepatitis*

GU: Hematuria
INTEG: Rash, dermatitis, urticaria, alopecia, pruritus
CNS: Fever
HEMA: Hemorrhage, agranulocytosis, leukopenia, eosinophilia

Contraindications: Hypersensitivity, hemophilia, leukemia with bleeding, peptic ulcer disease, thrombocytopenic purpura, hepatic disease (severe), severe hypertension, subacute bacterial endocarditis, acute nephritis, blood dyscrasias, pregnancy (D), eclampsia, preeclampsia, lactation

Precautions: Alcoholism, elderly

Pharmacokinetics:
PO: Onset 12-24 hr, peak 1½-3 days, duration 3-5 days, half-life 1½-2½ days, metabolized in liver, excreted in urine/feces (active/inactive metabolites), crosses placenta, 99% bound to plasma proteins

Interactions/ incompatibilities:
■ Increased action of warfarin: allopurinol, chloramphenicol, amiodarone, diflunisal, heparin, steroids, cimetidine, disulfiram, thyroid, glucagon, metronidazole, quinidine, sulindac, sulfinpyrazone, sulfonamides, clofibrate, salicylates, ethacrynic acids, indomethacin, mefenamic acid, oxyphenbutazones, phenylbutazone, cefamondole, chloral hydrate, cotrimoxazole, erythromycin, quinolone antibiotics, isoniazid, thrombolytic agents, tricyclic antidepressants

■ Decreased action of warfarin: barbiturates, griseofulvin, ethchlorvynol, carbamazepine, rifampin, oral contraceptives, phenytoin, estrogens, Vit K, cholestyramine, corticosteroids, mercaptopurine, sucralfate, Vit K foods, vit supplement
■ Increased toxicity: oral sulfonylureas, phenytoin
■ Incompatible with amikacin, dextrose, epinephrine, metaraminol, oxytocin, promazine, tetracycline, vancomycin

Lab test interferences:
Increase: T_3 uptake
Decrease: Uric acid

RESPIRATORY CARE CONSIDERATIONS:
Assess/evaluate:
■ Avoid or minimize arterial punctures for blood gas analysis.
■ Use sites accessible to manual compression for arterial punctures.
■ Use pressure dressings for arterial puncture after prolonged manual compression.
■ Monitor for bleeding from any puncture site.
■ Evaluate therapeutic effect in pulmonary embolism by assessing improvement in gas exchange: level of PCO_2 in relation to level of ventilation (V_E), and PaO_2 in relation to FIO2.
■ Assess possibility of bleeding with unexplained fall in hematocrit or BP.

Patient education:
■ Instruct patient to notify health care personnel of any swelling, hematoma, or bleeding at a puncture site.

italic = common side effects   **bold** = life-threatening reactions

xylometazoline HCl (nasal)

(xye-loe-met-az'oh-leen)
Otrivin, Otrivin Pediatric Nasal Drops, Xylometazoline HCl
Func. class.: Nasal decongestant
Chem. class.: Sympathomimetic amine, imidazoline

Action: Strong alpha-adrenergic stimulation produces vasoconstriction of nasal membrane, which decreases congestion

Uses: Nasal congestion

Dosage and routes:
■ *Adult and child >12 yr:* INSTILL 2-3 gtts or 2 sprays q8-10h (0.1%)
■ *Child <12 yr:* INSTILL 2-3 gtts or 1% spray q8-10h (0.05%)
Available forms: Sol 0.05%, 0.1%

Side effects/adverse reactions:
EENT: Irritation, burning, sneezing, stinging, dryness, rebound congestion
INTEG: Contact dermatitis

Contraindications: Hypersensitivity to sympathomimetic amines

Precautions: Pregnancy (C), glaucoma

Pharmacokinetics:
INSTILL: Onset 5-10 min, duration 5-6 hr

RESPIRATORY CARE CONSIDERATIONS:
Assess/evaluate:
■ Therapeutic response: decreased nasal congestion.
■ Assess subject's BP if using beta agonist bronchodilator

simultaneously, for possible increases.

Patient education:
■ Environmental humidification may help to decrease nasal congestion, dryness.
■ Warn patient that rebound nasal congestion can occur.
■ Use for short-term symptoms only; prolonged rhinitis should be evaluated by physician, ENT specialist, or allergist.

zalcitabine (ddC)

(zal-sit'-a-bin)
Hivid
Func. class.: Antiviral
Chem. class.: Synthetic pyrimidine nucleoside analog of 2'-deoxycytidine

Action: Inhibits HIV replication by the conversion of this drug by cellular enzymes to an active antiviral metabolite

Uses: Advanced HIV infections in adults and children >13 yr who have been unable to use zidovudine or who have not responded to treatment

Dosage and routes:
■ *Adult:* Combined with zidovudine in advanced HIV infection: 0.75 mg administered concomitantly with 200 mg zidovudine q8h; dosage reduction not necessary for patients weighing >30 kg; in presence of peripheral neuropathy initiate dose at 0.375 mg q8h of zalcitabine
Available forms: Tabs 0.375 and 0.75 mg

Side effects/adverse reactions:
GI: Pancreatitis, diarrhea, nausea, vomiting, abdominal pain, constipation, stomatitis, dysplasia, liver

abnormalities, oral ulcers, flatulence, taste perversion, dry mouth, oral thrush, melena, increased ALT, AST, alk phosphatase, amylase, increased bilirubin
GU: Uric acid, **toxic nephropathy,** *polyuria*
CNS: Headache, peripheral neuropathy, seizures, confusion, anxiety, hypertonia, abnormal thinking, asthenia, insomnia, CNS depression, pain, dizziness, chills, fever
RESP: Cough, pneumonia, dyspnea, asthma, hypoventilation
INTEG: Rash, pruritus, alopecia, sweating, acne
MS: Myalgia, arthritis, myopathy, muscular atrophy
CV: Hypertension, vasodilation, dysrhythmia, syncope, palpitation, tachycardia
EENT: Ear pain, otitis, photophobia, visual impairment
HEMA: **Leukopenia, granulocytopenia, thrombocytopenia,** anemia

Contraindications: Hypersensitivity

Precautions: Renal, hepatic disease, pregnancy (C), lactation, children (<13 yr), patients with peripheral neuropathy

Pharmacokinetics:
PO: Elimination half-life 1.62 hr, extensive metabolism is thought to occur; administration within 5 min of food will decrease absorption

Interactions/ incompatibilities:
■ Increased risk of pancreatitis with agents having potential to cause pancreatitis
■ Increased risk of peripheral neuropathy with other agents that can cause peripheral neuropathy: chloramphenicol, cis-

platin, dapsone, disulfiram, ethionamide, glutethimide, gold, hydralazine, iodoquinol, isoniazid, metronidazole, nitrofurantoin, phenytoin, ribavirin, vincristine; use with didenosine is not recommended
■ Decreased absorption: ketoconazole, dapsone, food
■ Do not administer with tetracyclines
■ Decreased concentrations of: fluoroquinolone antibiotics

RESPIRATORY CARE CONSIDERATIONS:
Assess/evaluate:
■ Practice infection control to prevent opportunistic infection in subjects.
■ Monitor subjects for respiratory infections, especially *P. carinii* pneumonia (PCP).
■ Assess and screen for concomitant TB infection.
■ Use isolation techniques (e.g., negative pressure booth or hood,) for any aerosol treatments. Nebulizers with one-way valves and expiratory filtration are preferred for aerosol drug delivery.

zidovudine (formerly azidothymidine, or AZT)
(zid-o'-vue-dine)
Retrovir
Func. class.: Antiviral
Chem. class.: Thymidine analog

Action: Inhibits replication of HIV virus by incorporating into cellular DNA by viral reverse transcriptase, thereby terminating the cellular DNA chain

Uses: Initial therapy of HIV positive adults with CD4

Z

lymphocytes of $\leqq$500/mm^3; treatment of children who are HIV positive with symptoms, or without symptoms but abnormal laboratory values indicating immunosuppression; IV management of adults with HIV symptoms, AIDS, advanced ARC with a history of confirmed PCP or an absolute CD4 count of less than 200/mm^3

Dosage and routes:
■ *Adult:* PO 200 mg q4h; may have to stop treatment if severe bone marrow depression occurs, and restart after bone marrow recovery; IV 1-2 mg/kg q4h initiate PO as soon as possible
Available forms: Caps 100 mg; Inj (IV)

Side effects/adverse reactions:
HEMA: Granulocytopenia, anemia
CNS: Fever, headache, malaise, diaphoresis, dizziness, *insomnia,* paresthesia, somnolence, chills, tremor, twitching, anxiety, confusion, depression, lability, vertigo, loss of mental acuity
GI: Nausea, vomiting, diarrhea, anorexia, cramps, *dyspepsia,* constipation, dysphagia, *flatulence,* rectal bleeding, mouth ulcer
RESP: Dyspnea
EENT: Taste change, hearing loss, photophobia
INTEG: Rash, acne, pruritus, urticaria
MS: Myalgia, arthralgia, muscle spasm
GU: Dysuria, polyuria, frequency, hesitancy

Contraindications: Hypersensitivity

Precautions: Granulocyte count <1000/mm^3 or Hgb <9.5 g/dl, pregnancy (C), lactation, children, severe renal disease, severe hepatic function

Pharmacokinetics:
PO: Rapidly absorbed from GI tract, peak $\frac{1}{2}$-$1\frac{1}{2}$ hr, metabolized in liver (inactive metabolites), excreted by kidneys

Interactions/ incompatibilities:
■ Toxicity: amphotericin B, dapsone, flucytosine, adriamycin, interferon vincristine, vinblastine, pentamidine, probenecid, experimental nucleoside analogs, benzodiazepines, cimetidine, morphine, sulfonamides
■ Granulocytopenia: acetaminophen, aspirin, indomethacin
■ Incompatible with blood, protein products

RESPIRATORY CARE CONSIDERATIONS:
Assess/evaluate:
■ Practice infection control to prevent opportunistic infection in subjects.
■ Monitor subjects for respiratory infections, especially *P. carinii* pneumonia (PCP).
■ Assess and screen for concomitant TB infection.
■ Use isolation techniques (e.g., negative pressure booth or hood) for any aerosol treatments. Nebulizers with one-way valves and expiratory filtration are preferred for aerosol drug delivery.

---

*Available in Canada only

I. SCIENTIFIC NOTATION

Scientific notation is a method for expressing very large or very small numbers using a single digit multiplied by a whole number power of 10.

To use scientific notation, place the decimal point of the number to the right of the first non-zero digit. Multiply the number by 10 raised to a power equal to the number of places moved by the decimal point. The exponent of 10 is positive for moves to the left and negative for moves to the right.

Large number, example: 2,292.0 is the same as 2.292×10^3

Small number, example: 0.002292 is the same as 2.292×10^{-3}

II. METRIC SYSTEM

This system is based on multiples or fractions of 10.

PREFIXES	SCALE
Kilo	10^3
Hecto	10^2
Deca	10^1
base unit	$10^0 = 1$
Deci	10^{-1}
Centi	10^{-2}
Milli	10^{-3}
Micro	10^{-6}
Nano	10^{-9}
Pico	10^{-12}

III. SI UNITS (INTERNATIONAL SYSTEM OF UNITS)
(Systeme International d'Unites)

SI Base units

Length:	meter, m
Mass:	kilogram, kg
Time:	second, s
Temperature:	kelvin, K
Amount of substance:	mole, mol

SI Derived units

Area:	square meter, m^2
Volume:	cubic meter, m^3
Concentration:	mole per cubic meter, mol/m^3

I. THE METRIC SYSTEM OF MEASURE

Length

1 Kilometer (km)	=	10^3 meters	=	1000 meters
1 Hectometer (Hm)	=	10^2 meters	=	100 meters
1 Decameter (Dm)	=	10^1 meters	=	10 meters
1 Meter (m)		**Base unit**		
1 Decimeter (dm)	=	10^{-1} meter	=	0.1 meter
1 Centimeter (cm)	=	10^{-2} meter	=	0.01 meter
1 Millimeter (mm)	=	10^{-3} meter	=	0.001 meter
1 Micrometer (μm)	=	10^{-6} meter	=	0.000001 meter

Volume (capacity)

1 Kiloliter (kl)	=	10^3 liters	=	1000 liters
1 Hectoliter (Hl)	=	10^2 liters	=	100 liters
1 Decaliter (Dl)	=	10^1 liters	=	10 liters
1 Liter (L)		**Base unit**		
1 Deciliter (dl)	=	10^{-1} liter	=	0.1 liter
1 Centiliter (cl)	=	10^{-2} liter	=	0.01 liter
1 Milliliter (ml)	=	10^{-3} liter	=	0.001 liter
1 Microliter (μl)	=	10^{-6} liter	=	0.000001 liter

Mass

1 Kilogram (kg)	=	10^3 grams	=	1000 grams
1 Hectogram (Hg)	=	10^2 grams	=	100 grams
1 Decagram (Dg)	=	10^1 grams	=	10 grams
1 gram		**Base unit**		
1 Decigram (dg)	=	10^{-1} gram	=	0.1 gram
1 Centigram (cg)	=	10^{-2} gram	=	0.01 gram
1 Milligram (mg)	=	10^{-3} gram	=	0.001 gram
1 Microgram (μg)	=	10^{-6} gram	=	0.000001 gram
1 Nanogram (ng)	=	10^{-9} gram	=	0.000000001 gram
1 Picogram (pg)	=	10^{-12} gram	=	0.000000000001 gram

II. THE APOTHECARY SYSTEM OF WEIGHT AND VOLUME

Weight

20 grains	=	1 scruple
3 scruples	=	1 dram
8 drams	=	1 ounce
12 ounces	=	1 pound (= 5760 grains, apothecary)

Volume

60 minims	=	1 fluid dram
8 fluid drams	=	1 fluid ounce
16 fluid ounces	=	1 pint
2 pints	=	1 quart
4 quarts	=	1 gallon

III. THE AVOIRDUPOIS SYSTEM OF WEIGHT

437.5 grains	=	1 ounce
16 ounces	=	1 pound (= 7000 grains, avoirdupois)

IV. EQUIVALENT MEASURES
Metric
   1 kilogram = 1000 grams (1 gram = .001 kilogram)
   1 gram = 1000 milligrams (1 milligram = .001 gram)
   1 milligram = 1000 micrograms (1 microgram = .001 milligram)
   1 cubic centimeter (cm^3, cc) = 1 milliliter (ml)

Metric-apothecary-avoirdupois (Approximate)
   Metric:
   1 milligram = 0.015 grain = 1/65 grain
   1 gram = 15 grains
   1 kilogram = 2.2 pounds (Avoir.)
   1 milliliter = 16 minims or 16 drops   (1 minim = 1 drop)*
   *This may vary for different liquids and different droppers.
   Apothecary:
   1 grain = 65 milligrams
   1 ounce (Apoth.) = 31.1, or about 30 grams
   1 fluid ounce (Apoth.) = 29.57 ml, or about 30 ml
   1 pint = 473.2 ml, or about 500 ml
   1 quart = 986.4 mL, or about 1000 ml
   1 minim = 1 drop = .062 ml
   Avoirdupois:
   1 pound = 454 grams (1 kg = 2.2 pounds)
   1 ounce = 28.3 grams

Household equivalents
   1 teaspoon (tsp) = 5 ml
   1 tablespoon (tbsp) = 15 ml
   1 cup = 240 ml

V. TEMPERATURE SCALES AND CONVERSIONS

SCALE	ABSOLUTE ZERO	FREEZING, WATER	BOILING, WATER
Kelvin	0 degrees	273 degrees	373 degrees
Centigrade	-273 degrees	0 degrees	100 degrees
Fahrenheit	-460 degrees	32 degrees	212 degrees

Conversion—Centigrade/Kelvin
   To convert from Kelvin to Centigrade:
      Centigrade, degrees = Kelvin − 273
   To convert from Centigrade to Kelvin:
      Kelvin, degrees = Centigrade + 273

Conversion—Centigrade/Fahrenheit
   To convert from Fahrenheit to Centigrade:
      Centigrade, degrees = 0.55 × (Fahrenheit − 32)
   To convert from Centigrade to Fahrenheit:
      Fahrenheit, degrees = (1.8 × Centrigrade) + 32

I. PREPARED STRENGTH DRUG CALCULATIONS

A prepared strength drug dosage form contains a certain amount of the drug in a unit amount of a formulation. For example, a drug may be available as 4 mg/ml. A calculation may be needed to determine how much of the drug vehicle to give in order to administer a certain amount of the drug.

Method of solution

1. Be sure the order for the drug amount and the prepared strength dosage form are in consistent units (e.g., both are in milligrams or grams).

2. Express the problem as a proportion:

$$\frac{\text{original dose}}{\text{per amount}} = \frac{\text{desired dose}}{\text{per amount}}$$

3. Solve for the amount needed to give the desired dose.

Example:

Beractant (Survanta), an exogenous surfactant, is available with 25 mg per ml of solution. How many milliliters would be needed to administer a dose of 100 mg?

$$\frac{25 \text{ mg}}{1 \text{ ml}} = \frac{100 \text{ mg}}{X \text{ ml}}$$

Solving for X, we would obtain:

$$X = 100 \text{ mg } (1 \text{ ml})/25 \text{ mg}$$

$$X = 4 \text{ ml}$$

Calculating drug doses from schedules

Some drug doses are given in schedules based on an amount per unit of body weight or body surface area. In this case, the needed dose must first be calculated.

1. Convert to consistent units.

2. Calculate the amount of the desired dose first.

$$\text{desired dose} = \frac{\text{drug amount}}{\text{per unit body weight}} \times \text{actual body weight}$$

3. Then calculate the amount of drug vehicle needed for the desired dose.

Example:

In the case of beractant, a dose schedule is 100 mg of drug per kilogram of body weight for an infant. The drug is available in a dose per amount of 25 mg/ml. If an infant weighs 1200 grams, what dose of beractant is needed?

First, convert to consistent units for body weight:

1200 g = 1.2 kg (1200 g × 1 kg/1000 g = 1.2 kg)

Next, calculate the desired or needed dose:

100 mg/kg × 1.2 kg = 120 mg

Since the drug is available as 25 mg/ml, we would next calculate the amount of solution needed for the desired dose of 120 mg:

$$\frac{25\ mg}{1\ ml} = \frac{120\ mg}{X\ ml}$$

Solving the proportion, we obtain an amount of:

X = 120 mg (1 ml)/25 mg

X = 4.8 ml

Thus, 4.8 ml of the drug formulation would give the desired dose. (Note: this could be calculated directly, since a schedule of 100 mg/kg and a strength of 25 mg/ml is the same as 4 ml/kg: 4 ml/kg × 1.2 kg = 4.8 ml)

II. SOLUTIONS AND PERCENTAGE STRENGTH CALCULATIONS

Drug concentrations may also be expressed as percentage strengths—for example, a 2% solution. It may be necessary to calculate the amount of a drug in milligrams or grams, given a certain percentage strength. The following formulas can be used.

Undiluted active drug:

$$decimal\ strength = \frac{active\ ingredient\ (g,\ cc)}{total\ solution\ (g,\ cc)}$$

Example:
How many milligrams of active ingredient are given with half a milliliter of albuterol 0.5% strength solution?

$$0.005 = \frac{X\ g}{0.5\ ml}$$

X = 0.005 (0.5 ml) = 0.0025 g = 2.5 mg

Dilute active drug:

$$\text{decimal strength} = \frac{\text{dilute ingredient} \times \text{ingredient strength}}{\text{total solution}}$$

Example:
How many milliliters of 20% strength acetylcysteine are needed to form 5 milliliters of an 8% strength solution?

$$0.08 = \frac{X \text{ ml} \times 0.20}{5 \text{ ml}}$$

$$0.2(X) = 0.08 \ (5 \text{ ml})$$

$$X = 2 \text{ ml}$$

Combine 2 ml of the 20% solution with normal saline in a quantity sufficient to make up 5 ml of total solution.

III. INTRAVENOUS INFUSION RATES
The previous knowledge of using prepared strength drug units and solutions allows relatively straightforward calculation of IV infusion rates. Intravenous infusion incorporates calculation of the *rate* of drug administration per unit time (e.g., milligrams per minute). Ultimately an infusion rate in drops per minute will be needed on the IV infusion set. This requires knowing the Standard Drop Factor for that IV administration set, which gives the number of drops equaling one milliliter in the drip chamber. This information can be found when the IV set is opened. The following formulas can be used, depending on the type of order to be followed.

Order for total solution amount over a total time:
Use these equations to determine the amount of solution to deliver over a certain time period.
Calculate rate of flow in milliliters per minute = total solution, ml/total time, min
Calculate rate of flow in drops per minute = Standard Drop Factor × ml/min

Example:
To give 1 liter in a 3-hour period:
Convert 1 liter and 3 hours to milliliters and minutes:
1 liter × 1000 ml/L = 1000 ml
3 hours × 60 min/hr = 180 min
Rate of flow, ml/min = 1000 ml/180 min = 5.56 ml/min, or 6 ml/min approximately
If the Standard Drop Factor for your infusion set is 15 drops per milliliter:
Rate of flow, drops/min = 15 drops/ml × 6 ml/min = 90 drops/min

An infusion rate of 90 drops per minute should deliver the desired 1 liter in about 3 hours.

Order for mass of drug per unit of time:

Here is how to determine rate of milligrams per minute to deliver.

Calculate concentration of drug solution in mass per milliliter = total drug mass/total volume, ml

Calculate rate of flow in milliliters per minute = mass/min × ml/mass

Calculate rate of flow in drops per minute = Standard Drop Factor × ml/min

Example:

What infusion rate is needed to deliver 10 µg/min of a drug, which comes in a solution of 500 µg per 250 ml? The Standard Drop Factor for the IV administration set is 15 drops per milliliter.

Concentration of drug, in µg/ml = 500 µg/250 ml = 2 µg/ml

Rate of flow, in milliliters per minute = 10 µg/min × 1 ml/2 µg = 5 ml/min

Rate of flow, in drops per minute = 15 drops/ml × 5 ml/min = 75 drops/min

An infusion rate of 75 drops per minute will deliver the desired drug dose of 10 µg/min.

Summary

1. Given the order and information on the drug solution, calculate how many milliliters per minute are needed.

2. Convert this flow rate of milliliters per minute into drops per minute, using the Standard Drop Factor obtained from the IV administration set.

Several rules apply to estimating a pediatric dose if an established dose is not provided by the pharmaceutical manufacturer or has not been established in the literature through dose-response studies.

Fried's Rule (infants under 1 year):

$$\text{infant dose} = \frac{\text{infant age, months}}{150 \text{ months}} \times \text{adult dose}$$

For a child of 12.5 years (150 months), the full adult dose would be given.

Young's Rule (1 to 12 years):

$$\text{child dose} = \frac{\text{child age, years}}{\text{child age} + 12 \text{ years}} \times \text{adult dose}$$

Clark's Rule:

$$\text{child dose} = \frac{\text{child weight, pounds}}{150 \text{ pounds}} \times \text{adult dose}$$

Body Surface Area (BSA):

$$\text{child dose} = \frac{\text{child BSA, meter}^2}{1.73 \text{ meter}^2} \times \text{adult dose}$$

(Body surface area may be obtained from nomograms using the child's height and weight.)

A variety of drugs can cause adverse effects on the pulmonary system, both direct (e.g., pulmonary fibrosis) and indirect (e.g., impaired ventilatory drive). The following list of agents is grouped by the general type of effect on the pulmonary system and is intended to alert the practitioner to the possible effect. The practitioner may then wish to consult a more complete description of the drug's activity and side effects. The adverse effects listed are not necessarily observed in every administration or patient.

I. DRUG-INDUCED HYPOVENTILATION
Narcotics
Barbiturates
Benzodiazepines (e.g., diazepam (Valium))
General anesthetics
Alcohol
Antihistamines (H_1-antagonists)
Sodium bicarbonate

II. DRUG-INDUCED NEUROMUSCULAR BLOCKADE
Aminoglycoside antibiotics (e.g., gentamicin)
Benzodiazepines
Calcium blockers (e.g., verapamil)
Macrolide antibiotics (e.g., azithromycin (Zithromax))
Neuromuscular blocking agents (e.g., d-tubocurarine, succinylcholine)
Polymyxin antibiotics (colistin, polymyxin B)
Tetracyclines

III. DRUG-INDUCED BRONCHOSPASM AND COUGH
Angiotensin-converting enzyme inhibitors (e.g., captopril, enalapril)
Aspirin, salicylates
Beta-blocking agents (e.g., propranolol, timolol)
Cholinesterase inhibitors (e.g., pyridostigmine)
Contrast media/radiopaque agents (e.g., diatrizoate meglumine)
Inhaled agents
   MDI formulations—possible reaction to CFC propellants, dispersants (oleic acid)
   SVN solutions—sulfite sensitivity
   Nebulized antibiotics—e.g., polymyxin B, gentamicin
   Pentamidine (NebuPent)
Neuromuscular blocking agents (e.g., d-tubocurarine)
Nitrofurantoin (an acute reaction)
Nonsteroidal antiinflammatory agents (e.g., indomethacin)
Protamine

IV. DRUG-INDUCED PULMONARY INJURY/TOXICITY

(Includes noncardiogenic pulmonary edema, interstitial pneumonitis, fibrosis)

Cytotoxic agents
  Azathioprine
  Bleomycin
  Busulfan
  Carmustine (BCNU)
  Chlorambucil
  Chlorozotocin
  Cyclophosphamide
  Cytosine arabinoside
  Lomustine (CCNU)
  Melphalan
  Methotrexate
  Mitomycin-C
  Neocarzinostatin
  Procarbazine
  Semustine (methyl-CCNU)
  Teniposide
  Vinblastine
  Vincristine
  Vindesine
Amphotericin B
Gold salts
Hydrochlorothiazide
Interleukin-2
Methysergide maleate
Naloxone
Oxygen
Penicillamine
Radiation therapy
Salicylates
Tocainide HCl
Tocolytic agents (albuterol, terbutaline, ritodrine)
Substance abuse agents
  Narcotics—heroin, cocaine
  Chlordiazepoxide (Librium)—IV abuse
  Hydrocarbon inhalation—diisocyanates, toluene, butane
  Marijuana
  Methylphenidate (Ritalin)—IV abuse
  Propoxyphene (Darvon)—IV abuse
  Tricyclic antidepressant—overdose

To calculate body surface area from subject's height and weight, place a straight edge connecting the subject's height in the left column with the weight in the right column. The point of intersection on the column for body surface area (SA) indicates the body surface area. Reproduced from Behrman RE and Vaughn VC, eds: *Nelson's textbook of pediatrics,* ed 12, Philadelphia: WB Saunders, 1983.

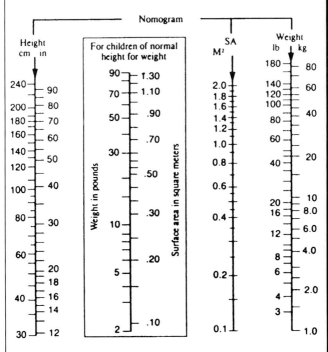

INDEX

Entries can be identified as follows: Trade Name, DRUG CATEGORY.

Entries can be identified as follows: Trade Name, DRUG CATEGORY.

Entries can be identified as follows: Trade Name, DRUG CATEGORY.

Entries can be identified as follows: Trade Name, DRUG CATEGORY.

Entries can be identified as follows: Trade Name, DRUG CATEGORY.

Entries can be identified as follows: Trade Name, DRUG CATEGORY.

Entries can be identified as follows: Trade Name, DRUG CATEGORY.

Entries can be identified as follows: Trade Name, DRUG CATEGORY.

Entries can be identified as follows: Trade Name, DRUG CATEGORY.

Entries can be identified as follows: Trade Name, DRUG CATEGORY.

Entries can be identified as follows: Trade Name, DRUG CATEGORY.

Entries can be identified as follows: Trade Name, DRUG CATEGORY.

Entries can be identified as follows: Trade Name, DRUG CATEGORY.

Entries can be identified as follows: Trade Name, DRUG CATEGORY.